Check it out

Are you doing the *G-Index Diet*? The *T-Factor Diet*? Following *Body Fueling* or *Eat More, Weigh Less*? Are you cross training, bodybuilding, running, cycling, or working out? Are you simply trying to cut back on fat and make carbohydrates the mainstay of your healthful diet?

Then you need the most complete, up-to-date carbohydrate gram counter you can buy. And Corinne T. Netzer, America's best-selling expert on the nutritional content of food, gives you all that, and more; *The Carbohydrate Gram Counter* includes all fresh and frozen produce, meats, and dairy products; all the brand-name items on your supermarket shelves, and menu items from the major fast-food chains and restaurants.

EAT A BAGEL OR A BURGER . . . BUT
MAKE SMART CHOICES AND INFORMED
DECISIONS WITH THE BEST REFERENCE BOOK
FOR TODAY'S GRAM-CONSCIOUS,
HEALTH-CONSCIOUS EATERS

**THE CORINNE T. NETZER
CARBOHYDRATE GRAM COUNTER**

Also by Corinne T. Netzer:

THE CORINNE T. NETZER CARBOHYDRATE GRAM COUNTER

Corinne T. Netzer

A DELL BOOK

Published by
Dell Publishing
a division of
Bantam Doubleday Dell Publishing Group, Inc.
1540 Broadway
New York, New York 10036

Copyright © 1994 by Corinne T. Netzer

The trademark Dell® is registered in the U.S. Patent and Trademark Office.

ISBN: 0-440-21665-6

Printed in the United States of America

Published simultaneously in Canada

June 1994

10 9 8 7 6 5 4 3 2 1

THE
CORINNE T. NETZER
CARBOHYDRATE
GRAM COUNTER

INTRODUCTION

The *Carbohydrate Gram Counter* is the largest compilation of carbo counts available under one cover. No matter what your aim or interest in carbohydrates might be, the information on all the foods—whether it be generic or brand name, fresh or frozen, even a fast-food favorite—can be found here.

Because this book is alphabetized, there is no index. I have tried to cross-reference as many items as possible; however, space does not allow this in every instance. If you do not find the item you are seeking in one place, please look for it under a category—i.e., if you don't find "caramel pudding" under "Caramel," look for it under "Pudding."

If you are making comparisons, remember to only compare foods that are similar in measure. Eight ounces is not necessarily equivalent to one eight-ounce cup. Eight ounces is a measure of how much the food weighs, while an eight-ounce cup is a measure of how much space the food occupies. For example, a cup of popcorn weighs about an ounce; thus, eight ounces of popcorn would fill quite a few cups.

The data contained herein is derived from information supplied by the various food producers, processors, distributors, and food chains, and from the United States Department of Agriculture. As we go to press, this information is the most complete and accurate available.

Good luck and good eating.

C.T.N.

Abbreviations & Symbols in This Book

" .... inch

lb. .... pound(s)

pkg. .... package(s)

oz. .... ounce(s)

tbsp. .... tablespoon(s)

tsp. .... teaspoon(s)

tr. .... trace

* .... prepared according to basic
package directions,
except as noted

A

Food and Measure	Carbohydrate Grams

Abalone, meat only, raw, 4 oz. 6.8
Acerola, fresh, trimmed, ½ cup 3.8
Acerola juice, 6 fl. oz. 8.7
Acorn squash:
baked, cubed, ½ cup 14.9
boiled, mashed, ½ cup 10.7
Adzuki beans, dry:
(Arrowhead Mills), 2 oz. 35.0
boiled, ½ cup 28.5
canned, *(Eden),* ½ cup 17.0
canned, sweetened, ½ cup 81.4
Agar, see "Seaweed"
Alfalfa seeds:
(Arrowhead Mills), 1 cup 4.0
Alfalfa seeds, sprouted, raw:
½ cup 6
1 tbsp. 1
(Shaw's), 2 oz. 2.0
Alfalfa and dill seeds, sprouted, raw *(Shaw's),*
2 oz. .... <1.0
Alfalfa and radish seeds, sprouted, raw *(Shaw's),*
2 oz. 2.0
Alfredo sauce:
mix *(Lawry's),* 1 pkg. 19.2
refrigerated *(Contadina Light),* 3.3 oz. 7.0
Algae, see "Seaweed"
Allspice *(Spice Islands),* 1 tsp. 1.4

Almond:
(Beer Nuts), 1 oz. 6.0
(Dole), 1 oz. 5.0
(Fisher), 1 oz. 6.0
dried:
  1 oz. 5.8
  slivered, 1 cup 27.5
  blanched, 1 oz. 5.3
dry-roasted, 1 oz. 6.9
honey-roasted, 1 oz. 7.9
oil-roasted:
  1 oz. 4.5
  salted *(Master Choice),* 1 oz. 5.0
  blanched, 1 oz. 5.1
toasted, 1 oz. 6.5
Almond butter:
1 tbsp. 3.4
(Erewhon), 1 tbsp. 2.0
(Roaster Fresh), 1 oz. 6.0
raw or toasted *(Hain* Natural), 2 tbsp. 3.0
honey cinnamon, 1 tbsp. 4.3
Almond meal, partially defatted, 1 oz. 8.2
Almond paste, 1 oz. 12.4
Amaranth:
raw, trimmed, 1/2 cup 6
boiled, drained, 1/2 cup 2.7
Amaranth, whole-grain, 1 oz. 18.8
Amaranth flakes *(Arrowhead Mills),* 1 oz. 21.0
Amaranth flour or seeds *(Arrowhead Mills),* 2 oz. 35.0
Anasazi beans, dry *(Arrowhead Mills),* 2 oz. 35.0
Anchovies, fresh or canned in oil 0
Angel hair pasta entree, frozen:
(Lean Cuisine), 10 oz. 38.0
(Weight Watchers Smart Ones), 8.55 oz. 18.0
Anise seed, 1 tsp. 1.1
Apple:
raw:
  unpeeled, 2¾"-diameter apple 21.1

unpeeled, sliced, ½ cup 8.4
peeled, 2¾″-diameter apple 19.0
peeled, sliced, ½ cup 8.2
cooked, peeled, boiled, sliced, ½ cup 11.7
cooked, peeled, microwaved, sliced, ½ cup 12.3
canned, sweetened, sliced, drained, ½ cup 17.0
dried, sulfured, uncooked, 2 oz. 37.4
dried, chunks *(Sun-Maid/Sunsweet)*, 2 oz. 42.0
Apple, escalloped, frozen *(Stouffer's)*, 6 oz. 41.0
Apple butter, all varieties *(Smuckers)*, 1 tsp. 3.0
Apple cider:
canned or frozen* *(Tree Top)*, 6 fl. oz. 22.0
sparkling *(Welch's)*, 6 fl. oz. 24.0
and spice *(R.W. Knudsen)*, 8 fl. oz. 28.0
Apple crisp, frozen:
(Pepperidge Farm Classic), 4 oz. 41.0
(Weight Watchers Sweet Celebrations), 3.5 oz. 40.0
Apple drink, canned *(Hi-C Jammin' Apple)*, 6 fl. oz. 23.0
Apple dumpling, frozen *(Pepperidge Farm)*, 3 oz. 33.0
Apple fritter, frozen *(Mrs. Paul's)*, 4 oz. 35.0
Apple fruit roll, see "Fruit snack"
Apple fruit square, frozen *(Pepperidge Farm)*,
   2.5 oz. 27.0
Apple juice:
unsweetened, 6 fl. oz. 21.7
(Minute Maid), 6 fl. oz. 21.0
(Mott's/Mott's Natural), 6 fl. oz. 20.0
(Ocean Spray 100%), 6 fl. oz. 23.0
(R.W. Knudsen Clear), 8 fl. oz. 22.0
(R.W. Knudsen Natural), 8 fl. oz. 21.0
(Red Cheek/Red Cheek Natural), 6 fl. oz. 20.0
(Tropicana), 6 fl. oz. 20.0
(Welch's), 6 fl. oz. 22.0
blend *(Juicy Juice)*, 6 fl. oz. 21.0
Gravenstein *(R.W. Knudsen)*, 8 fl. oz. 28.0
sparkling *(Welch's)*, 6 fl. oz. 24.0

Apple juice *(cont.)*
canned or frozen* *(Tree Top)*, 6 fl. oz. 22.0
chilled or frozen* *(Sunkist)*, 8 fl. oz. 19.4
frozen*, 6 fl. oz. 20.7
Apple pie spice *(Tone's)*, 1 tsp. 2.4
Apple punch:
(Red Cheek), 10 fl. oz. 47.0
chilled *(Minute Maid)*, 6 fl. oz. 23.0
Apple sticks, frozen *(Farm Rich)*, 4 oz. 44.0
Apple-apricot juice *(R.W. Knudsen)*, 8 fl. oz. 29.0
Apple-banana juice *(R.W. Knudsen)*, 8 fl. oz. 21.0
Apple-blackberry juice:
(R.W. Knudsen), 8 fl. oz. 24.0
(Santa Cruz Natural), 8 fl. oz. 29.0
Apple-blueberry juice drink *(Boku)*, 6 fl. oz. 22.0
Apple-boysenberry juice:
(R.W. Knudsen), 8 fl. oz. 28.0
(Santa Cruz Natural), 8 fl. oz. 29.0
Apple-cherry juice *(Red Cheek)*, 10 fl. oz. 47.0
Apple-citrus juice, canned or frozen* *(Tree Top)*,
   6 fl. oz. 22.0
Apple-cranberry drink *(Mott's)*, 11.5 fl. oz. 47.0
Apple-cranberry juice:
(R.W. Knudsen), 8 fl. oz. 28.0
(Master Choice), 6 fl. oz. 19.0
(Mott's), 6 fl. oz. 24.0
(Santa Cruz Natural), 8 fl. oz. 28.0
(Smucker's Naturally 100%), 8 fl. oz. 32.0
canned or frozen* *(Tree Top)*, 6 fl. oz. 25.0
cocktail *(Welch's)*, 6 fl. oz. 27.0
Apple-cranberry juice drink *(Tropicana)*, 6 fl. oz. 27.0
Apple-grape juice:
(Juicy Juice), 8.45 fl. oz. 29.0
(Mott's), 6 fl. oz. 23.0
(Red Cheek), 10 fl. oz. 45.0
canned or frozen* *(Tree Top)*, 6 fl. oz. 25.0
cocktail, canned or frozen* *(Welch's Orchard)*,
   6 fl. oz. 27.0

Apple-grape-cherry juice cocktail:
(Welch's), 6 fl. oz. 30.0
frozen* (Welch's Orchard), 6 fl. oz. 27.0
Apple-grape-raspberry juice cocktail:
(Welch's), 6 fl. oz. 30.0
frozen* (Welch's Orchard), 6 fl. oz. 27.0
Apple-orange-pineapple juice cocktail (Welch's/
Welch's Orchard), 6 fl. oz. 27.0
Apple-peach juice (R.W. Knudsen), 8 fl. oz. 34.0
Apple-peach juice drink (Boku), 6 fl. oz. 22.0
Apple-pear juice, canned or frozen* (Tree Top),
6 fl. oz. 22.0
Apple-raspberry drink (Mott's), 10.5 fl. oz. 43.0
Apple-raspberry juice:
(R.W. Knudsen), 8 fl. oz. 28.0
(Mott's), 6 fl. oz. 22.0
(Santa Cruz Natural), 8 fl. oz. 29.0
canned or frozen* (Tree Top), 6 fl. oz. 21.0
Apple-raspberry juice drink (Boku), 6 fl. oz. 22.0
Apple-strawberry juice:
(R.W. Knudsen), 8 fl. oz. 28.0
(Santa Cruz Natural), 8 fl. oz. 29.0
Apple-strawberry nectar (Kern's), 6 fl. oz. 26.0
Applesauce:
unsweetened, 1/2 cup 13.8
sweetened, 1/2 cup 25.5
(Mott's/Mott's Chunky), 4 oz. 22.0
(Mott's Natural), 4 oz. 12.0
(Stokely), 1/2 cup 23.0
(Tree Top Natural), 1/2 cup 15.0
regular or Gravenstein (Santa Cruz Natural), 4 oz. 14.0
original or cinnamon (Tree Top), 1/2 cup 21.0
cinnamon (Mott's), 4 oz. 23.0
Dutch, spice (Mott's), 4 oz. 21.0
Applesauce blends:
all blends (Santa Cruz Natural), 4 oz. 14.0
with mixed fruit, peach, or strawberry (Mott's Fruit
Pak), 3.9 oz. 18.0

Applesauce blends *(cont.)*
with pineapple *(Mott's* Fruit Pak), 3.9 oz. 21.0
Apricot:
fresh, 3 medium, 12 per lb. 11.8
fresh, pitted, halves, ½ cup 8.6
canned:
  in water *(Libby's),* ½ cup 9.0
  in juice, ½ cup 15.3
  in heavy syrup, with skin, ½ cup 27.7
  in heavy syrup *(Libby's),* ½ cup 28.0
dried *(Del Monte),* 2 oz. 35.0
frozen, sweetened, ½ cup 30.4
Apricot fruit roll, see "Fruit snack"
Apricot nectar:
6 fl. oz. 27.1
(Kern's), 6 fl. oz. 27.0
(R.W. Knudsen), 8 fl. oz. 24.0
(Libby's), 6 fl. oz. 26.0
Apricot-pineapple nectar *(Kern's),* 6 fl. oz. 27.0
Arby's, 1 serving:
breakfast dishes:
  biscuit, plain 34.0
  biscuit, with bacon 35.5
  biscuit, with ham 34.3
  biscuit, with sausage 35.0
  croissant, plain 28.0
  croissant, bacon and egg 28.8
  croissant, ham and cheese 29.3
  croissant, mushroom and cheese 34.0
  croissant, sausage and egg 29.3
  danish, cinnamon nut 60.0
  muffin, blueberry 40.0
  platter, scrambled egg 44.9
  platter, scrambled egg with bacon 51.0
  platter, scrambled egg with ham 45.3
  platter, scrambled egg with sausage 45.9
  Toastix 43.0

sandwiches:
  ArbyQ 48.2
  Bac'N Cheddar Deluxe 38.9
  Beef'N Cheddar 43.2
  chicken barbeque, grilled 46.7
  chicken, breast fillet or Cordon Bleu 52.1
  chicken deluxe, grilled 41.8
  fish fillet 50.0
  French dip 35.0
  French Dip'N Swiss 35.5
  Ham'N Cheese 34.5
  Italian sub 47.4
  light deluxe, roast beef, chicken, or turkey 33.0
  Philly Beef'N Swiss 38.2
  roast beef, giant 45.6
  roast beef, junior 22.8
  roast beef, regular 35.4
  roast beef, super 54.1
  roast beef sub 46.8
  roast chicken club 36.6
  tuna sub 50.2
  turkey sub 46.5
potatoes:
  cakes 19.8
  cheddar fries 46.2
  curly fries 43.2
  french fries 29.8
potatoes, baked:
  plain 50.2
  with butter and sour cream 52.7
  Broccoli'N Cheddar 55.0
  deluxe 58.9
  Mushroom'N Cheese 57.5
soups, 8 oz.:
  Boston clam chowder 17.5
  cream of broccoli 18.0
  lumberjack mixed vegetable 12.6
  old fashioned chicken noodle 14.8

Arby's, soups, 8 oz. *(cont.)*
  potato with bacon 20.0
  Wisconsin cheese.. 19.7
salads:
  chef 13.0
  garden.. 11.4
  roast chicken 12.2
  side 4.0
salad dressing, 2 oz.:
  blue cheese 2.5
  buttermilk ranch... 1.9
  honey French 21.8
  light Italian 3.5
  Thousand Island 9.8
sauces:
  au jus, 4 oz.. 1.0
  Arby's Sauce, .5 oz. 3.3
  Horsey Sauce, .5 oz. 2.6
desserts:
  apple turnover 27.5
  blueberry turnover 32.0
  cheesecake.. 21.3
  cherry turnover 25.4
  chocolate chip cookie 17.0
  Polar Swirl, Butterfinger 61.6
  Polar Swirl, Heath 76.3
  Polar Swirl, Oreo 65.8
  Polar Swirl, peanut butter cup 61.4
  Polar Swirl, Snickers 73.3
  shake, chocolate 76.5
  shake, jamocha 59.1
  shake, vanilla 46.2
Arrowhead:
raw, 2⅝"-diameter corm..................................... 2.4
boiled, 1"-diameter corm 1.9
Arrowroot flour, 1 cup 112.8

Artichoke, globe:

fresh, boiled, 1 medium, 10.6 oz.. 13.4

fresh, boiled, hearts, 1/2 cup 9.4

canned, hearts:

  with liquid *(Progresso),* 1/2 cup 5.0

  drained *(Progresso),* 1/2 cup 4.0

  marinated, with liquid *(Progresso),* 1/2 cup...................... 16.0

frozen, hearts *(Birds Eye Deluxe),* 3 oz. 7.0

frozen, hearts *(Seabrook),* 3 oz.. 4.0

Artichoke, Jerusalem, see "Jerusalem artichoke"

Arugula:

trimmed, 1 oz.. 1.0

trimmed, 1/2 cup 4

Asparagus:

fresh:

  raw, 4 spears, 3.8 oz. 2.6

  boiled, 4 spears, 1/2"-diameter base 2.5

  boiled, drained, cuts, 1/2 cup... 3.8

canned:

  (Stokely), 1/2 cup 3.0

  spears, green or white, or cut *(Green Giant),*

    1/2 cup... 3.0

  cut *(Green Giant 50% Less Salt),* 1/2 cup 3.0

frozen:

  boiled, 4 spears, approximately 2.1 oz. 2.9

  spears or spears and cuts *(Frosty Acres),* 3.3 oz. 4.0

  cuts *(Green Giant Harvest Fresh),* 1/2 cup...................... 4.0

Asparagus bean, see "Winged bean"

Asparagus pilaf, frozen *(Green Giant Garden*

  Gourmet Right for Lunch), 9.5 oz. 37.0

Au jus gravy:

canned *(Franco-American),* 2 oz. 2.0

canned *(Heinz Home-Style),* 2 oz. 2.0

mix:

  (French's), 1/8 packet 1.0

  (Lawry's), 1 packet 11.7

  (McCormick/Schilling), 1/4 cup*... 3.5

Au jus sauce mix, *(Knorr),* 1 serving.................................. 2.6

Au jus seasoning mix *(French's* Roasting Bag),
  ⅛ pkg. 2.0
Avocado, California:
1 medium, 8 oz. 12.0
trimmed, 1 oz. 2.0
pureed, ½ cup 8.0
cocktail *(Frieda's),* 1 oz. 1.8
Avocado dip *(Kraft),* 2 tbsp. 3.0

B

Food and Measure	Carbohydrate Grams

Bacon, cooked:

4.5 oz. (yield from 1 lb. raw)......................................8

turkey, see "Turkey bacon"

Bacon, Canadian, unheated, 1 oz. 5

"Bacon," vegetarian:

1 strip, .2 oz. 5

frozen *(Morningstar Farms* Breakfast Strips), 3 strips 4.0

frozen *(Worthington Stripples),* 4 strips.....................6.0

Bacon bits, real or imitation:

(Bac*Os), 2 tsp. 2.0

(Hormel), 1 oz..1.0

(McCormick/Schilling Bac'N Pieces), 1 tbsp........................2.0

(Oscar Mayer), 1 tbsp. 0

pieces *(Hormel),* 1 oz...<2.0

Bacon breakfast biscuit, frozen *(Swanson),* 3.2 oz. 22.0

Bacon horseradish dip:

(Breakstone's/Sealtest), 2 tbsp................................2.0

(Kraft), 2 tbsp. 3.0

(Kraft Premium), 2 tbsp..2.0

Bacon and onion dip:

(Breakstone's Gourmet), 2 tbsp..............................2.0

(Kraft Premium), 2 tbsp..2.0

Bagel:

plain *(Thomas'),* 1 piece...34.0

cinnamon raisin *(Thomas'),* 1 piece.......................36.0

egg *(Thomas'),* 1 piece 33.0

onion *(Thomas'),* 1 piece 35.0

Bagel, frozen:
plain:
   (Lender's), 1 piece.. 30.0
   (Lender's Bagelettes), 1 piece 14.0
   (Lender's Big'n Crusty), 1 piece...................................... 43.0
blueberry *(Lender's)*, 1 piece 38.0
cinnamon raisin *(Lender's)*, 1 piece................................... 39.0
cinnamon raisin *(Lender's Big'n Crusty)*, 1 piece 47.0
egg *(Lender's)*, 1 piece 30.0
egg *(Lender's Big'n Crusty)*, 1 piece................................. 44.0
oat *(Lender's)*, 1 piece... 36.0
onion *(Lender's)*, 1 piece 30.0
onion *(Lender's Big'n Crusty)*, 1 piece 43.0
poppy *(Lender's)*, 1 piece.. 30.0
pumpernickel *(Lender's)*, 1 piece 31.0
rye *(Lender's)*, 1 piece 30.0
sesame *(Lender's)*, 1 piece.. 29.0
soft *(Lender's* Original), 1 piece... 38.0
Bagel chips, cheese or toasted onion and garlic
   (Pepperidge Farm), ½ oz. 10.0
Bagel sandwich, see specific listings
Baked beans, canned:
(Allens), ½ cup 21.0
(Campbell's Home Style), 4 oz. 24.0
(Grandma Brown's), ½ cup 27.0
(Grandma Brown's Saucepan), ½ cup 26.2
(Green Giant/Joan of Arc), ½ cup 30.0
barbecue *(Campbell's)*, 4 oz.. 22.0
barbecue *(Campbell's* Old Fashioned), 4 oz. 26.0
with beef, ½ cup.. 22.5
brown sugar and bacon *(Campbell's)*, 4 oz. 25.0
brown sugar and bacon *(Hanover)*, ½ cup 27.0
brown sugar and molasses *(Campbell's* Old
   Fashioned), 4 oz. 27.0
with franks, in sauce *(Libby's Diner)*, 7.75 oz. 38.0
with honey *(B&M* Brick Oven), 8 oz. 50.0
with honey, Boston *(Health Valley* Fat Free), 7.5 oz. 41.0

maple *(B&M* Brick Oven/Friends), 8 oz. 52.0
with onions *(Bush's Best)*, 4 oz. 27.0
pea *(B&M* Brick Oven), 8 oz. 50.0
with pork:
   (Crest Top), 1/2 cup 18.0
   (Heinz), 8 oz. 44.0
   (Hunt's), 4 oz. 26.0
   (Wagon Master), 1/2 cup 24.0
   pea, small *(Friends)*, 8 oz. 53.0
   red kidney *(Friends)*, 8 oz. 55.0
   tomato *(B&M* Brick Oven), 8 oz. 48.0
   in tomato sauce *(Campbell's)*, 4 oz. 21.0
   in tomato sauce *(Green Giant/Joan of Arc)*, 1/2 cup 21.0
red kidney *(B&M* Brick Oven), 8 oz. 48.0
vegetarian:
   4 oz. 23.3
   (B&M 50% Less Sodium), 8 oz. 50.0
   (Bush's Deluxe), 4 oz. 25.0
   (Heinz), 8 oz. 50.0
   honey baked, with miso *(Health Valley)*, 7.5 oz. 38.0
   in tomato sauce *(Campbell's)*, 4 oz. 20.0
yellow eye *(B&M* Brick Oven), 8 oz. 50.0
Baking mix:
(Bisquick), 1/2 cup 37.0
(Bisquick Reduced Fat), 1/2 cup 39.0
whole wheat *(Hain)*, 1/3 cup 30.0
Baking powder *(Davis)*, 1 tsp. 2.0
Baking soda *(Tone's)*, 1 tsp. 0
Balsam pear, fresh:
leafy tips, raw, 1/2 cup 8
leafy tips, boiled, drained, 1/2 cup 2.0
pods, raw, 1/2″ pieces, 1/2 cup 1.7
pods, boiled, drained, 1/2″ pieces, 1/2 cup 2.7
Bamboo shoots:
fresh, raw, 1/2″ slices, 1/2 cup 4.0
fresh, boiled, drained, 1/2″ slices, 1/2 cup 1.2
canned, drained, 1/2 cup 2.1
canned *(La Choy)*, 1/4 cup 1.0

Banana:
fresh:
    whole, 1 lb. untrimmed 69.1
    1 medium, 8-3/4" long.. 26.7
    mashed, 1/2 cup 26.4
  dehydrated, 1/4 cup 22.1
Banana, baking, see "Plantain"
Banana, manzano (Frieda's), 1 oz. 6.3
Banana, red, 1 medium, 7-1/4" long................................... 30.7
Banana berry drink (Hi-C Stompin' Banana Berry),
  6 fl. oz.. 22.0
Banana flavor drink mix (Nestlé Quik), 2-1/2 heaping
  tsp. 21.0
Banana nectar (Libby's), 6 fl. oz. 26.0
Banana squash, baked (Frieda's), 1 oz. 4.4
Banana-pineapple nectar (Kern's), 6 fl. oz. 27.0
Barbecue sauce:
(Enrico's Original), 2 tbsp. 6.0
(Heinz Select), 2 tbsp.. 9.0
(Heinz Thick & Rich Chunky), 1 oz. 6.0
(Heinz Thick & Rich Original/Old Fashioned), 1 oz. 8.0
(Hunt's Homestyle), 1 tbsp. 6.0
(Hunt's Original), 1 tbsp.. 5.0
(Kraft), 2 tbsp. 10.0
(Kraft Thick'N Spicy Original), 2 tbsp. 12.0
(Lea & Perrins Original), 1 tbsp... 7.0
(Luzianne), 2 tbsp.. 19.0
(Maull's), 2 tbsp... 10.0
(Maull's Lite), 2 tbsp. 6.0
(Ott's Original), 2 tbsp.. 7.0
beer flavor (Maull's), 2 tbsp... 9.0
Cajun style (Heinz Thick & Rich), 1 oz. 8.0
chunky (Kraft Thick'N Spicy), 2 tbsp...................................... 13.0
country style (Hunt's), 1 tbsp. 5.0
Dijon and honey (Lawry's), 1/4 cup....................................... 27.0
fajita (Lawry's), 1 oz. 5.1
garlic (Kraft), 2 tbsp. 9.0
Hawaiian style (Heinz Thick & Rich), 1 oz............................. 10.0

hickory smoke:
  (Heinz Select/Thick & Rich), 1 oz. 8.0
  (Hunt's), 1 tbsp. 5.0
  (Kraft), 2 tbsp. 10.0
  (Kraft Thick'N Spicy), 2 tbsp. 12.0
  (Lea & Perrins), 1 tbsp. 7.0
with honey *(Hain)*, 1 tbsp. 1.0
with honey *(Kraft Thick'N Spicy)*, 2 tbsp. 13.0
hot, regular or hickory smoke *(Kraft)*, 2 tbsp. 9.0
hot, Texas *(Heinz* Thick & Rich), 1 oz. 7.0
hot and spicy *(Master Choice)*, 1 tbsp. 7.0
Italian seasonings *(Kraft)*, 2 tbsp. 10.0
Kansas City style:
  (Hunt's), 1 tbsp. 5.0
  (Kraft), 2 tbsp. 11.0
  (Kraft Thick'N Spicy), 2 tbsp. 13.0
  (Maull's), 2 tbsp. 15.0
mesquite:
  (Enrico's), 1 tbsp. 3.0
  smoke *(Heinz* Thick & Rich), 1 oz. 7.0
  smoke *(Kraft)*, 2 tbsp. 10.0
  smoke *(Kraft Thick'N Spicy)*, 2 tbsp. 12.0
mushroom *(Heinz* Thick & Rich), 1 oz. 6.0
New Orleans style *(Hunt's)*, 1 tbsp. 5.0
onion:
  (Heinz Thick & Rich), 1 oz. 7.0
  (Maull's), 2 tbsp. 9.0
  bits, plain or hickory smoke *(Kraft)*, 2 tbsp. 11.0
Oriental *(La Choy)*, 1 tbsp. 3.8
Oriental, stir-fry *(Lawry's)*, ¼ cup 19.6
Ozark recipe *(Ott's)*, 2 tbsp. 14.0
Silver Dollar City *(Ott's)*, 2 tbsp. 10.0
sloppy Joe, with beef *(Libby's)*, ⅓ cup 7.0
smoky *(Maull's)*, 2 tbsp. 10.0
smoky *(Ott's)*, 2 tbsp. 7.0
Southern or Western *(Hunt's)*, 1 tbsp. 5.0

Barbecue sauce *(cont.)*
sweet:
  (Maull's Sweet-N-Mild), 2 tbsp. 12.0
  (Maull's Sweet-N-Smokey), 2 tbsp. 13.0
  (Ott's Sweet-n-Mild), 2 tbsp. 10.0
sweet and sour *(Lawry's)*, ¼ cup 11.7
teriyaki *(Lawry's)*, 1 oz. 14.1
Texas style *(Hunt's)*, 1 tbsp. 6.0
Barley:
dry, 1 cup 135.2
dry *(Arrowhead Mills)*, 2 oz. 45.0
hulless *(Arrowhead Mills)*, 2 oz. 43.0
pearled, dry, 1 cup 155.5
pearled, cooked, 1 cup 44.3
Barley flakes *(Arrowhead Mills)*, 2 oz. 45.0
Barley flour *(Arrowhead Mills)*, 2 oz. 35.0
Barley malt *(Eden)*, ½ tsp. 2.0
Basella, see "Vine spinach"
Basil:
fresh:
  1 oz. 1.2
  5 medium leaves 1
  chopped, 2 tbsp. 2
dried, ground, 1 tbsp. 2.7
dried, ground, 1 tsp. 9
Baskin-Robbins:
ice cream, 1 regular scoop:
  chocolate, raspberry truffle *International Creams* or
    world class 35.0
  strawberry, very berry 30.0
  vanilla 24.0
Chilly Burger, vanilla, 1 piece 32.0
Tiny Toon Aventures, 1 piece:
  mint chocolate chip 19.0
  vanilla 18.0
  Toonwiches, chocolate 46.0
  Toonwiches, vanilla 45.0

cone, sugar, unfilled, 1 piece 11.0
cone, waffle, unfilled, 1 piece... 28.0
Bass, without added ingredients 0
Batter mix (see also specific listings):
(Golden Dipt), 1 oz.. 21.0
(Golden Dipt Corny Dog), 1 oz... 22.0
Bay leaf, dried, crumbled (Spice Islands), 1 tsp. 3
Bean dip:
(Chi-Chi's Fiesta), 1 oz. 4.0
hot (Hain), 2 tbsp. 5.0
jalapeño (Frito-Lay's), 1 oz... 4.0
jalapeño (Old El Paso), 1 tbsp. 2.0
Mexican (Hain), 2 tbsp. 5.0
onion (Hain), 2 tbsp. 5.0
Bean dishes, canned, see specific bean listings
Bean dishes mix* (see also specific bean listings):
(Hunt's Big John's Beans'n Fixin's), 4 oz. 26.0
Cajun, and sauce (Lipton), ½ cup...................................... 28.0
Bean salad, three bean, canned (Green Giant),
½ cup 18.0
Bean sprouts, see "Sprouts" and specific listings
Beans, see specific listings
Beans, snap or string, see "Green beans"
Beans and frankfurters, frozen (Morton), 8.5 oz. 39.0
Béarnaise sauce mix:
dry, .9-oz. packet... 14.8
(McCormick/Schilling McCormick Collection), ¼ cup* 6.0
Beechnuts, dried, shelled, 1 oz... 9.5
Beef, without added ingredients 0
Beef, corned (see also "Beef luncheon meat")
brisket, cooked, 4 oz. 5
Beef, corned, hash, canned:
(Dinty Moore Cup), 7.5 oz. 22.0
(Libby's), 7.5 oz.. 20.0
(Mary Kitchen), 1 oz... 2.0
Beef, dried:
cured, 1 oz. 4
sliced (Hormel), 1 oz.. 1.0

Beef, roast, hash, canned *(Mary Kitchen)*, 1 oz. 3.0
"Beef," vegetarian (see also " 'Hamburger,'
  vegetarian"):
canned:
  (Worthington Savory Slices), 2 slices 4.0
  steak *(Worthington Prime Stakes)*, 3.25-oz. piece 7.0
  steak *(Worthington Vegetable Steaks)*, 2½ pieces 5.0
  stew *(Worthington* Country Stew), 9.5 oz. 23.0
  Swiss steak *(LaLoma)*, 1 piece 7.0
frozen:
  (Worthington Beef Style Meatless), 4 slices 7.0
  (Worthington Stakelets), 1 piece 7.0
  corned *(Worthington)*, 4 slices 8.0
  pie *(Worthington)*, 1 pie 44.0
  smoked *(Worthington)*, 3 slices 7.0
  steak *(LaLoma* Griddle Steaks), 1 piece 4.0
Beef dinner, frozen:
(Banquet Extra Helping), 15.5 oz. 42.0
in barbecue sauce *(Swanson)*, 11 oz. 51.0
champignon *(Tyson* Premium), 10.5 oz. 31.0
chopped *(Banquet* Meals), 9.5 oz. 24.0
chopped steak *(Swanson Hungry Man)*, 16.75 oz. 41.0
enchilada, see "Enchilada dinner"
marinated, slow-cooked *(Le Menu New American
  Cuisine)*, 10.25 oz. 28.0
meat loaf, see "Meat loaf dinner"
patty, charbroiled *(Freezer Queen)*, 9.5 oz. 20.0
pepper steak *(Armour Classics Lite)*, 11.25 oz. 29.0
pepper steak *(Healthy Choice)*, 11 oz. 40.0
pot roast:
  (The Budget Gourmet Light and Healthy), 10 oz. 19.0
  old fashioned *(Le Menu New American Cuisine)*,
    10 oz. 22.0
  Yankee *(Freezer Queen)*, 9.25 oz. 35.0
  Yankee *(Healthy Choice)*, 11 oz. 36.0
  Yankee *(Swanson)*, 11.5 oz. 35.0
  Yankee *(Swanson Hungry Man)*, 16 oz. 49.0
roast, sandwich *(Swanson)*, 10.25 oz. 50.0

Salisbury steak:
  (Armour Classics), 11.25 oz. 26.0
  (Armour Classics Lite), 11.5 oz. 29.0
  (Banquet Extra Helping), 16.25 oz. 57.0
  (Freezer Queen), 9.5 oz. 19.0
  (Healthy Choice), 11.5 oz. 45.0
  (Swanson), 10.5 oz. 42.0
  (Swanson Hungry Man), 16.25 oz. 37.0
  chargrilled *(Le Menu New American Cuisine)*,
    10.5 oz. 30.0
  old fashioned *(Le Menu New American Cuisine
    Healthy)*, 10.25 oz. 37.0
  parmigiana *(Armour Classics)*, 11.5 oz. 32.0
  sirloin *(The Budget Gourmet Light and Healthy)*,
    11 oz. 30.0
short ribs *(Tyson Premium)*, 11 oz. 38.0
sirloin:
  with barbecue sauce *(Healthy Choice)*, 11 oz. 44.0
  chopped *(Swanson)*, 10.5 oz. 29.0
  smothered *(Le Menu New American Cuisine)*,
    10 oz. 60.0
  special recipe *(The Budget Gourmet Light and
    Healthy)*, 11 oz. 29.0
  wine sauce *(The Budget Gourmet Light and
    Healthy)*, 11 oz. 36.0
sirloin tips:
  (Healthy Choice), 11.25 oz. 29.0
  (Le Menu New American Cuisine), 7.7 oz. 25.0
  (Swanson), 7 oz. 18.0
  (Swanson Hungry Man), 15.75 oz. 50.0
sliced:
  (Banquet Meals), 9 oz. 19.0
  (Swanson), 11.25 oz. 37.0
  gravy and *(Freezer Queen)*, 9 oz. 18.0
Stroganoff *(Armour Classics Lite)*, 11.25 oz. 33.0
Swiss steak *(Swanson)*, 10 oz. 36.0
teriyaki *(The Budget Gourmet Light and Healthy)*,
  10.75 oz. 37.0

Beef entree, canned or packaged:
chow mein *(La Choy)*, ¾ cup 5.0
chow mein *(La Choy Bi-Pack)*, ¾ cup 8.0
pepper *(La Choy Bi-Pack)*, ¾ cup.................................... 10.0
pepper, Oriental *(La Choy)*, ¾ cup 12.0
roast, and gravy, with potatoes *(Dinty Moore*
    American Classics), 10 oz. 26.0
roast, tender *(Hormel Top Shelf)*, 10 oz. 19.0
Salisbury steak *(Hormel Top Shelf)*, 10 oz. 22.0
stew:
    (Dinty Moore Cup), 7.5 oz. 15.0
    (Healthy Choice), 7.5 oz. 16.0
    (Hormel Micro Cup), 7.5 oz. 11.0
    (Libby's), 7.5 oz. 17.0
    (Libby's Diner), 7.75 oz. 22.0
Beef entree, freeze-dried*:
Bourguignon *(Mountain House)*, 1 cup.............................. 20.0
and rice, with onions *(Mountain House)*, 1 cup 42.0
and rice, with pepper and onion sauce *(Mountain*
    House), 1 cup 32.0
stew *(Mountain House)*, 1 cup... 26.0
Stroganoff *(Mountain House)*, 1 cup 27.0
Beef entree, frozen:
Cantonese *(The Budget Gourmet)*, 9.1 oz. 31.0
Cantonese, with rice *(Weight Watchers Stir-Fry)*,
    9 oz. 27.0
champignon *(Tyson Gourmet Selection)*, 10.5 oz. 31.0
cheeseburger:
    (Hormel Quick Meal), 4.8 oz.. 35.0
    (MicroMagic), 4.75 oz... 29.0
    bacon *(Hormel Quick Meal)*, 5 oz. 32.0
    bacon *(MicroMagic)*, 4 oz. 31.0
    chili *(Hormel Quick Meal)*, 6 oz. 39.0
    double *(Hormel Quick Meal)*, 7.5 oz. 47.0
    mini *(Jimmy Dean)*, 1 burger 11.0
chop suey, without rice *(On-Cor)*, 8 oz. 9.0

creamed, chipped:
  (Banquet Cookin' Bag), 4 oz. 9.0
  (Freezer Queen Cook-in-Pouch), 4 oz. 9.0
  (Stouffer's), 5.5 oz. 9.0
  (Swanson), 9 oz. 17.0
enchilada, see "Enchilada entree"
hamburger *(Hormel Quick Meal)*, 4.3 oz. 34.0
hamburger *(MicroMagic)*, 4 oz. 26.0
jade garden *(Weight Watchers Stir-Fry)*, 9 oz. 17.0
London broil *(Weight Watchers Ultimate 200)*, 7.5 oz. 4.0
meat loaf, see "Meat loaf entree"
and noodles, with gravy and vegetables *(Stouffer's
  Homestyle)*, 8³⁄₈ oz. 26.0
Oriental *(The Budget Gourmet Light and Healthy)*,
  10 oz. 36.0
Oriental, with vegetables and rice *(Lean Cuisine)*,
  8⁵⁄₈ oz. 31.0
patty:
  charbroiled *(Freezer Queen Family)*, 7 oz. 9.0
  charbroiled *(On-Cor)*, 8 oz. 12.0
  charbroiled, mushroom gravy and *(Banquet
    Family)*, 7 oz. 12.0
  Italian, tomato sauce and *(On-Cor)*, 8 oz. 17.0
  and mushroom gravy *(Banquet Entree Express)*,
    7 oz. 12.0
  onion gravy and *(Banquet Family)*, 7 oz. 13.0
  onion gravy and *(Freezer Queen Family)*, 7 oz. 10.0
pepper Oriental *(Chun King)*, 13 oz. 53.0
pepper steak:
  (Healthy Choice), 9.5 oz. 36.0
  green, with rice *(Stouffer's)*, 10.5 oz. 35.0
  with rice *(The Budget Gourmet)*, 10 oz. 40.0
and peppers *(Freezer Queen)*, 9 oz. 30.0
pie:
  (Stouffer's), 10 oz. 37.0
  (Swanson), 7 oz. 38.0
  (Swanson Hungry Man), 14 oz. 51.0

Beef entree, frozen *(cont.)*

pot roast, with browned potatoes *(Stouffer's*
    Homestyle), 8⅞ oz. 24.0
pot roast, Yankee *(Freezer Queen)*, 9 oz. 20.0
ribs, barbecue *(Healthy Choice Homestyle Classics)*,
    11 oz. 40.0
Salisbury steak:
    (Banquet Healthy Balance), 10.5 oz. 31.0
    (Banquet Meals), 9.5 oz. 28.0
    (Dining Lite), 9 oz. 14.0
    (Freezer Queen), 9 oz. 21.0
    (On-Cor), 8 oz. 10.0
    and gravy *(Banquet Entree Express)*, 7 oz. 13.0
    gravy and *(Banquet Cookin' Bag)*, 5 oz. 8.0
    gravy and *(Banquet Family)*, 7 oz. 11.0
    gravy and *(Freezer Queen Family)*, 7 oz. 9.0
    gravy and *(Freezer Queen Cook-in-Pouch)*, 5 oz. 4.0
    with macaroni and cheese *(Lean Cuisine)*, 9.5 oz. 22.0
    with macaroni and cheese *(Stouffer's* Homestyle),
        9⅝ oz. 23.0
    with mushroom gravy *(Healthy Choice Homestyle*
        Classics), 11 oz. 35.0
    with mashed potatoes *(Swanson)*, 9 oz. 23.0
    sirloin *(The Budget Gourmet* Light and Healthy),
        9 oz. 24.0
sandwich, see "Beef sandwich"
sirloin:
    cheddar melt *(The Budget Gourmet)*, 9.4 oz. 29.0
    in herb sauce *(The Budget Gourmet* Light and
        Healthy), 9.5 oz. 21.0
    roast, supreme *(The Budget Gourmet)*, 9 oz. 28.0
sirloin tips:
    (Weight Watchers Ultimate 200), 7.5 oz. 20.0
    with mushroom gravy *(Healthy Choice)*, 9.5 oz. 34.0
    and noodles, with gravy *(Swanson)*, 7 oz. 18.0
    and country vegetables *(The Budget Gourmet)*,
        10 oz. 19.0

sliced:
  (On-Cor), 8 oz. 7.0
  gravy and *(Banquet Cookin' Bag)*, 4 oz. 5.0
  gravy and *(Banquet Family)*, 7 oz. 8.0
  gravy and *(Freezer Queen Cook-in-Pouch)*, 4 oz. 6.0
  gravy and *(Freezer Queen Family)*, 7 oz. 10.0
stew:
  (Banquet Family), 7 oz. 18.0
  (Freezer Queen), 7 oz. 15.0
  (On-Cor), 8 oz. 15.0
Stroganoff *(The Budget Gourmet Light and Healthy)*,
  8.75 oz. 27.0
Stroganoff, with parsley noodles *(Stouffer's)*, 9.75 oz. 30.0
Beef entree mix:
pepper steak *(La Choy Dinner Classics)*, 3/4 cup* 9.0
stew, hearty *(Stew Starter)*, 1/8 mix 20.0
Beef entree sauce, see "Entree sauces"
Beef gravy, canned:
2 oz. or 1/4 cup 2.8
(Franco-American), 2 oz. 4.0
(Pepperidge Farm Hearty), 2 oz. 3.0
Beef jerky (see also "Sausage sticks"):
(Frito-Lay's), .21 oz. 1.0
(Frito-Lay's Tender), .7 oz. 2.0
(Slim Jim/Slim Jim Big Jerk), 1 piece 1.0
(Slim Jim Giant Jerk), 1 piece 2.0
all varieties *(Pemmican)*, 1 oz. 2.0
plain or *Tabasco (Slim Jim Super Jerk)*, 1 piece 1.0
Beef luncheon meat:
corned:
  (Healthy Deli St. Paddy's), 1 oz. 1.1
  (Hillshire Farm Deli Select), 1 oz. .... <1.0
  (Hormel), 1 oz. .... <2.0
  cooked *(Healthy Deli)*, 1 oz. 7
  canned *(Libby's)*, 2.4 oz. 2.0
roast:
  (Healthy Deli), 1 oz. 4
  (Hormel Bread Ready), 1 oz. 1.0

Beef luncheon meat, roast *(cont.)*
(Oscar Mayer Deli-Thin), 5 slices 7
  Black Forest *(Healthy Deli),* 1 oz... .7
  Italian *(Healthy Deli),* 1 oz.. .3
  oven-roasted *(Weight Watchers),* 1 oz........................... <1.0
  oven-roasted, cured *(Hillshire Farm* Deli Select),
    1 oz. .... <1.0
smoked *(Healthy Deli),* 1 oz... .7
smoked *(Hillshire Farm* Deli Select), 1 oz. .... <1.0
Beef marinade seasoning mix *(Lawry's* Seasoning
  Blends), 1 pkg. 10.7
Beef pie, see "Beef entree, frozen"
Beef roll or stick, see "Beef jerky" and "Sausage
  sticks"
Beef sandwich, frozen:
barbecue *(Hormel Quick Meal),* 4.3 oz............................... 40.0
barbecue *(Tyson Microwave),* 1 piece 29.0
pocket:
  in BBQ sauce, *(Hot Pockets),* 4.5 oz. 47.0
  and broccoli, *(Hot Pockets),* 4.5 oz. 31.0
  and cheddar, *(Hot Pockets),* 4.5 oz. 36.0
Beef sandwich mix (see also "Sandwich sauce"):
and gravy *(Swift Premium Quick Fixin's),* 3.5 oz. 7.0
Italian sauce and *(Swift Premium Quick Fixin's),*
  3.5 oz. 4.0
Beef stew, see "Beef entree"
Beef seasoning mix:
stew:
  (French's), 1/7 pkg. 3.0
  (Lawry's Seasoning Blends), 1 pkg............................... 25.7
  (McCormick/Schilling), 1/4 pkg. 6.0
  (McCormick/Schilling Bag'n Season), 1 pkg. 11.0
Stroganoff *(McCormick/Schilling),* 1/4 pkg........................... 6.0
Beefalo, without added ingredients 0
Beer:
regular, 12 fl. oz. 13.2
light, 12 fl. oz. 4.8

Beer batter mix *(Golden Dipt)*, 1 oz..................................22.0
Beerwurst, see "Salami, beer"
Beet:
fresh:
   raw, 2 medium, 2" diameter, approximately 8.6 oz. 15.6
   raw, trimmed, sliced, ½ cup..6.5
   boiled, drained, 2 medium, 2" diameter 10.0
   boiled, drained, sliced, ½ cup 8.5
canned:
   with liquid, ½ cup 8.3
   drained, sliced, ½ cup...6.1
   cut and sliced *(Stokely)*, ½ cup 8.0
   Harvard, with liquid, ½ cup 22.4
   pickled, with liquid, ½ cup..18.5
Beet greens:
raw, 1" pieces, ½ cup 8
boiled, drained, 1" pieces, ½ cup 3.9
Berliner, pork and beef, 1 oz...7
Berry drink:
canned:
   (Hawaiian Punch Very Berry), 6 fl. oz...........................22.0
   (Hi-C Boppin' Berry), 6 fl. oz.......................................23.0
   wild *(Hi-C)*, 6 fl. oz..22.0
mix*:
   (Wyler's Bunch 'O Berries), 8 fl. oz.............................20.0
   mountain berry punch *(Kool-Aid)*, 8 fl. oz. 25.0
   mountain berry punch *(Kool-Aid* Presweetened)*,
     8 fl. oz. 18.0
Berry juice:
(Juicy Juice), 6 fl. oz. 22.0
(R.W. Knudsen Razzleberry), 8 fl. oz. 21.0
Berry juice drink:
(Tropicana Berries & Berries), 6 fl. oz. 23.0
blend *(Tang Fruit Box)*, 8.45 fl. oz. 36.0
Berry nectar *(Santa Cruz Natural)*, 8 fl. oz. 22.0
Berry punch *(Minute Maid)*, 6 fl. oz.................................23.0
Berry-grape juice drink, mixed berry *(Boku)*,
   8 fl. oz..29.0

Biscuit:
(Arnold Old Fashioned), 1 piece.. 8.0
(Wonder), 1 piece... 14.0
breakfast, whole wheat *(LaLoma Ruskets),* 2 pieces......... 22.0
country or square *(Awrey's 3"),* 2 oz................................... 23.0
round or square *(Awrey's 2"),* 1 oz..................................... 12.0
sliced or unsliced *(Awrey's),* 2 oz....................................... 23.0
frozen *(Bridgford),* 2 oz.. 28.0
mix* (see also "Baking mix") *(Robin Hood/Gold*
    Medal), 1 piece.. 14.0
Biscuit, refrigerated:
(Big Country Butter Tastin'), 1 piece 13.0
(1869 Brand Butter Tastin'), 1 piece................................... 12.0
(Grands! Butter Tastin'), 1 piece 22.0
(Pillsbury Big Premium Heat 'N Eat), 2 pieces.................... 32.0
(Pillsbury Country), 1 piece.. 10.0
plain or buttermilk *(Ballard Extra Lights Ovenready),*
    1 piece... 10.0
baking powder *(1869 Brand),* 1 piece 12.0
butter *(Pillsbury),* 1 piece.. 10.0
buttermilk:
    (Big Country), 1 piece 14.0
    (1869 Brand), 1 piece 12.0
    (Hungry Jack Extra Rich), 1 piece 9.0
    (Hungry Jack Flaky/Fluffy), 1 piece............................. 12.0
    (Pillsbury), 1 piece.. 10.0
    (Pillsbury Heat 'N Eat), 2 pieces 27.0
    (Pillsbury Tender Layer), 1 piece................................... 9.0
cinnamon raisin *(Grands!),* 1 piece..................................... 27.0
flaky:
    (Grands!), 1 piece 23.0
    (Hungry Jack), 1 piece 12.0
    (Hungry Jack Butter Tastin'), 1 piece............................ 11.0
    (Hungry Jack Honey Tastin'), 1 piece 13.0
fluffy *(Pillsbury Good 'N Buttery),* 1 piece........................... 11.0
grain, mixed *(Roman Meal),* 2 pieces................................. 33.6
honey nut oat bran *(Roman Meal),* 1 piece......................... 20.6
Southern style *(Big Country),* 1 piece 14.0

Southern style *(Hungry Jack* Flaky), 1 piece 12.0
white *(Roman Meal)*, 1 piece 18.8
Bitter melon, see "Balsam pear"
Black bean dishes:
canned, with tofu wieners *(Health Valley Tofu Fast
  Menu)*, 5 oz. 14.0
canned, Western, with vegetables *(Health Valley Fast
  Menu* Fat Free), 5 oz. 9.0
mix* *(Fantastic* Instant), ½ cup 23.0
mix*, and rice *(Fantastic* Caribbean), 10 oz. 41.0
Black beans:
dry *(Frieda's)*, 1 oz. 6.8
dry, boiled, ½ cup 20.4
canned:
  (Eden No Salt Added), ½ cup 17.0
  (Green Giant/Joan of Arc), ½ cup 21.0
  (Progresso), 4 oz. 19.0
Black beans, turtle soup:
dry:
  ½ cup 58.2
  (Arrowhead Mills), 2 oz. 35.0
  boiled, ½ cup 22.4
canned *(Hain)*, 4 oz. 15.0
Blackberries:
fresh, trimmed, ½ cup 9.2
canned in water *(Allens)*, ½ cup 4.0
canned in heavy syrup, ½ cup 29.6
frozen, unsweetened, ½ cup 11.8
Black-eyed peas, see "Cowpeas"
Blintz, frozen:
apple-raisin *(Golden)*, 2 pieces 32.0
blueberry *(Golden)*, 2 pieces 37.0
cheese:
  (Golden), 2 pieces 25.0
  (King Kold), 1 piece 18.9
  (King Kold No Salt), 1 piece 18.6
cherry *(Golden)*, 2 pieces 37.0
potato *(Golden)*, 2 pieces 29.0

Blood sausage, 1 oz. 4
Bloody Mary mixer:
(Libby's), 6 fl. oz. 8.0
regular or extra spicy *(Tabasco),* 6 fl. oz. 11.0
Blueberries:
fresh, 1/2 cup 10.2
canned in heavy syrup, 1/2 cup 28.2
frozen, unsweetened, 1/2 cup 9.4
frozen, sweetened, 1/2 cup 25.2
Blueberry nectar *(R.W. Knudsen),* 8 fl. oz. 34.0
Blueberry-cranberry drink *(Ocean Spray Cran-*
  Blueberry), 6 fl. oz. 31.0
Bluefish, without added ingredients 0
Boar, wild, without added ingredients 0
Bockwurst, raw, 1 oz. 1
Bok-choy, see "Cabbage, Chinese"
Bologna:
(Healthy Deli), 1 oz. 1.6
(Hillshire Farm Large/Ring), 1 oz. .... <1.0
(Oscar Mayer), 1 slice .... <1.0
(Oscar Mayer Healthy Favorites), 3 slices 4.0
(Oscar Mayer Light), 1 slice 2.0
(Oscar Mayer Wisconsin Ring), 2 oz. 1.0
all varieties *(Kahn's),* 1 slice 1.0
beef *(Oscar Mayer),* 1 slice .... <1.0
beef *(Oscar Mayer* Light), 1 slice 2.0
chicken, see "Chicken bologna"
garlic *(Oscar Mayer),* 1 slice 1.0
ham, see "Ham bologna"
turkey, see "Turkey bologna"
"Bologna," vegetarian, frozen *(Worthington*
  Bolono), 2 slices 2.0
Bonito, without added ingredients 5
Borage:
raw, 1″ pieces, 1/2 cup 1.4
boiled, drained, 4 oz. 4.0

Bouillon (see also "Soup"):
dry:
  all varieties (Herb-Ox Very Low Sodium), 1 packet.......... 2.0
  beef (Herb-Ox), 1 cube 1.0
  beef (Herb-Ox Instant), 1 tsp. 1.0
  beef, chicken, or vegetable vegetarian (Knorr),
    1 serving 1.0
  beef, chicken, or fish flavor (Knorr), 1 serving .... <1.0
  chicken (Herb-Ox), 1 cube .... <1.0
  chicken (Herb-Ox Instant), 1 tsp. 2.0
liquid, chicken or beef (Knorr), 2 tsp. 3.0
Boysenberry:
fresh, see "Blackberry"
canned in heavy syrup, ½ cup 28.6
frozen, unsweetened, ½ cup 8.1
Boysenberry juice (Smucker's Naturally 100%),
  8 fl. oz. 30.0
Boysenberry nectar (R.W. Knudsen), 8 fl. oz. 33.0
Brains, without added ingredients 0
Bran, see "Cereal" and specific listings
Bratwurst:
(Kahn's), 1 link 2.0
all varieties (Hillshire Farm), 2 oz. 1.0
pork, cooked, 1 oz. 6
Braunschweiger:
(Oscar Mayer Sliced/German Brand), 2 oz. .... <1.0
(Oscar Mayer Tube), 2 oz. 2.0
Brazil nuts, shelled, 1 oz., 6 large or 8 medium
  kernels 3.6
Bread:
apple walnut swirl (Pepperidge Farm), 1 slice 14.0
(Arnold/Brownberry Bran'nola), 1 slice 16.0
bran:
  (Arnold Bakery Light Country), 1 slice 7.0
  (Brownberry Light Country), 1 slice 10.0
  honey (Pepperidge Farm), 1 slice 18.0
  whole (Brownberry Natural), 1 slice 10.0
brown, see "Bread, brown"

Bread *(cont.)*
brown and serve:
  Austrian wheat *(Bread du Jour)*, 1 oz. 12.0
  French *(Bread du Jour)*, 1 oz. 13.0
  French *(DiCarlo's* Parisian), 1 oz. 12.0
  French, petite *(Bread du Jour)*, 1 loaf 44.0
  grain, mixed, stick, soft *(Roman Meal)*, 2.7 oz. 31.8
  grain, mixed, mini *(Roman Meal)*, 1/2 loaf 23.8
cinnamon:
  chip *(Arnold)*, 1 slice 13.0
  raisin *(Wonder)*, 1 slice 12.0
  swirl *(Pepperidge Farm)*, 1 slice 15.0
corn or date nut, see "Bread, sweet"
French:
  (Pepperidge Farm Fully Baked), 1 oz. 15.0
  (Wonder), 1 slice 13.0
  sliced or twin *(Pepperidge Farm)*, 1 oz. 15.0
  stick *(Francisco)*, 1 slice 12.0
  stick *(Savoni)*, 1 oz. 15.0
  twin *(Francisco)*, 2 oz. 27.0
grain, mixed:
  (Roman Meal Round Top), 1 slice 11.9
  (Roman Meal Sandwich), 1 slice 9.6
  with oat bran *(Roman Meal)*, 1 slice 11.9
  nutty *(Arnold/Brownberry Bran'nola)*, 1 slice 14.0
  7 *(Home Pride* ButterTop), 1 slice 12.0
  7 *(Pepperidge Farm* Hearty), 1 slice 18.0
  7 *(Pepperidge Farm* Light Style), 1 slice 10.0
  7 *(Roman Meal)*, 1 slice 11.9
  7 *(Roman Meal* Light), 1 slice 7.1
  with sunflower seeds *(Roman Meal* Sun Grain),
    1 slice 10.8
  12 *(Arnold* Natural), 1 slice 10.0
  12 *(Brownberry* Natural), 1 slice 11.0
  12 *(Roman Meal)*, 1 slice 11.6
  12 *(Roman Meal* Light), 1 slice 6.9
  whole *(Roman Meal* 100%), 1 slice 16.1
health nut *(Brownberry* Natural), 1 slice 11.0

(Hollywood Special Formula), dark or light, 1 slice 9.0
(Hollywood Special Formula), Fitness Blend, 1 slice........... 8.0
Italian:
  (Arnold Bakery Light), 1 slice 7.0
  (Brownberry Bakery Light), 1 slice................................... 9.0
  (Francisco Sliced), 1 slice 12.0
  (Pepperidge Farm Sliced), 1 slice.................................... 12.0
  (Wonder Family), 1 slice.. 13.0
  (Wonder Light), 1 slice 6.0
  sliced stick or loaf *(Francisco)*, 1 slice............................ 12.0
  stick *(Francisco)*, 1 oz. 17.0
oat:
  (Arnold/Brownberry Bran'nola Country), 1 slice 16.0
  (Roman Meal), 1 slice.. 12.5
  crunchy *(Pepperidge Farm* Hearty), 1 slice 17.0
oat bran:
  (Roman Meal Light), 1 slice.. 7.2
  honey *(Roman Meal)*, 1 slice... 11.8
  honey nut *(Roman Meal)*, 1 slice 11.2
oatmeal:
  (Arnold), 1 slice.. 12.0
  (Arnold Bakery Light), 1 slice 8.0
  (Brownberry Bakery Light), 1 slice 10.0
  (Brownberry Natural), 1 slice.. 11.0
  (Pepperidge Farm), 1 slice 17.0
  (Pepperidge Farm Light Style), 1 slice.............................. 9.0
  (Pepperidge Farm Thin), 1 slice 6.0
  with bran *(Oatmeal Goodness* Light), 1 slice.................... 6.0
  with bran, sunflower or wheat *(Oatmeal*
    Goodness), 1 slice 14.0
  raisin *(Arnold/Brownberry)*, 1 slice 12.0
  sandwich *(Brownberry* Natural), 1 slice 11.0
  soft *(Brownberry)*, 1 slice 12.0
  soft *(Pepperidge Farm)*, 1 slice.. 11.0
  with wheat *(Oatmeal Goodness* Light), 1 slice.................. 6.0
orange raisin *(Brownberry)*, 1 slice..................................... 13.0
pan de aqua *(Arnold Augusto)*, 1 oz. 14.0

Bread *(cont.)*

pita or pocket:

    oat bran *(Sahara)*, ½ piece 15.0

    wheat or white *(Arnold)*, ½ piece 16.0

    wheat, whole *(Sahara)*, 1 piece 23.0

    wheat, whole, mini *(Sahara)*, 1 piece 12.0

    white *(Pepperidge Farm* Wholesome Choice),

        1 piece 30.0

    white, mini *(Pepperidge Farm* Wholesome Choice),

        1 piece 15.0

    white *(Sahara)*, 1 mini or ½ regular 16.0

    white *(Sahara)*, ½ large 23.0

pumpernickel:

    (Arnold), 1 slice 15.0

    (August Bros. 1 lb.), 1 slice 14.0

    (August Bros. 24 oz.), 1 slice 18.0

    (Pepperidge Farm Family), 1 slice 15.0

    (Pepperidge Farm Party), 4 slices 12.0

raisin *(Arnold Sun-Maid)*, 1 slice 13.0

raisin cinnamon:

    (Arnold), 1 slice 13.0

    (Brownberry), 1 slice 12.0

    (Monk's), 1 oz. 10.0

    swirl *(Pepperidge Farm)*, 1 slice 16.0

raisin walnut *(Brownberry)*, 1 slice 10.0

rye:

    (Arnold Real Jewish Melba Thin), 1 slice 9.0

    (Beefsteak Hearty/Soft), 1 slice 11.0

    (Beefsteak Mild), 1 slice 12.0

    (Pepperidge Farm Party), 4 slices 12.0

    caraway *(Arnold* Real Jewish), 1 slice 13.0

    caraway *(Brownberry* Natural), 1 slice 15.0

    Dijon *(Arnold* Real Jewish), 1 slice 15.0

    Dijon *(Pepperidge Farm)*, 1 slice 9.0

    dill *(Arnold)*, 1 slice 10.0

    dill *(Brownberry* Natural), 2 slices 28.0

    onion *(August Bros.)*, 1 slice 14.0

    onion *(Beefsteak)*, 1 slice 11.0

pumpernickel *(Brownberry* Natural), 1 slice.................... 13.0
seeded *(Pepperidge Farm* Family), 1 slice 16.0
seeded or seedless *(August Bros.* 1 lb.), 1 slice............ 14.0
seeded or seedless *(August Bros.* 24 oz.), 1 slice......... 18.0
seeded or seedless *(Levy's* Real Jewish), 1 slice 16.0
seedless *(Arnold* Real Jewish), 1 slice 15.0
seedless *(August Bros.* Thin), 1 slice............................... 8.0
seedless *(Brownberry* Natural), 2 slices........................ 28.0
seedless *(Brownberry* Natural Thin), 1 slice 9.0
seedless *(Pepperidge Farm* Family), 1 slice 16.0
soft *(Arnold Bakery* Light), 1 slice................................... 7.0
soft *(Brownberry Bakery* Light), 1 slice.......................... 10.0
soft, seeded or unseeded *(Arnold Bakery),* 1 slice 14.0
rye and pumpernickel *(August Bros.),* 1 slice 18.0
sandwich, dark *(Brownberry* Natural), 1 slice 12.0
sourdough:
    (Francisco), 1 slice... 19.0
    (Roman Meal Light), 1 slice................................... 7.0
    (Wonder Light), 1 slice 6.0
    whole grain *(Roman Meal),* 1 slice...................................11.5
    whole grain *(Roman Meal* Light), 1 slice........................... 6.9
sunflower and bran *(Monk's),* 1 oz. 12.0
Vienna *(Pepperidge Farm* Light Style), 1 slice 10.0
wheat:
    (Arnold Brick Oven 1 lb.), 1 slice 9.0
    (Arnold Brick Oven 2 lb.), 1 slice 14.0
    (Arnold Natural), 1 slice.. 15.0
    (Beefsteak Hearty), 1 slice... 12.0
    (Brownberry Hearth), 1 slice 12.0
    (Brownberry Natural), 1 slice...................................... 14.0
    (Fresh & Natural), 1 slice 11.0
    (Home Pride ButterTop), 1 slice................................. 12.0
    (Home Pride Honey ButterTop), 1 slice 17.0
    (Home Pride Light), 1 slice... 7.0
    (Pepperidge Farm 1½ lb.), 1 slice 18.0
    (Pepperidge Farm Light Style), 1 slice........................ 9.0
    (Pepperidge Farm Family 2 lb.), 1 slice 13.0
    (Pepperidge Farm Very Thin), 2 slices........................ 7.0

Bread, wheat *(cont.)*

(*Roman Meal* Light), 1 slice.. 7.2
(*Thomas'* Light), 1 slice 6.0
(*Wonder* Country Style/Golden), 1 slice........................... 12.0
(*Wonder* Family), 1 slice.. 13.0
(*Wonder* Light), 1 slice 7.0
apple honey (*Brownberry*), 1 slice 11.0
cracked (*Pepperidge Farm* Thin), 2 slices 13.0
cracked (*Roman Meal*), 1 slice....................................... 15.3
cracked (*Wonder*), 1 slice 13.0
dark (*Arnold/Brownberry Bran'nola*), 1 slice................... 15.0
golden (*Arnold Bakery* Light), 1 slice............................. 7.0
golden (*Brownberry* Light), 1 slice................................. 8.0
hearty (*Arnold Brownberry Bran'nola*), 1 slice................ 15.0
hearty (*Roman Meal* Light), 1 slice 7.3
honey wheatberry (*Arnold*), 1 slice 13.0
honey wheatberry (*Roman Meal*), 1 slice....................... 12.3
sesame (*Pepperidge Farm* Hearty), 1 slice...................... 18.0
soft (*Brownberry*), 1 slice 14.0
sprouted (*Pepperidge Farm*), 2 slices............................. 11.0
wheatberry (*Roman Meal* Light), 1 slice 7.3
wheat, whole:
(*Arnold Brick Oven* Light 100%), 1 slice 6.0
(*Arnold* Stone Ground 100%), 1 slice.............................. 8.0
(*Monk's* 100% Stone Ground), 1 oz. 13.0
(*Pepperidge Farm* Thin), 2 slices 12.0
(*Roman Meal* Light 100%), 1 slice.................................. 6.8
(*Roman Meal* 100%), 1 slice 10.8
(*Wonder* Stoneground 100%), 1 slice.............................. 13.0
regular or soft (*Wonder* 100%), 1 slice........................... 10.0
white:
(*Arnold Bakery* Light Premium), 1 slice........................... 7.0
(*Arnold Brick Oven* 1 lb.), 1 slice 11.0
(*Arnold Brick Oven* 2 lb.), 1 slice 14.0
(*Arnold Brick Oven* Light), 1 slice 10.0
(*Arnold Brick Oven* Thin), 1 slice 7.0
(*Arnold* Country), 1 slice.. 18.0
(*Beefsteak* Robust), 1 slice.. 12.0

(Brownberry Country), 1 slice 19.0
(Brownberry Natural), 1 slice.. 11.0
(Home Pride ButterTop), 1 slice 12.0
(Home Pride Light), 1 slice... 7.0
(Monk's), 1 slice.. 10.0
(Pepperidge Farm Country), 2 slices 38.0
(Pepperidge Farm Large Family), 1 slice 13.0
(Pepperidge Farm Thin), 1 slice 14.0
(Pepperidge Farm Thin 8 oz.), 1 slice............................ 13.0
(Pepperidge Farm Very Thin), 1 slice 4.0
(Roman Meal Light), 1 slice.. 7.4
(Wonder), 1 slice.. 13.0
(Wonder Light), 1 slice 7.0
with buttermilk *(Wonder)*, 1 slice 13.0
extra fiber *(Arnold Brick Oven)*, 1 slice........................... 10.0
sandwich *(Brownberry)*, 1 slice 12.0
sandwich *(Pepperidge Farm)*, 2 slices........................... 24.0
soft *(Brownberry)*, 1 slice 13.0
toasting *(Pepperidge Farm)*, 1 slice 17.0
Bread, brown, canned:
(B&M/Friends), 1/2" slice 21.0
raisin *(B&M/Friends)*, 1/2" slice 22.0
Bread, frozen, garlic *(Pepperidge Farm)*, 1 oz. 11.0
Bread, sweet, date nut:
(Dromedary), 1/2" slice 13.0
(Thomas'), 1-oz. slice.. 18.0
Bread, sweet, mix*:
apple cinnamon *(Pillsbury)*, 1/12 loaf.................................... 31.0
banana *(Pillsbury)*, 1/12 loaf... 27.0
blueberry *(Pillsbury)*, 1/12 loaf.. 30.0
cornbread:
   (Ballard), 1/12 loaf 25.0
   (Dromedary), 2" square 20.0
   white *(Robin Hood/Gold Medal* Pouch), 1/6 recipe 22.0
   yellow *(Robin Hood/Gold Medal* Pouch), 1/6 recipe........ 23.0
cranberry *(Pillsbury)*, 1/12 loaf... 30.0
date *(Pillsbury)*, 1/12 loaf... 31.0
date nut *(Dromedary)*, 1/12 loaf.. 26.0

Bread, sweet, mix *(cont.)*
gingerbread, see "Cake mix"
nut *(Pillsbury)*, 1/12 loaf 27.0
oatmeal raisin *(Pillsbury)*, 1/12 loaf 30.0
Bread crumbs:
plain or Italian *(Arnold)*, 1/2 oz. 8.0
plain or Italian *(Progresso)*, 1/2 oz. 11.0
seasoned *(Contadina)*, 1 rounded tbsp. 7.0
Bread dough:
frozen, honey wheat or white *(Bridgford)*, 1 oz. 14.0
frozen, white *(Rich's)*, 2 slices 24.0
refrigerated:
  (Roman Meal), 1 oz. 13.2
  French, crusty *(Pillsbury)*, 1" slice 11.0
  twists, cornbread *(Pillsbury)*, 1 piece 8.0
  twists, country oatmeal *(Hearty Grains)*, 1 piece 15.0
  twists, wheat, cracked, and honey *(Hearty Grains)*,
    1 piece 14.0
  wheat or white *(Pipin' Hot)*, 1" slice 12.0
Bread shell, Italian:
(Boboli 6"), 1 piece 49.0
(Boboli 12"), 1 piece 196.0
Bread snacks, cinnamon raisin swirl or nacho
  cheese and corn *(Pepperidge Farm* Bread
  Bites), 1/2 oz. 9.0
Breadfruit:
1/2 cup 29.8
1/4 small, 3.4 oz. 26.0
Breadfruit seeds, 1 oz.:
raw[1], shelled 8.3
boiled[2], shelled 9.1
roasted, shelled 11.4
Breading mix, frying *(Golden Dipt)*, 1 oz. 20.0

---
[1] *South American cultivar.*
[2] *Pacific area cultivar.*

Breadstick:
plain *(Stella D'Oro/Stella D'Oro* Dietetic), 1 piece 7.0
cheddar *(Pepperidge Farm* Thin), ½ oz. 9.0
garlic and herb *(Master Choice)*, 1 piece 2.0
onion *(Stella D'Oro)*, 1 piece 6.0
onion *(Pepperidge Farm* Thin), ½ oz. 10.0
pizza *(Stella D'Oro)*, 1 piece 7.0
sesame *(Pepperidge Farm* Thin), ½ oz. 10.0
sesame *(Stella D'Oro/Stella D'Oro* Dietetic), 1 piece 6.0
wheat *(Stella D'Oro)*, 1 piece 6.0
refrigerated, soft *(Pillsbury)*, 1 piece 17.0
refrigerated, soft *(Roman Meal)*, 1 piece 18.2
Breakfast, see specific listings
Broad beans:
raw, ½ cup 6.4
boiled, drained, 4 oz. 11.5
Broad beans, mature:
dry *(Frieda's* Fava Beans), 1 oz. 1.9
dry, boiled, ½ cup 16.7
canned *(Progresso* Fava Beans), ½ cup 15.0
canned, with liquid, ½ cup 15.9
Broccoli:
fresh:
   raw, chopped, ½ cup 2.3
   raw, 1 spear, 8.7 oz. 7.9
   boiled, drained, chopped, ½ cup 3.9
   boiled, drained, 1 spear, 6.3 oz. 9.1
frozen:
   spears, 10-oz. pkg. 15.2
   spears *(Green Giant Harvest Fresh)*, ½ cup 4.0
   spears *(Green Giant Select)*, ½ cup 5.0
   spears, cuts or chopped *(Seabrook)*, 3.3 oz. 5.0
   spears, cuts or chopped *(Stilwell)*, ½ cup 4.0
   florets *(Frosty Acres)*, 3.3 oz. 5.0
   cuts *(Green Giant Polybag)*, ½ cup 5.0
   cuts *(Green Giant Harvest Fresh)*, ½ cup 3.0
   chopped, 10-oz. pkg. 13.6

Broccoli, frozen *(cont.)*
  in butter sauce, cut *(Green Giant* One Serving),
    4.5 oz. 7.0
  in butter sauce, spears *(Green Giant),* ½ cup 6.0
  in cheese sauce *(Birds Eye),* ½ cup 7.0
  in cheese sauce *(Freezer Queen Family),* 4.5 oz. 8.0
  in cheese sauce *(Green Giant),* ½ cup 9.0
  in cheese sauce, cut *(Green Giant* One Serving),
    5 oz. 13.0
Broccoli combinations, frozen:
carrots and rotini, in cheese sauce *(Green Giant* One
    Serving), 5.5 oz. 17.0
and cauliflower *(Frosty Acres* Swiss Mix), 3 oz. 5.0
and cauliflower, medley *(Green Giant Valley*
    Combinations), ½ cup 9.0
cauliflower and carrots:
    (Green Giant One Serving), 4 oz. 7.0
    in butter sauce *(Green Giant),* ½ cup 4.0
    in cheese sauce *(Birds Eye),* ½ cup 8.0
    in cheese sauce *(Green Giant* One Serving), 5 oz. 13.0
    in cheese sauce *(Green Giant),* ½ cup 9.0
fanfare *(Green Giant Valley Combinations),* ½ cup 14.0
pasta, cauliflower, carrots, cheese sauce *(Freezer*
    Queen Family), 4.5 oz. 13.0
and red peppers *(Green Giant Select),* ½ cup 4.0
Broccoli and cheese pastry, frozen *(Pepperidge*
    Farm), 1 piece 18.0
Brown gravy:
canned or in jars:
    (Heinz HomeStyle), 2 oz. or ¼ cup 3.0
    (La Choy), ½ tsp. 4.0
    with onions *(Heinz* HomeStyle), 2 oz. or ¼ cup 3.0
mix:
    (French's), ¼ pkg. 3.0
    (Hain), ¼ pkg. 3.0
    (Lawry's), 1 pkg. 13.2
    (McCormick/Schilling), ¼ cup* 3.5
    (McCormick/Schilling Lite), ¼ cup* 2.0

(Pillsbury), ¼ cup* 3.0
(Spatini), 1 cup* 16.4
vegetarian *(LaLoma Gravy Quik),* 2 tbsp.* 2.0
Brownie:
(Drake's Old Fashion), 1 piece..................................... 20.0
(Tastykake), 1 piece 53.0
all varieties *(Hostess Brownie Bites),* 5 pieces................... 31.0
butterscotch *(Rachel's),* 2.1 oz. 36.0
chocolate, double *(Rachel's),* 2.1 oz. 29.0
chocolate, double, with nuts *(Rachel's),* 2.1 oz. 30.0
fudge *(Drake's),* 1 piece.. 60.0
fudge *(Little Debbie),* 1 piece 38.0
fudge nut *(Awrey's* Sheet Cake), 1.2 oz........................... 16.0
fudge nut *(Frito-Lay's),* 3 oz. 56.0
fudge nut, iced *(Awrey's* Sheet Cake), 2.5 oz.................... 36.0
Brownie, frozen:
à la mode *(Weight Watchers Sweet Celebrations),*
   1 piece.. 35.0
chocolate *(Weight Watchers Sweet Celebrations),*
   1 piece.. 16.0
hot fudge *(Pepperidge Farm* Classic), 1 piece 46.0
fudge, all varieties *(Weight Watchers Sweet*
   Celebrations), 1 piece.. 18.0
Brownie mix*:
(Betty Crocker Supreme Original), 1 piece......................... 22.0
(Betty Crocker Supreme Party), 1 piece............................. 26.0
caramel *(Betty Crocker* Supreme), 1 piece 21.0
chocolate:
   double *(Pillsbury Great Additions),* 1 piece 19.0
   German *(Betty Crocker* Supreme), 1 piece..................... 24.0
   milk *(Duncan Hines* Brownies Plus), 1 piece.................. 20.0
chocolate chip *(Betty Crocker* Supreme), 1 piece 20.0
frosted *(Betty Crocker* Supreme), 1 piece......................... 26.0
frosted *(Betty Crocker* MicroRave), 1 piece 27.0
fudge:
   (Betty Crocker Family Size), 1 piece............................... 22.0
   (Betty Crocker Light), 1 piece 21.0
   (Duncan Hines), 1 piece 18.0

Brownie mix, fudge *(cont.)*
(Pillsbury 15 oz.), 1 piece.. 21.0
(Pillsbury 21.5 oz.), 1 piece... 20.0
(Pillsbury Lovin' Lites), 1 piece...................................... 19.0
(Pillsbury Microwave), 1 piece....................................... 25.0
(Robin Hood/Gold Medal Pouch), 1 piece.................... 15.0
with chocolate fudge frosting *(Pillsbury*
    Microwave), 1 piece.. 32.0
double *(Duncan Hines* Brownies Plus), 1 piece 22.0
Funfetti, frosted *(Pillsbury Great Additions),* 1 piece 23.0
with hot fudge topping *(Betty Crocker MicroRave*
    Singles), 1 piece... 54.0
peanut butter *(Duncan Hines* Brownies Plus), 1 piece 16.0
turtle *(Duncan Hines* Gourmet), 1 piece............................ 27.0
walnut:
(Betty Crocker Supreme), 1 piece................................. 18.0
(Duncan Hines Brownies Plus), 1 piece........................ 19.0
(Pillsbury Great Additions), 1 piece.............................. 16.0
Browning sauce *(Gravymaster),* 1 tsp............................... 2.4
Brussels sprouts:
fresh:
raw, ½ cup... 3.9
boiled, drained, 1 sprout, .7 oz.................................... 1.8
boiled, drained, ½ cup... 6.8
frozen:
boiled, drained, ½ cup... 6.5
(Birds Eye), 3.3 oz... 7.0
regular or baby *(Seabrook),* 3.3 oz............................... 7.0
in butter sauce *(Green Giant),* ½ cup.............................. 8.0
Buckwheat, whole-grain:
1 oz. 20.3
1 cup.. 121.6
Buckwheat flour:
1 oz. 20.0
1 cup... 84.7
(Arrowhead Mills), 2 oz.. 41.0

Buckwheat groats:
brown or white *(Arrowhead Mills)*, 2 oz.............................. 41.0
roasted, dry, 1 oz.. 21.2
roasted, cooked, 1 cup.. 39.5
Bulgur (see also "Tabouleh mix"):
dry, 1 oz. 21.5
dry, 1 cup 106.2
cooked, 1 cup.. 33.8
Bun, see "Rolls"
Bun, sweet (see also "Roll, sweet"):
honey:
   (Aunt Fanny's), 1 piece.................................... 42.0
   apple bear *(Aunt Fanny's)*, 1 piece 50.0
   creme-filled *(Aunt Fanny's Bogie)*, 1 piece...................... 49.0
   glazed *(Tastykake)*, 1 piece 42.0
   iced *(Tastykake)*, 1 piece 50.0
   jelly-filled *(Aunt Fanny's Birdie)*, 1 piece................. 53.0
   lemon bear *(Aunt Fanny's)*, 1 piece 52.0
   snow bear *(Aunt Fanny's)*, 1 piece 60.0
frozen, cinnamon *(Rich's Ever Fresh)*, 1 piece.................. 34.0
frozen, honey *(Rich's Ever Fresh)*, 1 piece.................... 29.0
Burbot, without added ingredients 0
Burdock root:
raw, pieces, 1/2 cup... 10.3
raw, 1 medium, 7.3 oz... 13.6
boiled, drained, 1" pieces, 1/2 cup.................................. 13.2
Burger King, 1 serving:
breakfast dishes:
   blueberry mini muffins.. 37.0
   Breakfast Buddy with sausage, egg, and cheese.......... 15.0
   Croissan'wich with bacon, egg, and cheese.................. 19.0
   Croissan'wich with ham, egg, and cheese.................. 20.0
   Croissan'wich with sausage, egg, and cheese 22.0
   French toast sticks.. 60.0
   hash browns 25.0
burgers and sandwiches:
   bacon double cheeseburger, regular or deluxe.............. 26.0
   BK Broiler chicken sandwich 29.0

Burger King, burgers and sandwiches (cont.)

BK Big Fish sandwich	58.0
cheeseburger	28.0
chicken sandwich	54.0
Chicken Specialty, American	57.0
Chicken Specialty, French	55.0
Chicken Specialty, Italian	61.0
double cheeseburger	29.0
hamburger	28.0
Whopper or Double Whopper	44.0
Whopper or Double Whopper with cheese	46.0
Whopper Jr.	28.0
Whopper Jr., with cheese	29.0

Chicken Tenders, 6 pieces	14.0
shrimp, butterfly	21.0

side dishes:

baked potato	48.0
dinner roll	13.0
french fries, medium	43.0
onion rings	38.0

salad, without dressing:

chef salad	7.0
chunky chicken or garden salad	8.0
dinner or side salad	5.0

salad dressings, 1.1 oz.:

bleu cheese	1.0
French	12.0
light Italian, low calorie	3.0
ranch	2.0
Thousand Island	8.0

sauces:

A.M. Express dipping, 1 oz.	21.0
barbecue dipping, 1 oz.	9.0
BK Broiler, .4 oz.	1.0
Bull's Eye barbecue sauce, .5 oz.	5.0
honey dipping, 1 oz.	23.0
ranch dipping, 1 oz.	2.0
sweet & sour dipping, 1 oz.	11.0

desserts:
  Dutch apple pie.. 39.0
  Snickers ice cream bar................................... 20.0
shakes, medium:
  chocolate 54.0
  chocolate, with syrup added 68.0
  strawberry, with syrup added 67.0
  vanilla.. 53.0
Burrito, frozen (see also "Burrito entree"):
beef *(Hormel),* 4 oz. 37.0
beef, nacho *(Patio Britos),* 3 oz............................ 25.0
beef and bean:
  (Patio Britos), 3 oz.. 28.0
  hot, red chili *(Patio),* 5 oz. 44.0
  medium, mild or hot, red or green chili *(Patio),*
    5 oz. 43.0
cheese *(Hormel),* 4 oz...................................... 43.0
cheese, nacho *(Patio Britos),* 3.63 oz................ 32.0
chicken and cheese, spicy *(Patio Britos),* 3 oz. 28.0
chili, red *(Hormel),* 4 oz.................................... 40.0
Burrito, breakfast, frozen:
(Swanson Original), 3.5 oz. 25.0
bacon *(Swanson),* 3.5 oz. 27.0
wlth home fries *(Swanson Fiesta),* 5.75 oz.......... 31.0
sausage *(Swanson),* 3.15 oz................................ 24.0
Burrito dinner mix:
(Tio Sancho Dinner Kit):
  seasoning, 3.25 oz. 49.3
  1 tortilla.. 24.0
Burrito entree, frozen:
bean and cheese *(Old El Paso),* 1 piece............ 44.0
beef and bean:
  hot or medium *(Old El Paso),* 1 piece 41.0
  medium or mild *(Healthy Choice* Quick Meal),
    5.4 oz. 42.0
  mild *(Old El Paso),* 1 piece............................ 42.0
chicken con queso, mild *(Healthy Choice* Quick
  Meal), 5.4 oz. 40.0

Burrito seasoning mix:
(*Lawry's* Seasoning Blends), 1 pkg. 23.3
(*Old El Paso*), ⅛ pkg. 3.0
Butter, salted or unsalted:
regular, 1 stick or 4 oz. 0
whipped, ½ cup or 1 stick .... <.1
Butter beans, see "Lima beans"
Butter flavor seasoning, all flavors (*McCormick/*
Shilling Best O'Butter), ½ tsp. .... <1.0
Butterbur:
fresh:
  raw, ½ cup 1.7
  raw, 1 stalk, .2 oz. 2
  boiled, drained, 4 oz. 2.4
canned, chopped, ½ cup 2
Butterfish, without added ingredients 0
Buttermilk, see "Milk" and "Milk, dry"
Butternut squash:
fresh, raw, cubed, ½ cup 8.1
fresh, baked, cubed, ½ cup 10.7
frozen:
  12-oz. pkg. 49.0
  boiled, drained, 4 oz. 11.4
  mashed, ½ cup 12.1
Butternuts, dried:
in shell, 1 lb. 14.8
shelled, 1 oz. 3.4
Butterscotch chips, baking (*Nestlé* Toll House
  Morsels), 1 oz. 19.0
Butterscotch topping:
(*Kraft*), 1 tbsp. 13.0
(*Smucker's/Smucker's* Special Recipe), 2 tbsp. 33.0

C

Food and Measure	Carbohydrate Grams

Cabbage:
raw, 5¾"-diameter head, 2.5 lb. 49.3
raw, shredded, ½ cup 1.9
boiled, drained, shredded, ½ cup 3.4
Cabbage, Chinese:
bok-choy:
  raw, whole, 1 lb. 8.7
  raw, shredded, ½ cup 8
  boiled, drained, shredded, ½ cup 1.5
napa, raw *(Frieda's)*, 1 oz. 9
pe-tsai:
  raw, whole, 1 lb. 13.6
  raw, shredded, ½ cup 1.2
  boiled, drained, shredded, ½ cup 1.4
Cabbage, red:
raw, whole, 1 lb. 22.2
raw, shredded, ½ cup 2.1
boiled, drained, shredded, ½ cup 3.5
Cabbage, savoy:
raw, whole, 1 lb. 22.1
raw, shredded, ½ cup 2.1
boiled, drained, shredded, ½ cup 4.0
Cabbage, stuffed, frozen:
(On-Cor), 8 oz. 15.0
with meat, in tomato sauce *(Lean Cuisine)*, 9.5 oz. 26.0
Cactus pear, see "Prickly pear"
Cajun sauce, see "Creole sauce"
Cajun seasoning *(Tone's)*, 1 tsp. 2.1

Cake (see also "Cake, snack"):
apple streusel *(Awrey's)*, 2" square 18.0
banana, iced *(Awrey's)*, 2" square........................ 17.0
Black Forest torte *(Awrey's)*, 1/14 cake................ 38.0
carrot, iced, supreme *(Awrey's)*, 2" square 23.0
carrot, 3-layer *(Awrey's)*, 1/12 cake 44.0
chocolate:
  double, iced *(Awrey's)*, 2" square 21.0
  double, 2-layer *(Awrey's)*, 1/12 cake.............. 38.0
  double, 3-layer *(Awrey's)*, 1/12 cake.............. 48.0
  double torte *(Awrey's)*, 1/14 cake.................... 51.0
  German, iced *(Awrey's)*, 2" square 19.0
  German, 3-layer *(Awrey's)*, 1/12 cake 46.0
  milk, yellow, 2-layer *(Awrey's)*, 1/12 cake 33.0
  white iced, 2-layer *(Awrey's)*, 1/12 cake 34.0
coconut, butter cream *(Awrey's)*, 2" square...... 19.0
coconut, yellow, 3-layer *(Awrey's)*, 1/12 cake 40.0
coffee, caramel nut *(Awrey's)*, 1/12 cake............ 15.0
coffee, long John *(Awrey's)*, 1/12 cake................ 19.0
devil's food, iced *(Awrey's)*, 2" square.............. 17.0
lemon, 3-layer *(Awrey's)*, 1/12 cake...................... 38.0
lemon, yellow, 2-layer *(Awrey's)*, 1/12 cake 33.0
Neapolitan torte *(Awrey's)*, 1/14 cake.................. 43.0
orange, iced, frosty *(Awrey's)*, 2" square 19.0
orange, iced, three-layer *(Awrey's)*, 1/12 cake 40.0
peanut butter torte *(Awrey's)*, 1/14 cake 44.0
pistachio torte *(Awrey's)*, 1/14 cake.................... 41.0
pound, golden *(Awrey's)*, 1/12 cake 19.0
raisin spice, iced *(Awrey's)*, 2" square 21.0
raspberry nut *(Awrey's)*, 1/16 cake 39.0
sponge *(Awrey's)*, 2" square.............................. 11.0
strawberry supreme or walnut torte *(Awrey's)*,
  1/14 cake 38.0
yellow, iced *(Awrey's)*, 2" square........................ 18.0
Cake, frozen (see also "Cake, snack, frozen"):
Boston creme *(Pepperidge Farm* Special Recipe),
  2 oz. 28.0

cheesecake, French *(Sara Lee),* 1/8 cake 23.0
cheesecake, New York *(Master Choice),* 1/6 cake 19.0
chocolate:
    double, layer *(Sara Lee),* 1/8 cake 33.0
    fudge layer *(Pepperidge Farm),* 1.7 oz. 23.0
    fudge stripe *(Pepperidge Farm),* 1.7 oz. 20.0
    German, layer *(Pepperidge Farm),* 1.7 oz. 22.0
chocolate mousse *(Pepperidge Farm* Special
    Recipe), 2 oz. 25.0
chocolate mousse *(Sara Lee),* 1/8 cake 23.0
coconut layer *(Pepperidge Farm),* 1.7 oz. 24.0
coconut layer *(Sara Lee Flaky),* 1/8 cake 33.0
devil's food or golden layer *(Pepperidge Farm),*
    1.7 oz. 24.0
lemon mousse *(Pepperidge Farm* Special Recipe),
    1.6 oz. 21.0
pineapple cream *(Pepperidge Farm* Special Recipe),
    2 oz. 28.0
pound, all butter *(Sara Lee),* 1/15 cake 14.0
pound cake, chocolate or golden *(Pepperidge Farm*
    Fat Free), 1 oz. 15.0
strawberry cream *(Pepperidge Farm* Special Recipe),
    2 oz. 30.0
strawberry stripe layer *(Pepperidge Farm),* 1.5 oz. 21.0
vanilla layer *(Pepperidge Farm),* 1.7 oz. 25.0
Cake, snack (see also "Cookies," "Donuts," and
    specific listings):
apple:
    (Little Debbie Apple Roos), 1.5-oz. piece 30.0
    filled *(Little Debbie* Apple Delights), 1.25-oz. piece 22.0
    pastry pocket *(Tastykake),* 1 piece 38.0
    spice *(Hostess Light),* 1 piece 29.0
    strudel *(Aunt Fanny's),* 3 oz. 38.0
banana:
    (Hostess Suzy Q's), 1 piece 38.0
    (Hostess Twinkies), 1 piece 26.0
    (Tastykake Creamie), 1 piece 25.0
    (Little Debbie Banana Twins), 1.1-oz. piece 18.0

Cake, snack *(cont.)*

butter pecan bites *(Barbara's Small Indulgences)*,
    1 oz. 16.0
butterscotch *(Tastykake Krimpets)*, 1 piece 19.0
cheese pastry pocket *(Tastykake)*, 1 piece 38.0
cherry:
    cordial *(Little Debbie)*, 1.31-oz. piece 23.0
    pastry *(Tastykake)*, 1 piece 41.0
    strudel *(Aunt Fanny's)*, 3 oz. 39.0
chocolate:
    (Hostess Choco Bliss), 1 piece 29.0
    (Hostess Choco-Diles), 1 piece 32.0
    (Hostess Ding Dongs), 1 piece 21.0
    (Hostess Grizzly Chomps), 1 piece 23.0
    (Hostess Ho Hos), 1 piece 16.0
    (Hostess Suzy Q's), 1 piece 37.0
    (Little Debbie Choco-Cake), 2.08-oz. piece 35.0
    (Little Debbie Choco-o-Jels), 1.16-oz. piece 20.0
    (Little Debbie Chocolate Twins), 1.18-oz. piece 21.0
    (Tastykake Creamie), 1 piece 24.0
    (Tastykake Junior), 1 piece 57.0
    (Tastykake Kandy Kakes), 1 piece 13.0
    cream filled *(Drake's Devil Dog)*, 1 piece 25.0
    cream filled *(Drake's Ring Ding)*, 1 piece 23.0
    roll, cream filled *(Drake's Yodel)*, 1 piece 16.0
chocolate chip *(Little Debbie)*, 1.2-oz. piece 21.0
chocolate chip crisps *(Barbara's Small Indulgences)*,
    1 oz. 18.0
coconut:
    (Little Debbie Cakes), 2.17-oz. piece 38.0
    (Little Debbie Rounds), 1.16-oz. piece 21.0
    (Tastykake Junior), 1 piece 60.0
    (Tastykake Kandy Kake), 1 piece 11.0
    covered *(Hostess Sno Balls)*, 1 piece 26.0
coffee cake:
    (Drake's Small), 1 piece 37.0
    (Tastykake Koffee Kake Junior), 1 piece 44.0
    apple streusel *(Little Debbie)*, 1-oz. piece 16.0

cinnamon crumb (Hostess 97% Fat Free), 1 piece........ 19.0
cream filled (Tastykake Koffee Kake), 1 piece 18.0
crumb (Hostess), 1 piece 19.0
crunch (Barbara's Small Indulgences), 1 oz. 18.0
crisp bars (Little Debbie Dutch Crisp), .71-oz. piece......... 13.0
cupcake:
    butter cream, cream filled (Tastykake), 1 piece 20.0
    chocolate (Tastykake), 1 piece 19.0
    chocolate (Tastykake Royale), 1 piece............................ 28.0
    chocolate, cream filled (Drake's Yankee Doodle),
        1 piece 16.0
    chocolate, creme filled (Hostess Lights), 1 piece........... 26.0
    creme (Tastykake Kreme Kup), 1 piece............................ 15.0
    golden, cream filled (Drake's Sunny Doodle),
        1 piece 16.0
    orange (Aunt Fanny's), 1 piece 54.0
    orange (Hostess), 1 piece 27.0
    vanilla, cream filled (Tastykake Tasty Too), 1 piece 21.0
date nut pastry (Awrey's), 1.6 oz......................................35.0
devil's food:
    (Little Debbie Devil Cremes), 1.62-oz. piece 28.0
    (Little Debbie Devil Squares), 1.1-oz. piece 19.0
    finger (Aunt Fanny's), 1 piece 49.0
(Drake's Funny Bone), 1 piece..18.0
fudge:
    (Little Debbie Rounds), 1.19-oz. piece 23.0
    crispy bars (Little Debbie), 1.14-oz. piece.................... 20.0
    macaroon (Little Debbie), 1.04-oz. piece........................ 18.0
golden, cream filled:
    (Hostess Twinkies), 1 piece... 27.0
    (Hostess Twinkies Lights), 1 piece.................................. 21.0
    (Little Debbie Golden Cremes), 1.47-oz. piece 24.0
(Hostess Dessert Cup), 1 piece..18.0
(Hostess Li'l Angels), 1 piece 14.0
(Hostess Tiger Tails), 1 piece 38.0
jelly (Tastykake Krimpets), 1 piece....................................... 19.0
jelly roll (Little Debbie), 2.17-oz. piece 41.0
lemon (Tastykake Junior), 1 piece...64.0

Cake, snack *(cont.)*
lemon almond delights *(Barbara's Small*
 Indulgences), 1 oz. 18.0
lemon stix *(Little Debbie)*, .78-oz. piece 15.0
(Little Debbie Zebra Cakes)*, 1 piece 22.0
marshmallow supreme *(Little Debbie)*, 1.13-oz. piece 22.0
mint *(Little Debbie* Sprints)*, .78-oz. piece 13.0
oatmeal *(Little Debbie* Oatmeal II)*, 1 piece 27.0
orange *(Tastykake* Junior)*, 1 piece 61.0
peanut butter:
    (Tastykake Kandy Kakes)*, 1 piece 11.0
    bar *(Little Debbie)*, .96-oz. piece 16.0
    and jelly sandwich *(Little Debbie)*, 1.13-oz. piece 21.0
    wafer *(Little Debbie* Nutty Bar)*, 1-oz. piece 17.0
peanut cluster *(Little Debbie)*, 1.38-oz. piece 22.0
pies, see "Pies, snack"
pound, all butter *(Drake's)*, 1 piece 37.0
pumpkin *(Little Debbie* Delights)*, 1.13-oz. piece 21.0
raspberry finger *(Aunt Fanny's)*, 1 piece 53.0
spice *(Little Debbie)*, 1.23-oz. piece 21.0
spice, finger *(Aunt Fanny's)*, 1 piece 49.0
strawberry *(Tastykake* Krumpets)*, 1 piece 20.0
strawberry filled *(Hostess Twinkies Fruit N Creme)*,
    1.5 oz. 27.0
Swiss cake rolls *(Little Debbie)*, 1.08-oz. piece 19.0
vanilla:
    (Hostess Grizzly Chomps), 1 piece 23.0
    (Little Debbie Snack Cakes)*, 1.3-oz. piece 22.0
    (Tastykake Creamie)*, 1 piece 25.0
    creme *(Little Debbie)*, 1.45-oz. piece 25.0
    finger *(Aunt Fanny's)*, 1 piece 50.0
Cake, snack, frozen (see also specific listings):
caramel fudge à la mode *(Weight Watchers Sweet*
 Celebrations), 1 piece 35.0
cheesecake:
    brownie *(Weight Watchers Sweet Celebrations)*,
     1 piece 34.0

strawberry *(Pepperidge Farm)*, 1 piece 41.0
strawberry *(Weight Watchers Sweet Celebrations)*,
   1 piece 28.0
chocolate, German *(Pepperidge Farm)*, 1 piece 29.0
coffee, cinnamon streusel *(Weight Watchers)*, 1 piece 27.0
fudge, double, or strawberry shortcake à la mode
   (Weight Watchers Sweet Celebrations), 1 piece............. 33.0
Cake, snack, mix* (see also "Dessert bar mix" and
   specific listings):
applesauce raisin *(Robin Hood/Gold Medal* Snackin
   Cake), 1 piece 28.0
banana, vanilla frosted *(Pillsbury* Microwave), 1 piece 26.0
banana walnut *(Robin Hood/Gold Medal* Snackin
   Cake), 1 piece 27.0
carrot, cream cheese frosting *(Pillsbury* Microwave),
   1 piece.. 25.0
chocolate, chocolate fudge frosted *(Pillsbury*
   MicroRave), 1 piece... 24.0
chocolate chip, golden *(Robin Hood/Gold Medal*
   Snackin Cake), 1 piece 26.0
chocolate chip fudge *(Robin Hood/Gold Medal*
   Snackin Cake), 1 piece 25.0
cupcake, frosted, chocolate *(Pillsbury Funfetti*
   Microwave), 1 piece 24.0
cupcake, frosted, yellow *(Pillsbury Funfetti*
   Microwave), 1 piece 28.0
Cake, mix*:
angel food:
   (Betty Crocker Traditional), 1/12 cake 30.0
   (Duncan Hines), 1/12 cake.. 30.0
   (Pillsbury Lovin' Loaf), 1/8 cake... 20.0
   confetti, lemon custard, or white *(Betty Crocker)*,
      1/12 cake.. 34.0
banana *(Duncan Hines)*, 1/12 cake 36.0
banana *(Pillsbury Plus)*, 1/12 cake 35.0
Black Forest cherry *(Pillsbury Bundt)*, 1/16 cake 41.0
blueberry *(Streusel Swirl)*, 1/16 cake 39.0
Boston cream *(Betty Crocker* Classics), 1/8 cake 50.0

Cake, mix *(cont.)*
Boston cream *(Pillsbury Bundt)*, 1/16 cake 42.0
butter pecan *(Betty Crocker SuperMoist)*, 1/12 cake 35.0
butter recipe:
  (Pillsbury Plus), 1/12 cake 35.0
  chocolate *(Betty Crocker SuperMoist)*, 1/12 cake 35.0
  chocolate *(Pillsbury Plus)*, 1/12 cake 32.0
  fudge *(Duncan Hines)*, 1/12 cake 34.0
  golden *(Duncan Hines)*, 1/12 cake 36.0
  yellow *(Betty Crocker SuperMoist)*, 1/12 cake 37.0
carrot:
  (Betty Crocker SuperMoist), 1/12 cake 36.0
  (Dromedary), 1/12 cake 23.0
  (Pillsbury Plus), 1/12 cake 34.0
cherry chip *(Betty Crocker SuperMoist)*, 1/12 cake 37.0
chocolate:
  (Simply Splendid), 3 oz. 43.0
  dark *(Pillsbury Plus)*, 1/12 cake 32.0
  fudge *(Betty Crocker SuperMoist)*, 1/12 cake 35.0
  fudge *(Pillsbury Bundt Tunnel of Fudge)*, 1/16 cake 42.0
  fudge, dark Dutch *(Duncan Hines)*, 1/12 cake 33.0
  German *(Betty Crocker SuperMoist)*, 1/12 cake 35.0
  German *(Pillsbury Plus)*, 1/12 cake 34.0
  German, with frosting *(Betty Crocker MicroRave)*,
    1/6 cake 37.0
  milk *(Betty Crocker SuperMoist)*, 1/12 cake 34.0
  mousse *(Pillsbury Bundt)*, 1/16 cake 37.0
  pudding *(Betty Crocker Classic)*, 1/6 cake 44.0
  Swiss *(Duncan Hines)*, 1/12 cake 33.0
chocolate caramel *(Pillsbury Bundt)*, 1/16 cake 43.0
chocolate chip:
  (Betty Crocker SuperMoist), 1/12 cake 35.0
  (Pillsbury Plus), 1/12 cake 34.0
  chocolate *(Betty Crocker SuperMoist)*, 1/12 cake 34.0
chocolate eclair *(Pillsbury Bundt)*, 1/16 cake 42.0
chocolate macaroon *(Pillsbury Bundt)*, 1/16 cake 37.0
cinnamon *(Streusel Swirl)*, 1/16 cake 38.0

devil's food:
    (Betty Crocker SuperMoist), 1/12 cake 35.0
    (Betty Crocker SuperMoist Light), 1/12 cake 36.0
    (Duncan Hines), 1/12 cake... 33.0
    (Pillsbury Lovin' Lites/Pillsbury Plus), 1/12 cake 32.0
    chocolate frosted *(Betty Crocker MicroRave)*,
      1/6 cake 36.0
fudge marble *(Betty Crocker SuperMoist)*, 1/12 cake 36.0
fudge marble *(Duncan Hines)*, 1/12 cake............................. 36.0
fudge swirl *(Pillsbury Plus)*, 1/12 cake 36.0
Funfetti (Pillsbury Plus), 1/12 cake...................................... 35.0
funnel cake *(Golden Dipt)*, 1/8 mix...................................... 20.0
gingerbread:
    (Betty Crocker Classic), 1/9 cake 35.0
    (Dromedary), 2" square 19.0
    (Pillsbury), 1/9 cake.. 32.0
lemon:
    (Betty Crocker SuperMoist), 1/12 cake 37.0
    (Pillsbury Bundt Tunnel of Lemon), 1/16 cake 44.0
    (Pillsbury Plus), 1/12 cake.. 34.0
    chiffon *(Betty Crocker Classic)*, 1/12 cake 36.0
    pudding *(Betty Crocker Classic)*, 1/6 cake....................... 45.0
    supreme *(Streusel Swirl)*, 1/16 cake................................. 37.0
lemon, orange, or pineapple supreme *(Duncan
    Hines)*, 1/12 cake 36.0
lemon-poppyseed or orange-walnut *(Simply
    Splendid)*, 3 oz. 37.0
pineapple creme *(Pillsbury Bundt)*, 1/16 cake 42.0
pineapple upside-down *(Betty Crocker Classic)*,
    1/9 cake... 43.0
pound *(Dromedary)*, 1/2" slice... 21.0
pound, golden *(Betty Crocker Classic)*, 1/12 cake............... 28.0
rainbow chip *(Betty Crocker SuperMoist)*, 1/12 cake........... 35.0
sour cream, chocolate *(Betty Crocker SuperMoist)*,
    1/12 cake 35.0
sour cream, white *(Betty Crocker SuperMoist)*,
    1/12 cake 36.0
spice or swirl *(Betty Crocker SuperMoist)*, 1/12 cake.......... 36.0

Cake, mix *(cont.)*
spice or strawberry supreme *(Duncan Hines),*
 1/12 cake 36.0
strawberry *(Pillsbury Plus),* 1/12 cake 35.0
vanilla:
 French *(Duncan Hines),* 1/12 cake 36.0
 golden *(Betty Crocker SuperMoist),* 1/12 cake 36.0
 sunshine *(Pillsbury Plus),* 1/12 cake 34.0
white:
 (Betty Crocker SuperMoist), 1/12 cake 34.0
 (Betty Crocker SuperMoist Light), 1/12 cake 37.0
 (Duncan Hines), 1/12 cake 36.0
 (Pillsbury Lovin' Lites), 1/12 cake 35.0
 (Pillsbury Plus), 1/12 cake 34.0
yellow:
 (Betty Crocker SuperMoist), 1/12 cake 36.0
 (Betty Crocker SuperMoist Light), 1/12 cake 37.0
 (Duncan Hines), 1/12 cake 36.0
 (Pillsbury Lovin' Lites), 1/12 cake 35.0
 (Pillsbury Plus), 1/12 cake 34.0
 butter *(Betty Crocker SuperMoist),* 1/12 cake 37.0
 with frosting *(Betty Crocker Microwave),* 1/6 cake 36.0
Calamansi punch *(R.W. Knudsen Rain Forest),*
 8 fl. oz. 27.0
Calves liver, see "Liver, veal"
Candy:
almond, candy coated *(Brach's Jordan),* 1 oz. 23.0
(Baby Ruth), 2.2 oz. 37.0
(Boyer Smoothie), .5-oz. pkg. 12.5
bridge mix *(Brach's),* 1 oz. 19.0
butter rum *(Pearson Nips),* 1 piece 6.0
(Butterfinger), 2.1 oz. 41.0
butterscotch *(Callard & Bowser),* 1 oz. 25.2
candy corn *(Heide/Heide Indian),* 1 oz. 27.0
caramel:
 (Kraft), 1 piece 6.0
 (Pearson Nips), 1 piece 6.0
 (Sugar Babies), 1 5/8-oz. pkg. 40.0

(Sugar Daddy), 1⅜-oz. pop................................. 33.0
chocolate coated *(Pom Poms)*, 1 oz. 15.0
chocolate coated, with cookies *(Twix)*, 1-oz. piece........ 19.0
milk chocolate coated *(Rolo)*, 1.93 oz. 37.0
with peanut, chocolate coated *(Oh Henry!)*, 2 oz........... 34.0
carob:
  almond *(Caroby)*, 4 sections 12.0
  milk or mint *(Caroby)*, 4 sections..................... 13.0
  milk-free *(Caroby)*, 4 sections 11.0
cherry, chocolate cream *(Brach's)*, 1 oz.............. 21.0
cherry, dark or milk chocolate coated *(Brach's)*, 1 oz....... 22.0
chocolate:
  (Heide Chocolate Babies), 1 oz. 27.0
  (Hershey's Special Dark), 1.45 oz. 24.0
  with almonds *(Golden Almond Solitaires)*, 1.4 oz. 18.0
  with almonds, candy coated *(Holidays)*, 1 oz........... 17.0
  candy coated *(M&M's)*, 1.69 oz. 33.0
  candy coated *(Holidays)*, 1 oz........................ 19.0
  chips, see "Chocolate, baking"
  French vanilla, semisweet *(Guittard)*, 1 oz.............. 17.0
  parfait *(Pearson Nips)*, 1 piece....................... 5.0
  with peanut butter, candy coated *(M&M's)*, 1 oz. 18.0
  with peanuts, candy coated *(Holidays)*, 1 oz. 17.0
  with peanuts, candy coated *(M&M's)*, 1.7 oz. 29.0
  white, with almonds *(Nestlé Alpine)*, 1.25 oz. 16.0
chocolate, milk:
  (Cadbury's Dairy Milk), 1 oz. 17.0
  (Guittard Old Dutch), 1 oz. 17.0
  (Hershey's), 1.55 oz................................... 25.0
  (Hershey's Kisses), 1 oz. or 6 pieces................ 16.0
  (Nabisco Stars), 1 oz. 19.0
  (Nestlé), 1.45 oz..................................... 25.0
  (Symphony), 1.4 oz.................................... 22.0
  with almonds *(Hershey's)*, 1.45 oz. 20.0
  with almonds *(Hershey's Kisses)*, 1 oz. or 6 pieces 14.0
  with almonds *(Nestlé)*, 1.45 oz....................... 19.0
  with almonds and toffee chips *(Symphony)*, 1.5 oz. 22.0
  with caramel *(Cadbury's Caramello)*, 1 oz..................... 18.0

Candy, chocolate, milk *(cont.)*
with crisps *(Krackel),* 1.45 oz. 25.0
with crisps *(Nestlé Crunch),* 1.4 oz. 24.0
with crisps and peanuts *(100 Grand),* 1.5 oz. 31.0
with fruit and nuts *(Chunky),* 1.4 oz. 21.0
with peanuts *(Mr. Goodbar),* 1.75 oz. 23.0
with pecan and caramel *(Demet's* Turtles), 1 piece 10.0
with raisins and almonds *(Cadbury's* Fruit & Nut),
   1 oz. 17.0
chocolate mint *(Pearson Nips),* 1 piece 6.0
chocolate coated, candy coated *(M&M's),* 1 oz. 20.0
coconut, chocolate coated:
   (Mounds), 1.9 oz. 31.0
   dark or milk chocolate *(Bounty),* 2.12 oz. 18.0
   with almonds *(Almond Joy),* 1.76 oz. 28.0
coconut, toasted *(Andes* Thins), 8 pieces 21.0
coffee *(Pearson Nips),* 1 piece 6.0
cough drops *(Beech-Nut),* 1 piece 3.0
cough drops *(Halls* Tablets), 1 piece 3.7
cream *(Heide* Harvest Creams), 1 oz. 27.0
fruit flavored, all flavors *(Skittles),* 2.3 oz. 60.0
fruit flavored, all flavors *(Starburst),* 2.07 oz. 48.0
fudge *(Kraft* Fudgies), 1 piece 6.0
grape *(Heide* Cool Grape), 1 oz. 28.0
gum, chewing, all flavors:
   (Beech-Nut), 1 piece 2.0
   (Big Red/Juicy Fruit), 1 piece... 2.3
   *(Care*Free/Care*Free* Bubble), 1 piece............................. 2.0
   (Doublemint/Freedent/Wrigley's Spearmint),
      1 piece 2.3
   (Freshen-Up), 1 piece.. 3.1
   bubble *(Bubble Yum),* 1 piece... 7.0
   bubble *(Bubblicious),* 1 piece.. 6.2
   bubble *(Hubba Bubba),* 1 piece... 5.8
   candy coated *(Chiclets),* 1 piece 1.5
hard, all flavors *(Jolly Rancher* Kisses), 1 piece................. 5.7
honey *(Bit-O-Honey),* 1.7 oz. 39.0
hot *(Heide* Hawaii), 1 oz. 28.0

hot *(Heide Red Hot Dollars)*, 1 oz. 25.0
(Hot Tamales), 1 piece 2.1
jellied and gummed:
   (Chuckles), 1 oz. 25.0
   (Heide Gummi Bears), 1 oz. 21.0
   (Jujubes), 1 oz. 26.0
   (Jujyfruits), 1 oz. 25.0
   eggs *(Heide)*, 1 oz. 28.0
   spice *(Heide* Mexican Hats), 1 oz. 25.0
   spearmint leaves *(Brach's)*, 1 oz. 24.0
   tropical *(Amazin' Fruit* Gummy Bears), 1 oz. 21.0
licorice:
   (Diamond), 1 oz. 26.0
   (Panda), 1.1 oz. bar 25.0
   (Pearson Nips), 1 piece 6.0
   (Switzer), 1 oz. 22.0
   candy coated *(Good & Fruity/Good & Plenty)*, 1 oz. 26.0
   cherry *(Y&S Cherry Nibs/Twizzlers Bites)*, 1 oz. 23.0
   raspberry *(Panda)*, 1.1 oz. bar 25.0
   soft *(Heide)*, 1 oz. 25.0
   strawberry *(Y&S Twizzlers)*, 1 oz. 23.0
lollipop, all flavors, except chocolate *(Tootsie Pop)*,
   1 oz. 26.4
lollipop, chocolate *(Tootsie Pop)*, 1 oz. 26.2
lozenge *(Listerine)*, 1 piece 2.0
malted milk balls *(Whoppers)*, 1 oz. 20.0
(Mars Bar), 1.76 oz. 30.0
marshmallow:
   (Funmallows), 1 piece 7.0
   (Kraft Jet-Puffed), 1 piece 6.0
   miniature *(Kraft)*, 10 pieces 5.0
(Mike & Ikes), 1 piece 2.1
(Milky Way), 2.15 oz. 42.0
(Milky Way Dark), 1.76 oz. 36.0
mint:
   (Mint Meltaway), .33-oz. piece 5.0
   all flavors *(Breath Savers)*, 1 piece 2.0

Candy, mint *(cont.)*
  all varieties, except crunch and parfait *(Andes
    Thins)*, 8 pieces.. 21.0
  butter or party *(Kraft)*, 1 piece 2.0
  chocolate coated *(After Eight)*, 1 piece 6.0
  chocolate coated *(York Peppermint Pattie)*, 1.5 oz. 34.0
  crunch or parfait *(Andes Frost Mint)*, 8 pieces.............. 22.0
(Munch), 1.42 oz. 19.0
nonpareils *(Nestlé Sno-Caps)*, 1 oz. 21.0
nougat, chocolate coated, all flavors *(Charleston
  Chew!)*, 1 oz. 22.0
(Pay Day), 1.85 oz. 28.0
peanut:
  (Tom's Peanut Plank), 1.7 oz.. 28.0
  chocolate coated *(Goobers)*, 1³⁄₈ oz. 16.0
  French burnt *(Brach's)*, 1 oz. 18.0
  roll *(Tom's)*, 1.75 oz. 29.0
peanut brittle *(Kraft)*, 1 oz. 20.0
peanut butter:
  (Snickers), 1.76 oz. 23.0
  (Tom's Peanut Butter Pals), 1.3 oz................................... 19.0
  candy coated *(Reese's Pieces)*, 1.63 oz............................ 28.0
  chocolate coated, with cookie *(Twix)*, .9-oz. piece 13.0
  cup, chocolate coated *(Reese's)*, 1.6 oz. 23.0
  cup, chocolate coated, crunchy *(Reese's)*, 1.8 oz. 24.0
  parfait *(Pearson)*, 1 piece 5.0
popcorn, caramel, see "Popcorn"
raisins, chocolate coated *(Nabisco)*, 1 oz. 21.0
raisins, chocolate coated *(Raisinets)*, 1³⁄₈ oz..................... 28.0
rock candy *(Brach's Cut Rock)*, 1 oz. 27.0
(Snickers), 2.07 oz.. 35.0
sesame, all varieties *(Joyva)*, 1 oz. 25.0
sour *(Heide Silly Sours)*, 1 oz. 28.0
sour balls *(Brach's)*, 1 oz. 27.0
taffy, all flavors *(Brach's Salt Water)*, 1 oz. 24.0
(3 Musketeers), 2.13 oz.. 44.0

toffee:
   (Callard & Bowser), 1 oz..................................19.2
   crunch *(Andes* Thins), 8 pieces.........................23.0
   English *(Heath)*, 1.4-oz. bar.............................25.0
(Tootsie Roll), 1 oz. 22.8
Cane syrup, 1 tbsp...13.4
Cannellini, see "Kidney beans"
Cannelloni entree, frozen:
beef, with tomato sauce *(Lean Cuisine)*, 9⅝ oz. 28.0
cheese *(Dining Lite)*, 9 oz. 38.0
cheese, with tomato sauce *(Lean Cuisine)*, 9⅛ oz...........27.0
Florentine *(Celentano)*, 12 oz....................................48.0
Cantaloupe:
pulp, cubed, ½ cup 6.7
½ of 5"-diameter melon 22.3
Capers, 1 tbsp. 0
Capon, without added ingredients............................0
Caponata, see "Eggplant appetizer"
Capocollo *(Healthy Deli* Cappy), 1 oz. 1.1
Cappuccino, bottled:
hot, cinnamon *(Maxwell House)*, 6 fl. oz. 11.0
hot, coffee or mocha *(Maxwell House)*, 6 fl. oz. 12.0
iced:
   cinnamon *(Chock o'ccino)*, 8 fl. oz. 22.0
   cinnamon *(Maxwell House Cappio)*, 8 fl. oz. 25.0
   coffee *(Chock o'ccino)*, 8 fl. oz...........................23.0
   coffee *(Maxwell House Cappio)*, 8 fl. oz. 23.0
   decaf *(Chock o'ccino)*, 8 fl. oz. 20.0
   mocha *(Chock o'ccino)*, 8 fl. oz. 24.0
   mocha *(Maxwell House Cappio)*, 8 fl. oz................25.0
   mocha *(Nescafé* Mocha Cooler)*, 8 fl. oz. 23.0
   vanilla nut *(Chock o'ccino)*, 8 fl. oz......................23.0
Captain D's, 1 serving:
dinner [1]:
   chicken, with salad..54.8
   fish, baked, with salad 61.9

---

[1] *Includes rice, green beans, and bread stick.*

Captain D's, dinner *(cont.)*
  orange roughy, with salad... 55.6
  shrimp, with slaw 56.2
side dishes:
  breadstick, 1 piece.. 17.0
  cole slaw, 4 oz. 11.8
  crackers, 4 pieces 8.0
  cracklins, 1 oz. 15.7
  dinner salad, without dressing... 3.3
  french fries, 3.5 oz. 49.6
  green beans, seasoned, 4 oz.. 4.9
  hushpuppy, 1 piece.. 19.9
  okra, fried, 4 oz. 34.1
  rice, 4 oz.. 27.5
  white beans, 4 oz. 22.2
dressings, 1 packet:
  blue cheese 2
  French... 4.0
  Italian, low calorie.. 2.2
  ranch.. .4
sauces, side portion:
  cocktail 8.4
  sweet and sour 13.1
  tartar 3.2
desserts, 1 slice:
  carrot cake.. 49.1
  cheesecake.. 30.0
  chocolate cake 48.9
  lemon pie.. 59.0
  pecan pie.. 64.2
Carambola:
fresh, 1 medium, 4.7 oz... 9.9
fresh *(Frieda's),* 1 oz. 2.3
dried *(Frieda's),* 1 oz. 5.6
Caramel, see "Candy"
Caramel, creme, see "Pudding mix"

Caramel topping:
(Kraft), 1 tbsp. 13.0
(Smucker's), 2 tbsp. 33.0
hot *(Smucker's)*, 2 tbsp. 28.0
Caraway seed, 1 tsp. 1.1
Cardamom, ground or seed *(Tone's)*, 1 tsp. 1.3
Cardoon:
raw, shredded, ½ cup 4.4
boiled, drained, 4 oz. 6.0
Carissa:
1 medium, .8 oz. 2.7
sliced, ½ cup 10.2
Carl's Jr., 1 serving:
breakfast:
  bacon, 2 strips 0
  breakfast burrito 29.0
  English muffin with margarine...................................... 30.0
  French toast dips, without syrup 59.0
  hash brown nuggets.. 27.0
  hot cakes with margarine, without syrup 61.0
  sausage, 1 patty.. 0
  scrambled eggs... 2.0
  Sunrise Sandwich 31.0
chicken strips, 6 pieces.. 11.0
sandwiches:
  Carl's Catch Fish Sandwich 54.0
  Carl's Original Hamburger 46.0
  Charbroiled BBQ Chicken Sandwich 34.0
  Charbroiled Chicken Club Sandwich 42.0
  Double Western Bacon Cheeseburger 58.0
  Famous Star Hamburger 42.0
  hamburger 33.0
  roast beef deluxe.. 46.0
  Santa Fe Chicken Sandwich 36.0
  Super Star hamburger.. 41.0
  turkey club.. 50.0
  Western Bacon Cheeseburger..................................... 59.0

Carl's Jr. (cont.)
Great Stuff potatoes:
  bacon or broccoli and cheese 60.0
  cheese 70.0
  chili.. 50.0
  lite 60.0
  sour cream and chive... 64.0
Entree Salads-To-Go, chicken 8.0
Entree Salads-To-Go, garden 4.0
salad dressing, 1 oz.:
  blue cheese 0
  French or Italian, reduced calorie 5.0
  house... 2.0
  Thousand Island... 4.0
side dishes:
  CrissCut Fries, regular... 27.0
  fries, regular... 54.0
  onion rings.. 63.0
  salsa, 1 oz. 2.0
  zucchini.. 38.0
bakery products:
  blueberry muffin.. 61.0
  bran muffin 52.0
  cheese Danish.. 75.0
  cheesecake.. 32.0
  chocolate cake 49.0
  chocolate chip cookie 41.0
  cinnamon roll... 70.0
  fudge moussecake 42.0
shake, regular... 61.0
Carob drink mix, powder, 3 tsp... 11.2
Carob flour, 1 cup 91.6
Carp, without added ingredients... 0
Carrot:
fresh, raw:
  whole, 7½" long, 2.8 oz... 7.3
  shredded, ½ cup... 5.6

baby, 1 medium, 2³/₄" long 8
mini *(Frieda's)*, 1 oz. 2.7
fresh, boiled, drained, sliced, ¹/₂ cup....................................... 8.2
canned, ¹/₂ cup:
  (Stokely) 7.0
  sliced, with liquid.. 6.2
  sliced, drained 4.0
  sliced *(Allen)* 7.0
frozen:
  boiled, drained, sliced, ¹/₂ cup 6.0
  (Seabrook), 3.3 oz. 9.0
  whole, baby *(Green Giant Harvest Fresh)*, ¹/₂ cup............ 5.0
  whole, baby *(Green Giant Select)*, ¹/₂ cup 7.0
  sliced *(Frosty Acres)*, 3.3 oz.. 9.0
Carrot chips *(Hain/Hain No Salt)*, 1 oz............................. 16.0
Carrot juice, canned:
6 fl. oz. 17.1
(Hollywood), 6 fl. oz. 13.0
Casaba:
¹/₁₀ of 7³/₄"-diameter melon... 10.2
pulp, cubed, ¹/₂ cup 5.3
Cashew butter:
1 oz. 7.8
(Roaster Fresh), 1 oz. 9.0
raw or toasted *(Hain)*, 2 tbsp.. 8.0
Cashews:
(Beer Nuts), 1 oz. 8.0
(Frito-Lay's), 1 oz. 9.0
(Tom's), 1 oz... 7.0
dry-roasted:
  1 oz. or 18 medium.. 9.3
  whole or halves, 1 cup... 44.8
  (Flavor House), 1 oz. 9.0
  whole *(Fisher)*, 1 oz. 8.0
honey-roasted, whole *(Fisher)*, 1 oz. 7.0
oil-roasted:
  1 oz. or 18 medium.. 8.1
  whole or halves, 1 cup... 37.1

Cashews, oil-roasted *(cont.)*
(Flavor House), 1 oz. 8.0
(Master Choice), 1 oz. 8.0
whole or halves *(Fisher)*, 1 oz. 8.0
Cassava (see also "Yuca"), trimmed, 1 oz. 7.6
Catfish, without added ingredients 0
Catfish, frozen *(Delta Pride)*, 4 oz. 4.8
Catfish entree, Cajun, frozen *(Gorton's)*, 1 piece 3.0
Catjang, boiled, ½ cup 17.5
Catsup:
(Hain Natural), 1 tbsp. 4.0
(Heinz), 1 tbsp. 4.0
(Heinz Hot), 1 tbsp. 3.0
(Heinz Lite), 1 tbsp. 2.0
(Hunt's), 1 tbsp. 4.0
(Hunt's No Salt Added), 1 tbsp. 5.0
(Smucker's), 1 tbsp. 6.0
(Stokely), 1 tbsp. 5.0
Cauliflower:
fresh:
raw, 3 florets 2.9
raw, 1" pieces, ½ cup 2.6
boiled, drained, 1" pieces, ½ cup 2.6
frozen:
boiled, drained, 1" pieces, ½ cup 3.4
(Frosty Acres), 3.3 oz. 5.0
cuts *(Green Giant)*, ½ cup 3.0
breaded *(Stilwell)*, 13 pieces 16.0
in cheese sauce *(Birds Eye)*, 5 oz. 8.0
in cheese sauce *(Green Giant)*, ½ cup 10.0
in cheese sauce *(Green Giant* One Serving),
5.5 oz. 14.0
Cauliflower, pickled, sweet *(Vlasic)*, 1 oz. 9.0
Cavatelli, frozen *(Celentano)*, 3.2 oz. 79.0
Caviar, granular (see also "Roe"):
black or red, 1 oz. 1.1
black or red, 1 tbsp. 6
Caviar spread, see "Taramosalata"

Cayenne, see "Pepper"
Ceci, see "Chickpeas"
Celeriac, fresh:
raw, ½ cup.. 7.2
boiled, drained, 4 oz.. 6.7
Celery:
raw, 7½"-stalk, 1.6 oz. 1.5
raw, diced, ½ cup.. 2.2
boiled, drained, diced, ½ cup 3.0
Celery, dried:
flakes or seeds *(Tone's),* 1 tsp.. .9
seeds, 1 tsp. 8
Celery salt *(Tone's),* 1 tsp.. .6
Cellophane noodles, see "Noodle, Chinese"
Celtus, raw, trimmed, 1 oz.. 1.0
Cereal, ready-to-eat (see also specific grains):
bran (see also "oat bran," below):
  (All Bran), 1 oz.. 21.0
  (Arrowhead Mills Bran Flakes), 1 oz. 20.0
  (Bran Buds), 1 oz.. 23.0
  (Bran Chex), 1 oz.. 24.0
  (Kellogg's Bran Flakes), 1 oz.. 22.0
  (Kellogg's Fiberwise), 1 oz. 23.0
  (Nabisco 100% Bran), 1 oz. 22.0
  (Post Bran Flakes), 1 oz... 23.0
  extra fiber *(Kellogg's All Bran),* 1 oz. 22.0
  with fruit *(Kellogg's Fruitful Bran),* 1 oz. cereal with
    .4 oz. fruit.. 31.0
  shredded, see "wheat, shredded," below
bran, with raisins:
  (Barbara's Raisin Bran), 1.5 oz....................................... 36.0
  (Erewhon Raisin Bran), 1 oz.. 22.0
  (General Mills Raisin Nut Bran), 1 oz. 21.0
  (Kellogg's Raisin Bran), 1 oz. cereal with .4 oz.
    raisins 31.0
  (Malt-O-Meal Raisin Bran), 1.4 oz. 30.0
  (Nutri-Grain), 1 oz. cereal with .4 oz. raisins 31.0
  (Post Raisin Bran), 1.4 oz... 31.0

Cereal, ready-to-eat, bran, with raisins *(cont.)*
  (Skinner's Raisin Bran), 1 oz. 19.0
  (Total Raisin Bran), 1.5 oz. 33.0
corn:
  (Arrowhead Mills Flakes), 1 oz. 25.0
  (Barbara's Corn Flakes), 1 oz. 24.0
  (Cocoa Puffs), 1 oz. 25.0
  (Corn Pops), 1 oz. 26.0
  (Country Corn Flakes), 1 oz. 25.0
  (Honeycomb), 1 oz. 25.0
  (Kellogg's Corn Flakes), 1 oz. 24.0
  (Kellogg's Frosted Flakes), 1 oz. 26.0
  (Malt-O-Meal), 1 oz. 25.0
  (Nut & Honey Crunch), 1 oz. 24.0
  (Nutri-Grain), 1 oz. 24.0
  (Post Toasties), 1 oz. 25.0
  (Total Corn Flakes), 1 oz. 24.0
  apple *(Arrowhead Mills* Apple Corns), 1 oz. 23.0
  golden *(Health Valley Fruit Lites),* 1/2 oz. 12.0
  maple *(Arrowhead Mills* Maple Corns), 1 oz. 23.0
  puffed *(Arrowhead Mills),* 1/2 oz. 11.0
  sugar frosted *(Malt-O-Meal),* 1 oz. 26.0
granola:
  (C.W. Post Hearty), 1 oz. 21.0
  all varieties *(Health Valley* Fat Free), 1 oz. 21.0
  all varieties, except sunflower crunch *(Erewhon),*
    1 oz. 17.0
  banana almond *(Sunbelt),* 1 oz. 20.0
  with bran *(Erewhon #9),* 1 oz. 17.0
  fruit and nut *(Sunbelt),* 1 oz. 19.0
  maple nut *(Arrowhead Mills),* 1 oz. 18.0
  sunflower crunch *(Erewhon),* 1 oz. 18.0
kamut flakes *(Erewhon),* 1 oz. 18.0
kashi, puffed *(Kashi),* 3/4 oz. 16.0
millet, puffed *(Arrowhead Mills),* 1/2 oz. 11.0
mixed grain and natural style:
  (Almond Delight), 1 oz. 23.0
  (Apple Jacks), 1 oz. 26.0

(Arrowhead Mills Arrowhead Crunch), 1 oz. 18.0
(Barbara's High 5), 1 oz. 23.0
(Basic 4), 1.3 oz. 28.0
(Cinnamon Toast Crunch), 1 oz. 22.0
(Clusters), 1 oz. 22.0
(Crispix), 1 oz. 25.0
(Crunchy Nut Oh!s), 1 oz. 21.5
(Double Dip Crunch), 1 oz. 23.0
(Erewhon Aztec/Right Start/Super-O's), 1 oz. 24.0
(Fiber One), 1 oz. 23.0
(Froot Loops), 1 oz. 25.0
(Fruit & Frosted O's), 1 oz. 25.0
(Grape Nuts), 1 oz. 23.0
(Grape Nuts Flakes), 1 oz. 23.0
(Honey Graham Chex), 1 oz. 25.0
(Honey Graham Oh!s), 1 oz. 22.6
(Just Right), 1 oz. 23.0
(Kix), 1 oz. 24.0
(Multi Grain Cheerios), 1 oz. 23.0
(Product 19), 1 oz. 24.0
(Quaker 100% Natural), 1 oz. 18.0
(Special K), 1 oz. 20.0
(Sunflakes Multi-Grain), 1 oz. 24.0
(Total), 1 oz. 23.0
(Triples), 1 oz. 24.0
(Uncle Sam), 1 oz. 20.0
all varieties *(Health Valley Fiber Flakes)*, 1 oz. 20.0
all varieties *(Health Valley O's Fat Free)*, 1 oz. 19.0
with almonds *(Honey Bunches of Oats)*, 1 oz. 22.0
almond raisin *(Nutri-Grain)*, 1 oz. cereal with .4 oz.
    nuts and fruit 31.0
with apple *(Erewhon Apple Stroodles)*, 1 oz. 23.0
apple and almond *(Kellogg's Mueslix Golden
    Crunch)*, 1 oz. 25.0
apple raisin *(Apple Raisin Crisp)*, 1 oz. cereal with
    .3 oz. fruit 32.0
with banana *(Erewhon Banana-O's)*, 1 oz. 24.0
with bananas and Hawaiian fruit *(Sprouts 7)*, 1 oz. 16.0

Cereal, ready-to-eat, mixed grain and natural style *(cont.)*
  cinnamon *(Kellogg's* Mini Buns), 1 oz. 25.0
  cinnamon and raisin *(Nature Valley)*, 1 oz. 20.0
  dates, raisins, walnuts *(Fruit & Fibre)*, 1.25 oz. 27.0
  with fiber nuggets *(Just Right)*, 1 oz. 24.0
  with fruit and nuts *(Kellogg's Mueslix Crispy
    Blend)*, 1.5 oz. 33.0
  fruit and nut *(Nature Valley)*, 1 oz. 19.0
  honey roasted *(Honey Bunches of Oats)*, 1 oz. 24.0
  peaches, raisins, almonds *(Fruit & Fibre)*, 1.25 oz. 26.0
  pecan, double *(Post Great Grains)*, 1.25 oz. 20.0
  pineapple, banana, and coconut *(Fruit & Fibre)*,
    1.25 oz. 27.0
  plain or raisin *(Heartland)*, 1 oz. 18.0
  with raisins *(Erewhon Right Start)*, 1 oz. 22.0
  raisin *(Grape Nuts)*, 1 oz. 23.0
  with raisins *(Sprouts 7)*, 1 oz. 16.0
  raisins, dates, nuts *(Just Right)*, 1 oz. cereal with
    .3 oz. fruit and nuts 30.0
  raisin, date, pecan *(Post Great Grains)*, 1.25 oz. 27.0
  trail mix *(Heartland)*, 1 oz. 19.0
muesli *(Master Choice)*, 2 oz. 40.0
muesli *(Sunbelt)*, 1 oz. 22.0
oat:
  (Alpha-Bits), 1 oz. 24.0
  (Cheerios), 1 oz. 20.0
  (Cinnamon Life), 1 oz. 18.9
  (General Mills Oatmeal Crisp), 1 oz. 21.0
  (Honey Bunches of Oats), 1 oz. 23.0
  (Honey Nut Cheerios), 1 oz. 23.0
  (Life), 1 oz. 18.7
  (Nut & Honey Crunch O's), 1 oz. 22.0
  (Toasty O's), 1 oz. 20.0
  with almonds *(Honey Bunches of Oats)*, 1 oz. 23.0
  apple cinnamon *(Cheerios)*, 1 oz. 22.0
  apple and cinnamon *(Toasty O's)*, 1 oz. 22.0
  honey bran *(Kellogg's Oatbake)*, 1 oz. 21.0
  honey and nut *(Toasty O's)*, 1 oz. 23.0

marshmallow *(Alpha-Bits)*, 1 oz. 25.0
with raisins *(General Mills* Oatmeal Raisin Crisp),
   1.2 oz. 25.0
raisin nut *(Kellogg's Oatbake)*, 1 oz. 21.0
toasted *(Nature Valley)*, 1 oz. 20.0
toasted, rings *(Skinner's)*, 1 oz. 22.0
oat bran:
   (Arrowhead Mills Flakes), 1 oz. 20.0
   (Common Sense), 1 oz. 22.0
   (Cracklin' Oat Bran), 1 oz. 21.0
   (Post Oat Flakes), 1 oz. 21.0
   (Skinner's), 1 oz. 18.0
   with raisins *(Common Sense)*, 1 oz. cereal with
      .3 oz. raisins 29.0
   with toasted wheat germ *(Erewhon)*, 1 oz. 18.0
oatmeal, toasted *(Quaker)*, 1 oz. 22.0
oatmeal, honey nut *(Quaker)*, 1 oz. 20.0
rice:
   (Erewhon Poppets), 1 oz. 24.0
   (Frosted Krispies), 1 oz. 26.0
   (Rice Krispies), 1 oz. 25.0
   chocolate *(Cocoa Krispies)*, 1 oz. 25.0
rice, brown:
   (Health Valley Fruit Lites), 1/2 oz. 12.0
   crisps *(Barbara's)*, 1 oz. 26.0
   crispy *(Erewhon/Erewhon* Low Sodium), 1 oz. 24.0
   crispy *(Kellogg's Kenmei)*, 1 oz. 24.0
rice, puffed:
   (Arrowhead Mills), 1/2 oz. 11.0
   (Malt-O-Meal), 1/2 oz. 12.0
   (Quaker), 1/2 oz. 12.5
wheat:
   (Kellogg's Smacks), 1 oz. 25.0
   (Malt-O-Meal Sugar Puffs), 1 oz. 25.0
   (Nutri-Grain), 1 oz. 23.0
   (Total), 1 oz. 22.0
   (Wheat Chex), 1 oz. 23.0
   (Wheaties), 1 oz. 23.0

Cereal, ready-to-eat, wheat *(cont.)*
(*Wheaties Honey Gold*), 1 oz. 25.0
apple cinnamon filled (*Kellogg's Apple Cinnamon
    Squares*), 1 oz. 23.0
blueberry filled (*Kellogg's Blueberry Squares*),
    1 oz. 23.0
flakes (*Erewhon*), 1 oz. 22.0
with fruit (*Erewhon Fruit'n Wheat*), 1 oz. 21.0
golden (*Health Valley Fruit Lites*), 1/2 oz. 11.0
with raisins (*Crispy Wheat 'N Raisins*), 1 oz. 23.0
raisin filled (*Kellogg's Raisin Squares*), 1 oz. 23.0
strawberry filled (*Kellogg's Strawberry Squares*),
    1 oz. 23.0
wheat, puffed (*Arrowhead Mills*), 1/2 oz. 11.0
wheat, puffed (*Malt-O-Meal*), 1/2 oz. 10.0
wheat, shredded:
    (*Barbara's*), 2 biscuits, 1.4 oz. 31.0
    (*Kellogg's Frosted Mini-Wheats*), 1 oz. 24.0
    (*Nabisco*), 1 piece... 19.0
    (*Nutri-Grain*), 1 oz. 22.0
    (*S.W. Graham*), 1 oz. 23.0
    (*Sunshine*), 1 piece... 19.0
    bite size (*Sunshine*), 2/3 cup.................................. 22.0
    bran (*Nabisco Shredded Wheat'n Bran*), 1 oz.......... 23.0
    cinnamon (*S.W. Graham*), 1 oz. 24.0
    mini (*Nabisco Spoon Size*), 1 oz............................. 23.0
    whole grain (*Kellogg's*), 1 oz. 23.0
Cereal, cooking[1] (see also specific grains):
bran (*H-O Brand* Super Bran), 1/3 cup........................... 18.0
farina, see "wheat," below
granola (*H-O Brand*), 1/2 cup...................................... 43.0
mixed grain:
    (*Arrowhead Mills* Seven Grain), 1 oz....................... 17.0
    (*Erewhon* Organic Barley Plus), 1 oz. 22.0
    (*Roman Meal* Original), 1 oz.................................. 15.3

---
[1] *Uncooked, except as noted.*

apple cinnamon *(Roman Meal)*, 1.2 oz. 18.2
with oats *(Roman Meal* Original), 1.2 oz........................ 18.7
oat bran:
(*Arrowhead Mills*), 1 oz.. 17.0
(*Roman Meal*), 1 oz. 12.7
with toasted wheat germ *(Erewhon* Oat Bran),
1 oz. 18.0
oatmeal and oats:
(*Arrowhead Mills* Instant), 1 oz............................. 18.0
(*H-O Brand* Quick/Instant), 1 packet or ⅓ cup............. 18.0
(*Instant Quaker*), 1 packet 18.0
apple cinnamon *(Erewhon* Instant), 1.25 oz. 25.0
apple cinnamon *(Instant Quaker)*, 1 packet.................... 26.0
apple cinnamon *(Quaker Oat Cups)*, 5.5 oz.
container 27.0
apple, date, and almond *(Arrowhead Mills* Instant),
1 oz. 23.0
apple raisin *(Erewhon* Instant), 1.3 oz. 27.0
apple spice *(Arrowhead Mills* Instant), 1 oz. 23.0
bananas or blueberries and cream *(Instant
Quaker)*, 1 packet 26.0
cinnamon raisin and almond *(Arrowhead Mills*
Instant), 1 oz. 23.0
with fiber *(H-O Brand* Instant), 1 packet 18.0
with fiber *(H-O Brand* Instant Box), ⅓ cup 15.0
with fiber, apple and bran *(H-O Brand* Instant),
1 packet 26.0
with fiber, raisin and bran *(H-O Brand* Instant),
1 packet 32.0
maple brown sugar *(H-O Brand* Instant), 1 packet........ 32.0
maple brown sugar *(Instant Quaker)*, 1 packet 31.0
maple spice *(Erewhon* Instant), 1.2 oz. 24.0
with oat bran *(Erewhon* Instant), 1.25 oz...................... 23.0
peaches and cream *(Instant Quaker)*, 1 packet.............. 26.0
raisin, date, and walnut *(Erewhon* Instant), 1.2 oz. 24.0
strawberries and cream *(Instant Quaker)*, 1 packet 26.0
sweet'n mellow *(H-O Brand* Instant), 1 packet 30.0

Cereal, cooking, oatmeal and oats *(cont.)*
   with wheat, date, raisin, and almond *(Roman
    Meal)*, 1.3 oz. 23.9
   with wheat, honey, coconut, and almond *(Roman
    Meal)*, 1.3 oz. 22.0
  rice, brown *(Arrowhead Mills Rice & Shine)*, ¼ cup 35.0
  rice cream, brown *(Erewhon* Organic), 1 oz. 23.0
  rye, cream of *(Roman Meal)*, 1.3 oz. 20.3
  wheat:
    (Arrowhead Mills Bear Mush), 1 oz. 21.0
    (Malt-O-Meal), 1 oz. 21.0
    (Wheatena), 1 oz. 21.0
    bulgur *(Arrowhead Mills)*, 2 oz. 43.0
    chocolate *(Malt-O-Meal)*, 1 oz. 22.0
    cracked *(Arrowhead Mills)*, 2 oz. 40.0
    farina *(Pillsbury)*, ⅔ cup cooked 18.0
    farina, cream *(H-O Brand)*, 3 tbsp. 26.0
    maple and brown sugar *(Malt-O-Meal)*, 1 oz. 22.0
    with oat bran *(Malt-O-Meal* Plus 40%), 1.3 oz. 25.0
Cereal, freeze-dried*, granola, with blueberries and
  milk *(Mountain House)*, ½ cup 38.0
Cereal bars, see "Granola and cereal bars"
Cereal beverage, see "Coffee substitute"
Cervelat, see "Thuringer cervelat"
Chayote:
raw:
  1 medium, 7.2 oz. 11.0
  1″ pieces, ½ cup 3.6
  (Frieda's), 1 oz. 2.0
boiled, drained, 1″ pieces, ½ cup 4.1
Cheddarwurst *(Hillshire Farm* Bun Size/Links), 2 oz. 1.0
Cheese:
all varieties *(Heluva* Good), 1 oz. 1.0
American, processed:
  (Alpine Lace), 1 oz. 2.0
  (Alpine Lace Free'N Lean), 1 oz. 1.0
  (Kraft Deluxe Loaf or Slices), 1 oz. 1.0

plain or sharp *(Borden* Premium), 1 oz............................ 1.0
plain or sharp *(Land O'Lakes)*, 1 oz................................ 1.0
hot pepper *(Sargento)*, 1 oz. .... <.5
sharp *(Old English* Loaf or Slices), 1 oz. 1.0
American and Swiss, processed *(Land O'Lakes)*,
  1 oz.. 1.0
asiago *(Frigo)*, 1 oz. 1.0
babybel *(Laughing Cow)*, 1 oz..................................... 0
(Bel Paese), 1 oz. 0
blue:
  (Frigo), 1 oz... 1.0
  (Kraft), 1 oz. 1.0
  (Sargento), 1 oz. 1.0
Bonbel *(Laughing Cow)*, 1 oz. 0
brick *(Kraft)*, 1 oz. 0
brick *(Land O'Lakes)*, 1 oz....................................... 1.0
Brie *(Sargento)*, 1 oz. .... <.5
burger *(Sargento)*, 1 oz. .... <.5
Cajun *(Sargento)*, 1 oz. .... <.5
Camembert *(Sargento)*, 1 oz. .... <.5
cheddar:
  (Alpine Lace Ched-R-Lo), 1 oz. 1.0
  (Frigo/Frigo Lite), 1 oz.. 1.0
  (Kraft), 1 oz. 1.0
  (Land O'Lakes/Land O'Lakes Chedarella), 1 oz.............. <1.0
  (Sargento), 1 oz. .... <.5
  extra sharp, processed *(Land O'Lakes)*, 1 oz. 1.0
  mild *(Kraft* Light Naturals), 1 oz. 0
  processed *(Alpine Lace Free'N Lean)*, 1 oz..................... 1.0
  sharp, New York *(Master Choice* Special Reserve),
    1 oz. 0
cheddar and bacon, processed *(Land O'Lakes)*, 1 oz......... 1.0
Cheshire, 1 oz. 1.4
colby:
  (Alpine Lace Colbi-Lo), 1 oz.................................... 1.0
  (Kraft), 1 oz. 1.0
  (Kraft Light Naturals), 1 oz. 0

Cheese, colby *(cont.)*
  (Land O'Lakes), 1 oz. 1.0
  (Sargento), 1 oz. 1.0
colby jack *(Sargento)*, 1 oz. .... <.5
colby and Monterey jack, shredded *(Kraft* Light
  Naturals), 1 oz. 1.0
cottage cheese, 4% fat, creamed:
  (Bison), 1/2 cup 4.0
  (Breakstone's), 4 oz. 3.0
  (Friendship California), 1/2 cup 4.0
  large or small curd *(Knudsen)*, 4 oz. 4.0
  with pineapple *(Breakstone's)*, 4 oz. 14.0
  with pineapple *(Friendship)*, 1/2 cup 15.0
cottage cheese, dry curd *(Breakstone's)*, 4 oz. 6.0
cottage cheese, lowfat:
  2% fat *(Breakstone's)*, 4 oz. 4.0
  2% fat *(Knudsen)*, 4 oz. 4.0
  2% fat *(Sealtest)*, 4 oz. 4.0
  1% fat *(Bison)*, 1/2 cup 4.0
  1% fat *(Light n' Lively)*, 4 oz. 4.0
  all varieties, without fruit *(Friendship)*, 1/2 cup 4.0
  apple, spiced, 2% fat *(Knudsen)*, 6 oz. 20.0
  fruit cocktail, 2% fat *(Knudsen)*, 4 oz. 16.0
  garden salad, 1% fat *(Light n' Lively)*, 4 oz. 5.0
  mandarin orange, 2% fat *(Knudsen)*, 4 oz. 11.0
  peach, 2% fat *(Knudsen)*, 6 oz. 19.0
  peach and pineapple, 1% fat *(Light n' Lively)*,
    4 oz. 12.0
  pear, 2% fat *(Knudsen)*, 4 oz. 12.0
  pineapple, 1% fat *(Friendship)*, 1/2 cup 15.0
  pineapple, 2% fat *(Knudsen)*, 6 oz. 18.0
  strawberry, 2% fat *(Knudsen)*, 6 oz. 19.0
cottage cheese, nonfat:
  (Bison), 1/2 cup 4.0
  (Friendship), 1/2 cup 5.0
  (Knudsen), 4 oz. 3.0

cream cheese:
   regular, all varieties *(Philadelphia Brand)*, 1 oz................. 1.0
   soft, all varieties, except with pineapple,
      strawberries, or smoked salmon *(Philadelphia*
      Brand), 1 oz. 2.0
   soft, with pineapple or strawberries *(Philadelphia*
      Brand), 1 oz. 4.0
   soft, with smoked salmon *(Philadelphia Brand)*,
      1 oz. 1.0
   whipped, plain or with chives *(Philadelphia Brand)*,
      1 oz. 1.0
   whipped, with onion or smoked salmon
      (Philadelphia Brand), 1 oz............................... 2.0
Edam:
   (Kraft), 1 oz. 0
   (Land O'Lakes), 1 oz. .... <1.0
   (Laughing Cow), 1 oz. 0
   (Sargento), 1 oz. .... <.5
farmer *(Friendship/Friendship* No Salt), ½ cup 4.0
feta:
   (Frigo), 1 oz.. 1.0
   (Sargento), 1 oz. 1.0
   imported *(Krinos)*, 1 oz... 0
fontina *(Sargento)*, 1 oz. .... <.5
gjetost *(Sargento)*, 1 oz.. 12.0
goat cheese:
   hard type, 1 oz. 6
   semisoft type, 1 oz... .7
   soft type, 1 oz. 3
Gouda:
   (Kraft), 1 oz. 0
   (Land O'Lakes), 1 oz. 1.0
   (Laughing Cow), 1 oz. 0
   (Sargento), 1 oz. 1.0
Gruyère, 1 oz. 1
havarti *(Casino)*, 1 oz. 0
havarti *(Sargento)*, 1 oz.. <.5
hoop *(Friendship)*, ½ cup 2.0

Cheese *(cont.)*

Impastata *(Frigo)*, 1 oz. 1.0
Italian style, grated *(Sargento)*, 1 oz. 1.0
jalapeño jack, processed *(Land O'Lakes)*, 1 oz. 1.0
Jarlsberg *(Sargento)*, 1 oz. 1.0
Jarlsberg, smoked *(Norseland)*, 1 oz. 1.0
limburger *(Mohawk Valley* Little Gem)*, 1 oz. 0
limburger *(Sargento)*, 1 oz. .... <.5
mascarpone *(Galbani* Imported)*, 1 oz. 1.2
Monterey jack:
    (Alpine Lace Monti-Jack-Lo), 1 oz. 1.0
    (Kraft/Kraft Light Naturals)*, 1 oz. 0
    (Sargento), 1 oz. .... <.5
    with caraway or jalapeños *(Kraft)*, 1 oz. 1.0
    plain or hot pepper *(Land O'Lakes)*, 1 oz. .... <1.0
    with peppers *(Kraft* Light Naturals)*, 1 oz. 1.0
mozzarella:
    (Alpine Lace Free'N Lean), 1 oz. 0
    (Kraft Light Naturals)*, 1 oz. 4.0
    whole milk or part skim *(Frigo/Frigo* Lite)*, 1 oz. 1.0
    whole milk or part skim *(Kraft)*, 1 oz. 1.0
    whole milk or part skim *(Polly-O)*, 1 oz. 1.0
    whole milk or part skim *(Sargento)*, 1 oz. 1.0
    part skim *(Alpine Lace)*, 1 oz. 1.0
    part skim *(Land O'Lakes)*, 1 oz. 1.0
    processed *(Alpine Lace Free'N Lean)*, 1 oz. 0
Muenster:
    (Alpine Lace), 1 oz. 1.0
    (Land O'Lakes), 1 oz. .... <1.0
    red rind *(Sargento)*, 1 oz. .... <.5
Neufchâtel *(Philadelphia Brand* Light)*, 1 oz. 1.0
Parmesan:
    (Kraft), 1 oz. 1.0
    fresh *(Sargento)*, 1 oz. 1.0
    grated, 1 tbsp. 2
    grated *(Frigo/Frigo* Lite)*, 1 oz. 1.0
    grated *(Progresso)*, 1 tbsp. .... <1.0
    grated *(Sargento)*, 1 oz. 2.0

Parmesan and Romano, grated *(Sargento),* 1 oz. 1.0
Parmesan and Romano, grated, dry or fresh *(Frigo),*
  1 oz. 1.0
pimento, processed *(Kraft* Deluxe), 1 oz. 1.0
pizza, shredded *(Frigo),* 1 oz. 1.0
Port du Salut, 1 oz. 2
pot cheese *(Sargento),* 1 oz. 1.0
provolone:
  (Alpine Lace Provo-Lo), 1 oz. 1.0
  (Frigo/Frigo Lite), 1 oz. 1.0
  (Kraft), 1 oz. 1.0
  (Land O'Lakes), 1 oz. 1.0
  (Sargento), 1 oz. 1.0
queso blanco *(Sargento),* 1 oz. 3
queso de papa *(Sargento),* 1 oz. 4
ricotta:
  (Sargento Lite), 1 oz. 1.0
  whole milk, ½ cup 3.8
  whole milk or part skim *(Frigo),* 1 oz. 1.0
  whole milk or part skim *(Polly-O),* 1 oz. 1.0
  fat free *(Frigo),* 1 oz. 2.0
Romano:
  (Kraft Natural), 1 oz. 1.0
  (Sargento), 1 oz. 1.0
  grated *(Polly-O),* 1 oz. 1.0
  grated *(Progresso),* 1 tbsp. .... <1.0
  grated, fresh or dry *(Frigo)* 1.0
Roquefort, 1 oz. 6
smoked *(Sargento* Smokestick), 1 oz. 1.0
string:
  (Frigo/Frigo Lite), 1 oz. 1.0
  (Polly-O Stick), 1 oz. 2.0
  part skim, with jalapeños *(Kraft),* 1 oz. 1.0
  plain or smoked *(Sargento),* 1 oz. 1.0
Swiss:
  (Alpine Lace Swiss-Lo), 1 oz. 1.0
  (Casino), 1 oz. 1.0
  (Frigo), 1 oz. 1.0

Cheese, Swiss *(cont.)*
  (Land O'Lakes), 1 oz. 1.0
  (Sargento), 1 oz. 1.0
  all varieties, natural or processed *(Kraft),* 1 oz. 1.0
  baby *(Cracker Barrel* Natural), 1 oz. 0
  Finland *(Sargento),* 1 oz. .... <.5
  processed *(Borden* Premium), 1 oz. 1.0
taco:
  (Sargento), 1 oz. .... <.5
  shredded *(Frigo),* 1 oz. 1.0
  shredded *(Kraft),* 1 oz. 1.0
taleggio *(Tal-Fino* Brand Imported), 1 oz. 2
Tilsit *(Sargento),* 1 oz. 1.0
Tybo, red wax *(Sargento),* 1 oz. .... <.5
Cheese, imitation and substitute:
all varieties *(Smartbeat),* 1 slice 2.0
American *(Heluva* Good), 1 oz. 1.0
cheddar or mozzarella, imitation *(Frigo),* 1 oz. 1.0
cheddar or mozzarella, imitation *(Sargento),* 1 oz. .... <.5
cheese food *(Cheeztwin),* 1 oz. 3.0
mozzarella, 1 oz. 6.7
Parmesan, Italian, grated *(Country Cottage Farms),*
  1 tbsp. 2.0
Cheese dip:
(Chi-Chi's Fiesta), 1 oz. 3.0
blue cheese or nacho *(Kraft* Premium), 2 tbsp. 2.0
cheddar *(Frito-Lay's),* 1 oz. 3.0
nacho, jalapeño *(Price's),* 1 oz. 2.0
Cheese food:
(Heluva Good), 1 oz. 1.0
(Land O'Lakes), 1 oz. 2.0
American:
  (Borden Singles), 1 oz. 3.0
  (Kraft Singles), 1 oz. 2.0
  grated *(Kraft),* 1 oz. 8.0
  sharp *(Borden* Singles), 1 oz. 2.0
with bacon *(Cracker Barrel),* 1 oz. 3.0
with bacon *(Kraft Cheez'N Bacon),* 1 oz. 2.0

cheddar:
   port wine *(Wispride* Lite), 1 oz. 4.0
   port wine or sharp *(Cracker Barrel)*, 1 oz. 4.0
   extra sharp *(Cracker Barrel)*, 1 oz. 3.0
with garlic *(Kraft)*, 1 oz. 2.0
Italian herb *(Land O'Lakes)*, 1 oz. 2.0
with jalapeños:
   (Kraft/Kraft Singles), 1 oz. 2.0
   (Land O'Lakes), 1 oz. 2.0
   hot or mild *(Velveeta* Mexican), 1 oz. 3.0
Monterey jack *(Kraft* Singles), 1 oz. 2.0
(Nippy), 1 oz. 2.0
onion *(Land O'Lakes)*, 1 oz. 2.0
pepperoni *(Land O'Lakes)*, 1 oz. 1.0
pimento *(Kraft* Singles), 1 oz. 2.0
port wine, cold pack *(Wispride)*, 1 oz. 3.0
salami *(Land O'Lakes)*, 1 oz. 2.0
sharp *(Kraft* Singles) 1.0
shredded *Velveeta)*, 1 oz. 3.0
Swiss *(Borden* Singles), 1 oz. 2.0
Swiss *(Kraft* Singles), 1 oz. 2.0
Cheese nuggets, mozzarella, frozen *(Banquet Hot
   Bites)*, 2.5 oz. 15.0
Cheese-nut ball or log:
ball, with almonds:
   port wine or sharp cheddar *(Wispride)*, 1 oz. 5.0
   sharp cheddar *(Cracker Barrel)*, 1 oz. 4.0
   sharp cheddar, mini *(Wispride)*, 1 ball 5.0
log, with almonds:
   port wine or sharp cheddar *(Sargento)*, 1 oz. 3.0
   sharp or smoky cheddar *(Cracker Barrel)*, 1 oz. 4.0
   Swiss almond *(Sargento)*, 1 oz. 2.0
Cheese product:
(Kraft Free Singles), 1 oz. 4.0
all varieties *(Borden* Fat Free Singles), 1 oz. 4.0
all varieties *(Lite-Line)*, 1 oz. 1.0

Cheese product *(cont.)*
American flavor:
  (Alpine Lace), 1 oz... 2.0
  (Borden Light), 1 oz.. 1.0
  (Harvest Moon), 1 oz... 2.0
American or sharp cheddar flavor *(Kraft Light)*, 1 oz. 2.0
American or sharp cheddar flavor *(Light n' Lively)*,
  1 oz.. 2.0
cheddar flavor, all varieties *(Spreadery)*, 1 oz..................... 3.0
cheddar flavor, sharp *(Borden* Light), 1 oz. 2.0
cream cheese, light *(Philadelphia Brand)*, 1 oz.................... 2.0
Mexican, with jalapeños or nacho *(Spreadery)*, 1 oz........... 3.0
Neufchâtel:
  French onion or garden vegetables *(Spreadery)*,
    1 oz... 2.0
  garlic and herb *(Spreadery)*, 1 oz. 1.0
  garlic and herb or garden vegetable *(Wispride*
    Cheese Snack), 1 oz... 2.0
  ranch *(Spreadery* Classic), 1 oz... 1.0
pizza topping *(Lunch Wagon)*, 1 oz.. 1.0
port wine *(Spreadery)*, 1 oz. 3.0
sandwich slices *(Lunch Wagon)*, 1 oz. 2.0
Swiss flavor *(Kraft Light)*, 1 oz... 2.0
Swiss flavor *(Light n' Lively)*, 1 oz. 2.0
(Velveeta Light), 1 oz... 3.0
Cheese sauce mix:
(French's), 1/4 pkg.. 4.0
(McCormick/Schilling), 1/4 pkg... 3.5
nacho *(McCormick/Schilling)*, 1/4 pkg. 4.5
Cheese spread (see also "Cheese" and "Cheese
  Product"):
(Heluva Good), 1 oz. 2.0
all varieties *(Cheez Whiz)*, 1 oz.. 2.0
all varieties *(Easy Cheese)*, 1 oz. 2.0
all varieties *(Squeez-A-Snak)*, 1 oz....................................... 1.0
all varieties *(Velveeta)*, 1 oz... 3.0

American, processed:
  (Borden Cheese Loaf), 1 oz. 3.0
  (Kraft), 1 oz. 2.0
  with pimento or sharp *(Sargento* Cracker Snacks),
    1 oz. .... <.5
with bacon *(Kraft)*, 1 oz. 1.0
blue *(Roka)*, 1 oz. 2.0
brick or Swiss *(Sargento* Cracker Snacks), 1 oz. 1.0
cheddar:
  sharp or port wine, cold pack *(Wispride* Lite), 1 oz. 4.0
  (Kraft), 1 oz. 3.0
  loaf *(Kraft)*, 1 oz. 2.0
(Land O'Lakes Golden Velvet), 1 oz. 2.0
limburger *(Mohawk Valley)*, 1 oz. 0
olive and pimento *(Kraft)*, 1 oz. 2.0
pimento *(Kraft)*, 1 oz. 3.0
pineapple *(Kraft)*, 1 oz. 4.0
sharp *(Old English)*, 1 oz. 1.0
Cheese sticks, cheddar or mozzarella, frozen
  (Stilwell), 1 piece 5.0
Cheesecake, see "Cake, frozen" and "Cake, snack,
  frozen"
Cheeseburger, see "Beef entree, frozen"
Cherimoya:
1 medium, 1.9 lb. 131.3
(Frieda's), 1 oz. 6.8
Cherry:
fresh, sour, red:
  with pits, 1 oz. 3.5
  with pits, ½ cup 6.3
  pitted, ½ cup 9.4
fresh, sweet, with pits, ½ cup 12.0
fresh, sweet, 10 medium, 2.6 oz. 11.3
canned, sour, pitted:
  sour, pitted, in water *(Stokely)*, ½ cup 10.0
  sour, pitted, in heavy syrup, ½ cup 29.8
  sweet in heavy syrup, ½ cup.. 27.4
  dark, with pits *(Del Monte)*, ½ cup.................................. 23.0

Cherry, canned, sour, pitted *(cont.)*
   dark or light, pitted *(Del Monte)*, ½ cup 24.0
   light, with pits *(Del Monte)*, ½ cup 26.0
dried, bing *(Frieda's)*, 1 oz. 19.8
frozen, sour, red, unsweetened, 4 oz. 12.5
frozen, sweet, sweetened, 4 oz. 25.4
Cherry, maraschino, in jars, with liquid, 1 oz. 8.3
Cherry cider *(R. W. Knudsen)*, 8 fl. oz. 24.0
Cherry drink:
(Hi-C), 6 fl. oz. 24.0
(Kool-Aid Kool Bursts), 6.75 oz. 28.0
mix*:
   (Kool-Aid Presweetened), 8 fl. oz. 18.0
   regular or black *Kool-Aid)*, 8 fl. oz. 25.0
   wild *(Wyler's)*, 8 fl. oz. 21.0
Cherry fruit concentrate, black *(Hain)*, 2 tbsp. 17.0
Cherry fruit roll, see "Fruit snack"
Cherry juice:
(R. W. Knudsen Cherry Tart), 8 fl. oz. 30.0
black *(R. W. Knudsen)*, 8 fl. oz. 38.0
black *(Smucker's Naturally 100%)*, 8 fl. oz. 31.0
blend *(Juicy Juice)*, 6 fl. oz. 23.0
cocktail *(Welch's Orchard)*, 6 fl. oz. 45.0
Cherry juice drink:
(Kool-Aid Koolers), 8.45 fl. oz. 38.0
(Tang Fruit Box), 8.45 fl. oz. 34.0
Cherry-grape juice drink *(Boku)*, 8 fl. oz. 29.0
Chervil, dried, 1 tsp. 3
Chestnut, California *(Frieda's)*, 1 oz. 11.9
Chestnut, Chinese, shelled:
raw, 1 oz. 13.9
dried, 1 oz. 22.7
boiled or steamed, 1 oz. 9.6
roasted, 1 oz. 14.9
Chestnut, European:
raw, in shell, 1 lb. 152.8
raw, shelled, unpeeled, 1 cup or 13 kernels 66.0
dried, peeled, 1 oz. 22.3

boiled, 1 oz. 7.9
roasted, peeled, 1 oz. 15.0
roasted, peeled, 1 cup or 17 kernels 75.7
Chestnut, Japanese:
raw, 1 oz. 9.9
dried, 1 oz. 23.1
boiled or steamed, 1 oz. 3.6
roasted, 1 oz. 12.8
Chick-fil-A, 1 serving:
sandwiches:
  chicken 28.1
  chicken, chargrilled 23.7
  chicken, chargrilled, deluxe 25.5
  chicken deluxe 29.8
  chicken salad 26.4
  Chick-N-Q 40.9
chicken dishes:
  garden salad, chargrilled 8.3
  Grilled'n Lites, 2 skewer 4
  Nuggets, 8-pack 12.5
  salad plate 9.8
side dishes:
  carrot and raisin salad, cup 17.9
  chicken soup, breast of, hearty, cup 11.1
  coleslaw, cup 11.2
  potato salad, cup 13.9
  tossed salad 4.2
  tossed salad, with blue cheese dressing 6.0
  tossed salad, with honey French dressing 21.0
  tossed salad, with lite Italian dressing 7.0
  tossed salad, with lite ranch dressing 13.2
  tossed salad, with ranch dressing 6.0
  tossed salad, with Thousand Island dressing 12.0
  Waffle Fries, small 33.0
desserts:
  fudge brownie, with nuts 45.0
  cheesecake 24.7

Chick-fil-A, desserts *(cont.)*
   cheesecake, with blueberry topping 37.3
   cheesecake, with strawberry topping 35.2
   Icedream, small cup 18.9
   lemon pie 63.8
lemonade, small 34.2
Chicken, without added ingredients 0
Chicken, boneless and luncheon meat:
bologna, see "Chicken bologna"
breast:
   (Longacre Gourmet), 1 oz. 9
   hickory smoked *(Louis Rich),* 1 oz. .... <1.0
   hickory smoked or honey flavored *(Tyson),* 1 slice 8
   roast *(Oscar Mayer Deli-Thin),* 5 slices 2.0
breast, oven roasted:
   (Longacre Premium), 1 oz. 1.0
   (Louis Rich Thin Sliced), 5 slices 1.0
   (Louis Rich Deluxe), 1 oz. .... <1.0
   (Oscar Mayer), 1 slice .... <1.0
   (Oscar Mayer Healthy Favorites), 5 slices 1.0
   (Tyson), 1 slice 8
   (Weight Watchers), 1 oz. 1.0
   mesquite *(Tyson),* 1 slice 8
breast, smoked:
   (Hillshire Farm Deli Select), 1 oz. .... <1.0
   (Louis Rich Thin Sliced), 5 slices 1.0
   (Oscar Mayer) .... <1.0
roll:
   (Tyson), 1 slice 1.4
   breast *(Longacre),* 1 oz. 6
   light meat, 1 oz. 7
white, oven roasted *(Louis Rich),* 1 oz. .... <1.0
Chicken, canned, chunk:
all varieties *(Hormel),* 2.5 oz. 0
regular or white *(Swanson* Premium), 2.5 oz. 0
style *(Swanson* Mixin' Chicken), 2.5 oz. 1.0

"Chicken," vegetarian:
canned:
(Worthington Fri-Chik), 2 pieces 4.0
diced (Worthington), ¼ cup 2.0
fried, with gravy (LaLoma), 2 pieces.................... 4.0
sliced (Worthington), 2 slices 2.0
frozen:
(Worthington Chicketts), ½ cup 6.0
(Worthington Chik Stiks), 1 stick 4.0
(Morningstar Farms/Morningstar Farms Country
    Crisps Patties), 1 patty 13.0
diced (Worthington Meatless), ½ cup................... 5.0
fried (LaLoma), 1 piece...................................... 2.0
nuggets (LaLoma), 5 pieces................................ 8.0
nuggets (Worthington Crispy Chik), 6 pieces 17.0
patties (Worthington Crispy Chik), 1 patty............ 13.0
pie (Worthington), 1 pie..................................... 43.0
sliced (Worthington), 2 slices 3.0
mix, supreme (LaLoma), ¼ cup............................ 4.0
Chicken bologna:
(Perdue), 1-oz. slice... 2.0
(Tyson), 1 slice... 3.7
Chicken dinner, frozen:
à la king (Armour Classic Lite), 11.25 oz. 38.0
baked (Swanson Hungry Man), 15 oz. 57.0
with barbecue sauce (Healthy Choice), 12.75 oz. 57.0
barbecue (Tyson Healthy Portion), 12.5 oz. 56.0
boneless (Swanson Hungry Man), 17.25 oz.............. 71.0
breast, herbed, with fettuccine (The Budget Gourmet
    Light and Healthy), 11 oz................................ 30.0
breast, mesquite (The Budget Gourmet Light and
    Healthy), 11 oz. 33.0
Burgundy (Armour Classic Lite), 10 oz................... 25.0
Cordon Bleu, grilled (Le Menu New American
    Cuisine), 10.5 oz.. 34.0
Dijon (Healthy Choice), 11 oz. 40.0
Français (Tyson Premium), 9.5 oz.......................... 20.0

Chicken dinner, frozen *(cont.)*
fried:
  (Banquet Extra Helping), 14.25 oz. 68.0
  barbecue flavored *(Swanson)*, 10 oz. 61.0
  dark meat *(Swanson,* 4 Compartment), 9.75 oz............ 55.0
  dark meat *(Swanson Hungry Man)*, 14.25 oz. 77.0
  Southern *(Banquet Extra Helping)*, 13.25 oz. 75.0
  thigh meat *(Freezer Queen)*, 10 oz. 39.0
  white meat *(Banquet Extra Helping)*, 14.25 oz. 69.0
  white meat *(Freezer Queen)*, 10 oz. 47.0
  white meat *(Swanson)*, 10.25 oz. 59.0
  white meat *(Swanson Hungry Man* Mostly White),
    14.25 oz. 80.0
garlic *(Swanson Hungry Man)*, 16.5 oz. 55.0
glazed:
  (Armour Classics), 10.75 oz. 24.0
  golden *(Le Menu New American Cuisine* Healthy),
    11 oz. 52.0
  with sauce *(Tyson* Premium), 9.25 oz. 29.0
grilled:
  (Tyson Premium), 7.75 oz. 22.0
  (Swanson Hungry Man), 17 oz. 78.0
  with almonds *(Swanson)*, 10 oz. 39.0
herb:
  (Tyson Healthy Portion), 13.75 oz. 43.0
  roasted *(Healthy Choice)*, 11.5 oz. 56.0
  roasted *(Le Menu New American Cuisine* Healthy),
    10 oz. 43.0
honey mustard *(Tyson* Healthy Portion), 13.75 oz. 52.0
honey mustard, grilled *(Le Menu New American
  Cuisine)*, 9 oz. 50.0
honey roasted *(Tyson* Premium), 9 oz. 23.0
Italian, grilled *(Tyson* Premium), 9 oz. 19.0
Italian style *(Tyson* Healthy Portion), 13.75 oz. 38.0
Kiev *(Tyson* Premium), 9.25 oz. 39.0
marinara *(Tyson* Healthy Portion), 13.75 oz. 37.0
Marsala *(Armour Classics Lite)*, 10.5 oz. 27.0
Marsala *(Tyson* Premium), 9 oz. 19.0

mesquite:
   (Armour Classics), 9.5 oz. 42.0
   (Healthy Choice), 10.5 oz. 54.0
   (Le Menu New American Cuisine Healthy),
      10.25 oz. 48.0
   (Tyson Healthy Portion), 13.25 oz. 38.0
   (Tyson Premium), 9 oz. 39.0
and noodles *(Armour Classic)*, 11 oz. 23.0
nuggets:
   (Freezer Queen), 6 oz. 33.0
   (Swanson), 8.75 oz. 48.0
   with barbecue or sweet and sour sauce *(Banquet*
      Extra Helping), 10 oz. 68.0
Oriental *(Armour Classics Lite)*, 10 oz. 24.0
Oriental *(Healthy Choice)*, 11.25 oz. 32.0
parmigiana:
   (Armour Classics), 11.5 oz. 27.0
   (Healthy Choice), 11.5 oz. 41.0
   (Swanson 4 Compartment), 11.5 oz. 42.0
   (Tyson Premium), 11.25 oz. 37.0
   breast *(The Budget Gourmet* Light and Healthy),
      11 oz. 30.0
   breast *(Le Menu New American Cuisine)*, 10.25 oz. 28.0
and pasta divan *(Healthy Choice)*, 12.1 oz. 41.0
pasta primavera *(Le Menu New American Cuisine)*,
   11.5 oz. 40.0
patty *(Freezer Queen)*, 7.5 oz. 29.0
picante *(Tyson* Premium), 9 oz. 26.0
picatta *(Tyson* Premium), 9 oz. 18.0
roast, homestyle gravy *(The Budget Gourmet* Light
   and Healthy), 11 oz. 36.0
roasted *(Tyson* Premium), 9 oz. 21.0
salsa:
   (Healthy Choice), 11.25 oz. 36.0
   (Le Menu New American Cuisine Healthy),
      10.75 oz. 45.0
   (Tyson Healthy Portion), 13.75 oz. 52.0

Chicken dinner, frozen *(cont.)*

Santa Fe style, grilled *(Le Menu New American*
    Cuisine), 10 oz. 37.0
sesame *(Tyson* Healthy Portion), 13.5 oz. 59.0
Southwestern style *(Healthy Choice)*, 12.5 oz. 51.0
supreme *(Tyson* Premium), 9 oz. 23.0
sweet and sour:
    (Armour Classics Lite), 11 oz. 39.0
    (Healthy Choice), 11.5 oz. 52.0
    (Le Menu New American Cuisine), 11.25 oz. 47.0
    (Tyson Premium), 11 oz. 50.0
teriyaki *(The Budget Gourmet* Light and Healthy),
    11 oz. 41.0
teriyaki *(Healthy Choice)*, 12.25 oz. 39.0
tomato garden *(Le Menu New American Cuisine)*,
    10 oz. 24.0
with wine and mushroom sauce *(Armour Classics)*,
    10.75 oz. 24.0

Chicken entree, canned or packaged:

à la king *(Hormel Top Shelf)*, 10 oz. 49.0
à la king *(Swanson)*, 5.25 oz. 9.0
breast, glazed *(Hormel Top Shelf)*, 10 oz. 19.0
breast, with Spanish rice *(Hormel Top Shelf)*, 10 oz. 38.0
cacciatore *(Hormel Top Shelf)*, 10 oz. 25.0
chow mein:
    (La Choy), ³⁄₄ cup 5.0
    (La Choy Bi-Pack), ³⁄₄ cup 8.0
    (La Choy Dinner), ¹⁄₂ pkg. 29.0
and dumplings *(Dinty Moore)*, 7.5 oz. 17.0
and dumplings *(Swanson)*, 7.5 oz. 19.0
stew *(Dinty Moore)*, 7.5 oz. 15.0
stew *(Swanson)*, 7.6 oz. 15.0
sweet and sour *(La Choy)*, ³⁄₄ cup 47.0
sweet and sour *(La Choy* Bi-Pack), ³⁄₄ cup 18.0
teriyaki *(La Choy* Bi-Pack), ³⁄₄ cup 8.0

Chicken entree, freeze-dried*:

à la king or Polynesian *(Mountain House)*, 1 cup 33.0
stew *(Mountain House)*, 1 cup 30.0

Chicken entree, frozen:

à la king:
- (Dining Lite), 9 oz. 30.0
- (Freezer Queen Cook-in-Pouch), 4 oz. 7.0
- (Stouffer's Lunch Express), 9⅞ oz. 41.0
- with rice (Stouffer's), 9.5 oz. 38.0

à l'orange (Healthy Choice), 9 oz. 38.0
à l'orange, with almond rice (Lean Cuisine), 8 oz. 33.0
au gratin (The Budget Gourmet Light and Healthy),
- 9.1 oz. 23.0

barbecue:
- (Banquet Meals), 9 oz. 37.0
- glazed (Weight Watchers Ultimate 200), 6.5 oz. 16.0
- sauce, with pilaf (Lean Cuisine), 8.75 oz. 32.0

breast:
- baked, nuggets, patties, or tenders (Banquet
  Healthy Balance), 2.25 oz. 8.0
- baked, whipped potatoes (Stouffer's Homestyle),
  8⅞ oz. 18.0
- batter dipped (Weaver), 4.4 oz. 13.0
- breaded, Parmesan (Lean Cuisine), 10⅞ oz. 25.0
- chunks (Tyson), 3 oz. 10.0
- fillet (Tyson), 3 oz. 15.0
- fillet (Weaver), 4.5 oz. 18.0
- fillet, barbecue (Tyson), 3 oz. 6.0
- fillet, grilled (Tyson), 2.75 oz. 4.0
- fillet, mesquite (Tyson), 2.75 oz. 3.0
- fillet, Southern fried (Tyson), 3 oz. 15.0
- fillet strips (Tyson), 3.3 oz. 14.0
- fried (Weaver Crispy Dutch Frye), 4.5 oz. 17.0
- fried, whipped potato (Stouffer's Homestyle),
  7⅛ oz. 30.0
- glazed (Healthy Choice), 8.5 oz. 27.0
- grilled, barbecue sauce (Stouffer's Homestyle),
  7⅝ oz. 14.0
- Marsala, with vegetables (Lean Cuisine), 8⅛ oz. 13.0
- oven baked, breaded (Lean Cuisine), 8 oz. 21.0
- patties (Tyson), 2.6 oz. 11.0

Chicken entree, frozen, breast *(cont.)*
patties *(Weaver)*, 3 oz... 14.0
patties, Southern fried *(Tyson)*, 2.6 oz. 9.0
portions, fried *(Banquet)*, 5.75 oz. 13.0
strips, mesquite *(Tyson)*, 2.75 oz. 2.0
breast tenders:
(*Banquet Hot Bites*), 2.25 oz.. 12.0
(*Tyson*), 3 oz. 13.0
(*Tyson* Microwave), 3.5 oz... 19.0
(*Weaver* Premium), 3 oz. 11.0
breaded, O'Brien potatoes *(Stouffer's* Homestyle),
8⅜ oz.. 46.0
honey batter *(Weaver)*, 3 oz. 14.0
hot barbecue or mesquite *(Tyson)*, 2.75 oz. 4.0
Southern fried *(Banquet Hot Bites)*, 2.25 oz. 13.0
with spaghetti swirls *(On-Cor)*, 8 oz. 29.0
cacciatore, with vermicelli *(Lean Cuisine)*, 10⅞ oz. 31.0
cannelloni, see "Cannelloni entree"
with cheddar *(Tyson* Chick'n Cheddar), 2.6 oz. 11.0
chow mein:
(*Banquet* Meals), 9 oz. 29.0
(*Chun King*), 13 oz.. 53.0
(*Dining Lite*), 9 oz. 31.0
(*Healthy Choice*), 9 oz. 29.0
(*Stouffer's Lunch Express*), 10⅝ oz.................................. 47.0
(*Weight Watchers Smart Ones*), 9 oz................................. 27.0
with rice *(Stouffer's)*, 10.75 oz. 39.0
with rice *(Lean Cuisine)*, 9 oz... 34.0
chunks:
(*Country Skillet*), 3 oz. 17.0
(*Tyson* Chick'n Chunks), 2.6 oz. 11.0
(*Tyson* Microwave), 3.5 oz.. 11.0
Southern fried *(Country Skillet)*, 3 oz............................... 15.0
Southern fried *(Tyson* Chick'n Chunks), 2.6 oz. 11.0
Cordon Bleu *(Weight Watchers Ultimate 200)*, 7.7 oz. 15.0
creamed *(Stouffer's)*, 6.5 oz. 8.0
croquettes *(Freezer Queen Family)*, 7 oz. 20.0

croquettes, with gravy *(Weaver)*, 2 croquettes,
½ gravy cup 26.0
diced *(Tyson)*, 3 oz. 1.0
Divan *(Stouffer's)*, 8 oz. 11.0
drumsticks:
  (Banquet Drum-Snackers), 2.5 oz. 12.0
  crispy or herb and spice *(Weaver Mini Drums)*,
    3 oz. 13.0
  and thighs, batter dipped *(Weaver)*, 3 oz. 11.0
  and thighs, fried *(Weaver Crispy Dutch Frye)*,
    3.5 oz. 14.0
dumplings and *(Banquet Family)*, 7 oz. 28.0
and dumplings *(Banquet Meals)*, 10 oz. 35.0
enchilada, see "Enchilada entree"
escalloped, with noodles *(Stouffer's)*, 10 oz. 30.0
fajita, see "Fajita entree"
fettuccine, see "Fettuccine entree"
with fettuccine *(The Budget Gourmet)*, 10 oz. 29.0
fiesta *(Lean Cuisine)*, 8.5 oz. 30.0
fiesta *(Weight Watchers Smart Ones)*, 8 oz. 37.0
Français *(Weight Watchers Smart Ones)*, 8.5 oz. 18.0
French recipe *(The Budget Gourmet Light and
  Healthy)*, 10 oz. 21.0
fried:
  (Banquet Meals), 9 oz. 41.0
  (Swanson Plump & Juicy), 3.25 oz. 16.0
  breast half *(Swanson Plump & Juicy)*, 4.5 oz. 21.0
  hot'n spicy *(Banquet)*, 6.4 oz. 29.0
  hot'n spicy *(Banquet Snack'n)*, 3.75 oz. 8.0
  nibbles *(Swanson)*, 3.25 oz. 19.0
  original or Southern *(Banquet)*, 5.6 oz. 26.0
  and whipped potatoes *(Swanson)*, 7 oz. 34.0
  spicy *(Swanson Take-Out)*, 3.25 oz. 17.0
  thighs and drumsticks *(Banquet)*, 6.25 oz. 14.0
ginger, vegetable Hunan and *(Weight Watchers Stir-
  Fry)*, 9 oz. 21.0
glazed, with vegetable rice *(Lean Cuisine)*, 8.5 oz. 24.0

Chicken entree, frozen (cont.)
grilled, glazed (Weight Watchers Ultimate 200),
  7.5 oz. 17.0
honey mustard (Healthy Choice), 9.5 oz. 37.0
honey mustard (Lean Cuisine), 7.5 oz. 30.0
Imperial (Chun King), 13 oz. 54.0
Imperial (Weight Watchers Ultimate 200), 8.5 oz. 25.0
Italiano, with fettuccine and vegetables (Lean
  Cuisine), 9 oz. 33.0
Kiev (Weight Watchers Ultimate 200), 7 oz. 22.0
mandarin (The Budget Gourmet Light and Healthy),
  10 oz. 38.0
mandarin (Healthy Choice), 10 oz. 35.0
Marsala (The Budget Gourmet), 9 oz. 31.0
mesquite (Banquet Healthy Balance), 10.5 oz. 36.0
mirabella (Weight Watchers Smart Ones), 9.2 oz. 26.0
nibbles, with french fries (Swanson), 4.25 oz. 30.0
and noodles:
  (Banquet Entree Express), 8.5 oz. 23.0
  (Dining Lite), 9 oz. 28.0
  (Stouffer's Homestyle), 10 oz. 21.0
  (Swanson), 9 oz. 30.0
  (Weight Watchers), 9 oz. 25.0
  egg noodles (The Budget Gourmet), 10 oz. 28.0
nuggets:
  (Banquet Hot Bites), 2.5 oz. 10.0
  (Banquet Meals), 6.75 oz. 38.0
  (Country Skillet), 3 oz. 14.0
  (Freezer Queen Family), 7 oz. 16.0
  (Swanson), 3 oz. 14.0
  (Weaver), 2.6 oz. 10.0
  (Weight Watchers), 5.9 oz. 23.0
  with cheddar or hot'n spicy (Banquet Hot Bites),
    2.5 oz. 10.0
  with french fries (Swanson), 4.75 oz. 30.0
  Southern fried (Banquet Hot Bites), 2.5 oz. 12.0
orange glazed (The Budget Gourmet Light and
  Healthy), 9 oz. 46.0

orange glazed, with rice *(Weight Watchers* Stir-Fry),
  9 oz. 25.0
Oriental:
  (Banquet Meals), 9 oz. 37.0
  (Freezer Queen), 8.5 oz. 21.0
  with peanut sauce *(Healthy Choice)*, 9.5 oz. 31.0
  with vegetables *(The Budget Gourmet)*, 9 oz. 44.0
  with vegetables and vermicelli *(Lean Cuisine)*,
    9 oz. 31.0
Parmesan *(Banquet Healthy Balance)*, 10.8 oz. 34.0
parmigiana:
  (Banquet Meals), 9.5 oz. 27.0
  (Celentano), 9 oz. 17.0
  (Freezer Queen), 8.5 oz. 42.0
  (On-Cor), 8 oz. 26.0
  and pasta Alfredo *(Stouffer's* Homestyle), 10⅝ oz. 31.0
patties:
  (Banquet Hot Bites), 2.5 oz. 11.0
  (Country Skillet), 3 oz. 14.0
  (Tyson Thick & Crispy), 2.6 oz. 13.0
  Southern fried *(Banquet Hot Bites)*, 2.5 oz. 12.0
  Southern fried *(Country Skillet)*, 3 oz. 14.0
piccata, lemon herb *(Weight Watchers Smart Ones)*,
  7.5 oz. 25.0
pie:
  (Freezer Queen Family), 7 oz. 25.0
  (Stouffer's), 10 oz. 37.0
  (Swanson), 7 oz. 35.0
  (Swanson Deluxe), 9 oz. 39.0
  (Swanson Hungry Man), 16 oz. 57.0
Polynesian *(Weight Watchers* Stir-Fry), 9 oz. 34.0
primavera *(Celentano)*, 11.5 oz. 27.0
rondolet:
  original *(Weaver)*, 3 oz. 13.0
  cheese *(Weaver)*, 2.6 oz. 12.0
  Italian *(Weaver)*, 2.6 oz. 11.0

Chicken entree, frozen *(cont.)*
sandwich, see "Chicken sandwich"
sesame, with lo mein noodles *(Weight Watchers Stir-Fry)*, 9 oz. 23.0
skinless *(Weaver Crispy Light)*, 2.9 oz. 9.0
sliced, gravy and *(Freezer Queen Cook-in-Pouch)*,
   4 oz. 4.0
Southern baked *(Weight Watchers Ultimate 200)*,
   6.3 oz. 10.0
sticks *(Banquet Hot Bites)*, 2.5 oz. 10.0
stir-fry, with pasta *(Healthy Choice Extra Portion)*,
   12 oz. 42.0
sweet and sour:
   (Banquet Healthy Balance), 10.25 oz. 47.0
   (The Budget Gourmet), 10 oz. 55.0
   (Freezer Queen), 9 oz. 46.0
   with rice *(Lean Cuisine)*, 9 oz. 39.0
tenderloins, in herb cream sauce *(Lean Cuisine)*,
   9.5 oz. 19.0
tenderloins, in peanut sauce *(Lean Cuisine)*, 9 oz. 33.0
teriyaki *(Weight Watchers Ultimate 200)*, 7.6 oz. 7.0
teriyaki, with spring vegetables *(Weight Watchers Stir-Fry)*, 9 oz. 16.0
thighs and drumsticks *(Swanson Plump & Juicy)*,
   3.25 oz. 17.0
and vegetables:
   (Freezer Queen), 9 oz. 30.0
   (Healthy Choice), 11.5 oz. 39.0
   primavera *(Banquet Cookin' Bag)*, 4 oz. 14.0
   primavera *(Banquet Family)*, 7 oz. 18.0
   with vermicelli *(Lean Cuisine)*, 11.75 oz. 30.0
walnut, crunchy *(Chun King)*, 13 oz. 49.0
wings:
   (Banquet Meals), 8.75 oz. 37.0
   all varieties *(Tyson)*, 3.5 oz. 0
   batter dipped *(Weaver)*, 4 oz. 20.0
   fried *(Weaver Crispy Dutch Frye)*, 4 oz. 20.0
   hot *(Weaver)*, 2.7 oz. 1.0

Chicken entree, mix*:
broccoli, cheesy *(Skillet Chicken Helper)*, 7 oz. 34.0
creamy *(Skillet Chicken Helper)*, 8.25 oz. 29.0
fettuccine Alfredo *(Skillet Chicken Helper)*, 7.5 oz. 27.0
mushroom, creamy *(Skillet Chicken Helper)*, 8 oz. 31.0
stir-fried *(Skillet Chicken Helper)*, 7 oz. 36.0
sweet and sour *(La Choy Dinner Classics)*, ¾ cup 30.0

Chicken entree, refrigerated:
barbecue, all varieties, except drumstick *(Perdue
   Done It!)*, 1 oz. 1.0
barbecue, drumstick *(Perdue Done It!)*, 1 oz. 2.0
breast cutlet *(Perdue Done It!)*, 3.5 oz. 17.0
breast nugget, chicken or chicken and cheese
   (Perdue Done It!), 1 piece 3.0
breast tenders *(Perdue Done It!)*, 1 oz. 4.0
blue cheese, Italian *(Chicken By George)*, 5 oz. 2.0
Cajun *(Chicken By George)*, 5 oz. 4.0
Caribbean grill *(Chicken By George)*, 5 oz. 10.0
lemon herb *(Chicken By George)*, 5 oz. 6.0
lemon oregano *(Chicken By George)*, 5 oz. 4.0
mesquite barbecue *(Chicken By George)*, 5 oz. 6.0
mustard dill *(Chicken By George)*, 5 oz. 3.0
roasted:
   breast half *(Perdue Done It!)*, 1 oz. 1.0
   drumstick *(Perdue Done It!)*, 1 oz. 0
   thigh *(Perdue Done It!)*, 1 oz. .... <1.0
   whole or half, dark or white meat *(Perdue Done
      It!)*, 1 oz. .... <1.0
teriyaki *(Chicken By George)*, 5 oz. 9.0
tomato herb with basil *(Chicken By George)*, 5 oz. 7.0
wings, hot and spicy *(Perdue Done It!)*, 1 oz. 1.0

Chicken fat 0

Chicken frankfurter:
(Longacre), 1 oz. 0
(Perdue), 2-oz. link 3.0
(Tyson), 1 link 1.0
cheese *(Tyson)*, 1 link 1.0

Chicken giblets:
simmered, 4 oz. 1.1
simmered, chopped, 1 cup 1.4
Chicken gravy:
canned, 2 oz. or 1/4 cup:
  plain or giblet *(Franco-American)*, 1/4 cup 3.0
  plain or with mushroom and onion *(Heinz*
    HomeStyle), 2 oz. 3.0
  golden *(Pepperidge Farm)*, 2 oz. 3.0
mix:
  (Lawry's), 1/6 pkg. 5.0
  (McCormick/Schilling), 1/4 cup* 3.7
  (McCormick/Schilling Lite), 1/4 cup* 2
  (Pillsbury), 1/4 cup* 4.0
"Chicken" gravy, vegetarian, mix* *(LaLoma Gravy*
  Quik), 2 tbsp. 2.0
Chicken luncheon meat, see "Chicken, boneless
  and luncheon meat"
Chicken pie, see "Chicken entree, frozen"
Chicken salad:
(Longacre), 1 oz. 3.0
(Longacre Lite), 1 oz. 3.3
spread *(Libby's Spreadables)*, 1.9 oz. 5.0
Chicken sandwich, frozen:
(Hormel Quick Meal), 1 piece 40.0
(MicroMagic), 4.5-oz. piece 42.0
barbecue *(Tyson Microwave)*, 4-oz. piece 27.0
biscuit *(Hormel Quick Meal)*, 1 piece 36.0
breast *(Tyson Microwave)*, 4.25-oz. piece 33.0
breast, grilled *(Tyson)*, 3.5-oz. piece 2.0
grilled:
  (Hormel Quick Meal), 1 piece 35.0
  (Tyson), 3.5-oz. piece 25.0
  (Weight Watchers Ultimate 200), 1 piece 22.0
pocket:
  and cheddar with bacon *(Hot Pockets)*,
    4.5-oz. piece 35.0
  fajita *(Lean Pockets)*, 4.5-oz. piece 33.0

glazed (*Lean Pockets* Supreme), 4.5-oz. piece 32.0
Oriental (*Lean Pockets*), 4.5-oz. piece 33.0
Parmesan (*Lean Pockets*), 4.5-oz. piece 31.0
Chicken sauce, canned, see "Entree sauce"
Chicken sauce mix* (see also specific listings):
cacciatore (*McCormick/Shilling* Sauce Blends),
   1 serving 17.0
Creole (*McCormick/Shilling* Sauce Blends), 1 serving 16.0
curry, creamy (*McCormick/Shilling* Sauce Blends),
   1 serving 9.0
Dijon (*McCormick/Shilling* Sauce Blends), 1 serving 8.0
Italian marinade (*McCormick/Shilling* Sauce Blends),
   1 serving 3.0
mesquite (*McCormick/Shilling* Sauce Blends),
   1 serving 4.0
Parmesan (*McCormick/Shilling* Sauce Blends),
   1 serving 6.0
Southwest style (*McCormick/Shilling* Sauce Blends),
   1 serving 4.0
stir fry (*McCormick/Shilling* Sauce Blends), 1 serving 18.0
sweet and sour (*McCormick/Shilling* Sauce Blends),
   1 serving 20.0
teriyaki (*McCormick/Shilling* Sauce Blends), 1 serving........ 7.0
Chicken seasoning:
fried (*McCormick/Schilling* Spice Blends), 1 tsp.................... .6
mix, Southwest (*Lawry's* Seasoning Blends), 1 pkg.......... 16.0
Chicken seasoning and coating mix:
(*French's* Roasting Bag), 1/5 pkg............................... 4.0
(*McCormick/Schilling* Bag'n Season), 1 pkg.................... 22.0
(*Shake'n Bake*), 1/4 packet..................................... 14.0
barbecue (*Shake'n Bake*), 1/4 packet 18.0
batter, Cajun (*Tone's*), 1 tsp. 2.6
country (*McCormick/Shilling* Bag'n Season), 1 pkg. 19.0
extra crispy (*Oven Fry*), 1/4 packet............................ 21.0
frying (*Golden Dipt*), 1 oz..................................... 20.0
homestyle (*Oven Fry*), 1/4 packet 15.0
hot and spicy (*Shake'n Bake*), 1/4 packet 15.0

Chicken spread, chunky, canned:
(Swanson), 1 oz.. 2.0
(Underwood/Underwood Light), 2¹/₈ oz...................... 2.0
Chicken and fish seasoning *(McCormick/Schilling*
   Grillmates), 1 tsp. 2.0
Chickpea flour *(Arrowhead Mills),* 2 oz................ 35.0
Chickpeas:
dry *(Arrowhead Mills),* 2 oz... 35.0
dry, boiled, ¹/₂ cup 22.5
canned:
   with liquid, ¹/₂ cup 27.1
   (Allens), ¹/₂ cup 18.0
   (Eden/Eden No Salt Added), ¹/₂ cup 17.0
   (Hain), 4 oz. 18.0
   (Old El Paso), ¹/₂ cup 16.0
   (Progresso), 4 oz. 22.0
Chicory, witloof:
5–7"-long head, 2.1 oz. 2.1
¹/₂ cup.. 1.8
Chicory greens:
trimmed, 1 oz.. 1.3
chopped, ¹/₂ cup 4.2
Chicory root:
1 medium, 2.6 oz... 10.5
1" pieces, ¹/₂ cup 7.9
Chili, canned or packaged:
with beans:
   (Gebhardt), 1 cup 47.0
   (Hormel), 7.5 oz. 27.0
   (Hormel Micro Cup), 7.5 oz... 23.0
   (Just Rite), 4 oz. 16.0
   (Libby's), 7.5 oz. 25.0
   (Libby's Diner), 7.75 oz. 29.0
   (Old El Paso), 1 cup 17.0
   chunky *(Hormel),* 7.5 oz. 25.0
   hot *(Gebhardt),* 1 cup... 47.0
   hot *(Hormel),* 7.5 oz.. 27.0

hot *(Hormel Micro Cup)*, 7.5 oz. 24.0
hot *(Just Rite)*, 4 oz. 16.0
spicy, and turkey *(Healthy Choice)*, 7.5 oz. 26.0
without beans:
  (Gebhardt), 1 cup 20.0
  (Hormel), 7.5 oz. 14.0
  (Hormel Micro Cup), 7.4 oz. 15.0
  (Just Rite), 4 oz. 9.0
  (Libby's), 7.5 oz. 11.0
  hot *(Hormel)*, 7.5 oz. 14.0
with chicken, spicy *(Hain)*, 7.5 oz. 19.0
turkey, with beans *(Healthy Choice)*, 7.5 oz. 20.0
vegetarian:
  (Natural Touch), ²/₃ cup 19.0
  (Worthington), ²/₃ cup 15.0
  mild, three bean *(Health Valley* Fat Free), 5 oz. 12.0
  mild or spicy, with black beans *(Health Valley* Fat
    Free), 5 oz. 23.0
  spicy *(Hain)*, 7.5 oz. 29.0
  spicy *(Hain* Reduced Sodium), 7.5 oz. 31.0
  tempeh, spicy *(Hain)*, 7.5 oz. 24.0
with macaroni *(Hormel Micro Cup Chili Mac)*, 7.5 oz. 18.0
Chili, freeze-dried*, with beans or beef *(Mountain
  House)*, 1 cup 30.0
Chili, frozen (see also "Chili entree"):
with beans, meatless *(Bodin's)*, 4 oz. 14.0
turkey *(Banquet Cookin' Bag)*, 4 oz. 11.0
Chili, mix*:
(Fantastic Cha-Cha Chili), 10 oz. 38.0
(Hunt's Manwich Chili Fixin's), 8 oz. 20.0
black bean *(Aunt Patsy's Souper Black Bean)*, 8 oz. 30.0
lentil *(Aunt Patsy's Pantry)*, 8 oz. 27.0
vegetarian *(Fantastic)*, 4 oz. 18.0
Chili beans, canned:
(Gebhardt), 4 oz. 21.0
(Green Giant/Joan of Arc 50% Less Salt), ½ cup 21.0
(Hunt's), 4 oz. 18.0
extra spicy *(Green Giant/Joan of Arc)*, ½ cup 21.0

Chili beans (cont.)
hot (Campbell's), 4 oz. 19.0
spicy (Green Giant/Joan of Arc), ½ cup 21.0
Chili dip:
(La Victoria), 2 tbsp. 2.0
mix, caliente (Knorr), 1 serving dry 8
Chili entree, frozen:
con carne (Swanson Homestyle), 8.25 oz. 26.0
con carne, with beans (Stouffer's), 8¾ oz. 28.0
vegetarian (Right Course), 9¾ oz. 45.0
Chili powder:
1 tbsp. 4.1
1 tsp. 1.4
(Gebhardt), 1 tsp. 3.0
Chili sauce:
(Bennett's), 1 tbsp. 4.0
(Heinz), 1 oz. 7.0
(Tabasco 7 Spice), 1 oz. 2.5
hot dog (Gebhardt), 2 tbsp. 4.0
hot dog (Just Rite), 2 oz. 6.0
red (Las Palmas), ½ cup 3.0
spicy (Tabasco 7 Spice), 1 oz. 2.4
Chili seasoning mix:
(French's Chili O), ⅙ pkg. 5.0
(Gebhardt Chili Quik), 1 tsp. 2.0
(Lawry's Seasoning Blends), 1 pkg. 26.6
(McCormick/Schilling), ¼ pkg. 4.5
(Old El Paso), ⅕ pkg. 4.0
(Tio Sancho), 1.23 oz. 60.9
medium (Hain), ¼ pkg. 5.0
onion, real (French's Chili O), ⅙ pkg. 7.0
Texas style (French's Chili O), ¼ pkg. .... <1.0
Chimichanga, frozen:
beef (Old El Paso), 1 piece 35.0
chicken (Old El Paso), 1 piece 34.0
Chimichanga entree, beef and bean, frozen
  (Banquet Meals), 9.5 oz. 60.0
Chitterlings, pork 0

Chives:
fresh, 1 oz. 1.2
fresh, chopped, 1 tbsp. 1
freeze-dried, ¼ cup 5
freeze-dried, 1 tbsp. 1
Chocolate, see "Candy"
Chocolate, baking:
bar:
   semisweet (Hershey's Premium), 1 oz. 16.0
   semisweet (Nestlé), 1 oz. 16.0
   unsweetened (Baker's), 1 oz. 9.0
   unsweetened (Hershey's Premium), 1 oz. 7.0
   unsweetened (Nestlé), 1 oz. 9.0
   white (Nestlé Premier), 1 oz. 16.0
chips:
   milk (Hershey's), ¼ cup... 27.0
   milk (Nestlé Toll House Morsels), 1 oz........................ 19.0
   milk, maxi (Guittard), 1 oz. 18.0
   mint (Hershey's), ¼ cup... 28.0
   rainbow (Nestlé Toll House Morsels), 1 oz. 20.0
   semisweet (Guittard), 1 oz. 19.0
   semisweet (Nestlé Merry Morsels), 1 oz....................... 21.0
   semisweet or mint (Nestlé Toll House Morsels/
     Mini), 1 oz. 14.0
   semisweet, regular or mini (Hershey's), ¼ cup 27.0
   vanilla (Hershey's), ¼ cup.. 25.0
chunks:
   milk (Hershey's), 1 oz. 16.0
   milk (Nestlé Treasures), 1 oz. 17.0
   semisweet (Hershey's), 1 oz.. 15.0
   semisweet (Nestlé Treasures), 1 oz............................... 18.0
   white (Nestlé Treasures), 1 oz. 15.0
premelted, unsweetened, 1-oz. packet 9.6
shreds (Tone's), 1 tsp.. 2.2
Chocolate flavor drink:
canned (Frostee), 1 cup.. 30.0
chilled (Hershey's), 1 cup... 28.0

Chocolate flavor drink mix:

regular or malt *(Carnation* Instant Breakfast),
  1 packet 27.0
(Hershey's), 3 heaping tsp. 22.0
(Nestlé Quik), ¾ oz. 20.0
(Pillsbury Instant Breakfast), 1 packet 27.0
malt *(Pillsbury* Instant Breakfast), 1 packet 25.0
Chocolate milk:
(Hershey's), 1 cup 28.0
(Nestlé Quik), 1 cup 30.0
lowfat *(Nestlé Quik)*, 1 cup 29.0
lowfat *(Hershey's)*, 1 cup 29.0
Chocolate mousse, see "Mousse" and "Mousse
  mix"
Chocolate sauce, see "Chocolate syrup" and
  "Chocolate topping"
Chocolate soufflé mix *(Knorr)*, 1 serving dry 5.4
Chocolate syrup:
(Hershey's), 2 tbsp. 25.0
(Nestlé Quik), 1⅔ heaping tsp. 22.0
(Smucker's), 2 tbsp. 27.0
Chocolate topping:
(Barbara's Chocolate Mountain Chocolate Sauce),
  2 tbsp. 20.0
(Kraft), 1 tbsp. 11.0
(Smucker's Magic Shell), 2 tbsp. 16.0
dark *(Smucker's* Special), 2 tbsp. 31.0
fudge:
  (Hershey's), 2 tbsp. 17.0
  (Smucker's), 2 tbsp. 31.0
  (Smucker's Magic Shell), 2 tbsp. 16.0
fudge, hot:
  (Kraft), 1 tbsp. 11.0
  (Smucker's), 2 tbsp. 18.0
  (Smucker's Light), 2 tbsp. 19.0
  (Smucker's Special), 2 tbsp. 23.0
  Swiss milk chocolate *(Smucker's)*, 2 tbsp. 31.0
  toffee *(Smucker's)*, 2 tbsp. 18.0

nut *(Smucker's Magic Shell)*, 2 tbsp. 25.0
Chops, vegetarian, canned *(Worthington Choplets)*,
  2 slices.. 4.0
Chow mein, see specific entree listings
Chow mein noodles, see "Noodles, Chinese"
Chrysanthemum garland:
raw, 1″ pieces, ½ cup 5
boiled, drained, 1″ pieces, ½ cup... 2.2
Churro, frozen *(Tio Pepe's)*, 1 piece.................................. 16.0
Cilantro, see "Coriander"
Cinnamon, ground *(Tone's)*, 1 tsp. 1.8
Cisco, without added ingredients 0
Citrus grill marinade *(Lawry's)*, 2 tbsp. 3.4
Citrus juice *(Santa Cruz Natural)*, 8 fl. oz........................ 29.0
Citrus juice drink:
(Hi-C Citrus Cooler), 6 fl. oz. 23.3
chilled or frozen* *(Five Alive)*, 6 fl. oz. 22.0
berry, frozen* *(Five Alive)*, 6 fl. oz....................................... 22.0
tropical, chilled or frozen* *(Five Alive)*, 6 fl. oz. 21.0
Citrus punch *(Minute Maid)*, 6 fl. oz.................................. 23.0
Citrus-cranberry juice drink *(Ocean Spray*
  Refreshers), 6 fl. oz. 26.0
Citrus-peach juice drink *(Ocean Spray Refreshers)*,
  6 fl. oz.. 23.0
Clam, meat only:
raw, 4 oz. 2.9
raw, 9 large or 20 small, 6.3 oz.. 4.6
boiled, poached, or steamed, 4 oz. 5.8
Clam, canned, chopped or minced:
(Gorton's), ½ can 4.0
with liquid *(Doxsee/Snow's)*, 6.5 oz...................................... 8.0
with liquid *(Progresso)*, ½ cup... 1.0
drained *(Progresso)*, ½ cup .... <1.0
Clam entree, frozen:
fried *(Mrs. Paul's)*, 2.5 oz.. 21.0
strips, crunchy *(Gorton's Microwave)*, 2.9 oz. 20.0
Clam chowder, see "Soup"

Clam dip:
(Breakstone's/Sealtest), 2 tbsp. 2.0
(Breakstone's Gourmet Chesapeake), 2 tbsp. 2.0
(Kraft), 2 tbsp. 3.0
(Kraft Premium), 2 tbsp. 2.0
Clam juice *(Doxsee/Snow's)*, 3 fl. oz. 0
Clam sauce, canned:
red *(Ferrara)*, 4 oz. 8.0
red *(Progresso)*, ½ cup 7.0
white *(Ferrara)*, 4 oz. 4.0
white *(Progresso)*, ½ cup 1.0
Cloves, ground:
1 tbsp. 4.0
1 tsp. 1.3
Cobbler:
apple, deep dish *(Awrey's)*, ⅛ pie 48.0
blueberry, deep dish *(Awrey's)*, ⅛ pie 45.0
frozen:
  apple *(Stilwell)*, ½ cup 55.0
  apple, blueberry, or strawberry *(Pet-Ritz)*, ⅙ pkg. 50.0
  apricot or cherry *(Stilwell)*, ½ cup 54.0
  blackberry *(Pet-Ritz)*, ⅙ pkg. 39.0
  blackberry or strawberry *(Stilwell)*, ½ cup 53.0
  cherry or peach *(Pet-Ritz)*, ⅙ pkg. 46.0
  peach *(Stilwell)*, ½ cup 51.0
  pecan *(Stilwell)*, ½ cup 88.0
mix*, apple crumb *(Dromedary)*, ⅛ cake 41.0
mix*, cherry crumb *(Dromedary)*, ⅛ cake 42.0
Cocktail sauce:
(Bennett's), 1 tbsp. 4.0
(Sauceworks), 1 tbsp. 3.0
seafood:
  (Heinz), ¼ cup 13.0
  hot *(Bennett's)*, 1 tbsp. 7.0
  regular or extra hot *(Golden Dipt)*, 1 tbsp. 5.0
Cocoa powder:
(Bensdorp), 1 oz. 8.0
(Hershey's), 1 oz. 12.0

(Nestlé), 1 oz. 5.0
European *(Hershey's)*, 1 oz. 8.0
Cocoa mix:
(Swiss Miss Lite), 1 packet 17.0
all varieties *(Alba 66)*, .68 oz. 10.0
chocolate:
  all varieties *(Carnation)*, 1 packet 24.0
  Bavarian *(Swiss Miss)*, 1 packet 20.0
  double rich *(Swiss Miss)*, 1 packet 22.0
  milk *(Swiss Miss)*, 1 packet 24.0
  rich, plain or with marshmallow *(Nestlé)*, 1 packet 23.0
  with mini marshmallows *(Swiss Miss)*, 1 packet 23.0
Coconut, shelled:
fresh, 1 oz. 4.3
fresh, shredded or grated, 1 cup not packed 12.2
canned, sweetened, flaked, 1/3 cup 10.5
canned *(Baker's Angel Flake)*, 1/3 cup 10.0
dried, toasted, 1 oz. 12.6
packaged:
  sweetened, flaked, 1/2 cup 11.8
  (Baker's Angel Flake), 1/2 cup 10.0
  (Baker's Premium Shred), 1/2 cup 12.0
Coconut cream, canned, sweetened:
1 tbsp. 1.6
(Coco Lopez), 2 tbsp. 20.0
(Holland House), 2 fl. oz. 36.0
Coconut milk[1], 1 tbsp. 8
Coconut nectar *(R. W. Knudsen)*, 8 fl. oz. 29.0
Coconut water[2], 1 tbsp. 6
Coconut-pineapple nectar *(Kern's)*, 6 fl. oz. 26.0
Cod, without added ingredients 0
Cod, canned or dried, salted 0
Cod entree, frozen:
breaded *(Van de Kamp's Light)*, 1 piece 20.0
breaded *(Mrs. Paul's Light)*, 4.25 oz. 22.0

---

[1] *Liquid expressed from mixture of grated coconut and water.*
[2] *Liquid from coconuts.*

Cod entree, frozen *(cont.)*
lemon thyme *(Gorton's* Select), 1 piece...............................5.0
minced, nuggets, crunchy *(Frionor Bunch O'Crunch)*,
    8 nuggets, 4 oz. 19.0
Cod liver oil, regular or flavored...0
Coffee:
brewed, 6 fl. oz. 8
instant, regular, 1 rounded tsp.*..................................... .7
freeze-dried, all varieties *(Taster's Choice)*, 1 cup*.............. 1.0
Coffee, flavored* (see also "Cappuccino"):
café Amaretto *(General Foods* International), 6 fl. oz. 7.0
café Français *(General Foods* International), 6 fl. oz. 6.0
café Français *(Hills Bros.)*, 6 fl. oz................................... 8.0
café Vienna *(General Foods* International), 6 fl. oz. 10.0
café Vienna *(Hills Bros.)*, 6 fl. oz................................... 9.0
chocolate, double Dutch or Viennese *(General Foods*
    International), 6 fl. oz... 8.0
hazelnut, Belgian *(General Foods* International),
    6 fl. oz... 10.0
hazelnut, Belgian *(Hills Bros.)*, 6 fl. oz............................... 9.0
mocha, Suisse *(General Foods* International), 6 fl. oz. 7.0
mocha, Swiss *(Hills Bros.)*, 6 fl. oz..................................... 8.0
orange cappuccino *(General Foods* International),
    6 fl. oz... 10.0
vanilla, French *(General Foods* International), 6 fl. oz. 9.0
Coffee creamer, see "Cream" and "Creamer,
    nondairy"
Coffee flavored drink mix *(Carnation* Instant
    Breakfast), 1 packet 28.0
Coffee liqueur:
53 proof, 1 fl. oz. 16.3
with cream, 34 proof, 1 fl. oz. 6.5
Coffee substitute, cereal grain:
powder, 1 tsp... 1.9
(Kaffree Roma), 1 tsp.. 1.0
all varieties *(Postum* Instant), 6 fl. oz.*.................................. 3.0
Cold cuts, see specific listings

Collards:
fresh:
  raw, 1 oz.. 2.0
  raw, chopped, ½ cup... 1.3
  boiled, drained, chopped, ½ cup 3.9
canned *(Allens/Sunshine)*, ½ cup.................................. 2.0
frozen, chopped:
  boiled, drained, ½ cup.. 6.1
  (Seabrook), 3.3 oz. 4.0
  (Southern), 3.5 oz. 4.6
Cookie:
almond:
  (Frieda's), 1 piece... 8.0
  (Stella D'Oro Breakfast Treats), 1 piece 15.0
  (Stella D'Oro Chinese Dessert), 1 piece 19.0
  biscuit *(Almondina)*, 1 piece..................................... 5.5
  toast *(Stella D'Oro Mandel)*, 1 piece..................... 10.0
all varieties *(Barbara's Cookies & Creme)*, 1 oz.,
  2 pieces 18.0
animal cookies/crackers:
  (Sunshine), 13 pieces 21.0
  (Tom's), 2.5-oz. pkg.. 54.0
  candied *(Grandma's)*, 5 pieces 20.0
  vanilla *(Barbara's)*, 1 oz., 8 pieces 18.0
anise:
  (Stella D'Oro Anisette Sponge), 1 piece 10.0
  (Stella D'Oro Anisette Toast), 1 piece 9.0
  (Stella D'Oro Anisette Toast Jumbo), 1 piece......... 23.0
apple:
  bar *(Apple Newtons)*, 1 piece 15.0
  bar, Dutch *(Stella D'Oro)*, 1 piece.......................... 19.0
  bar, fat free *(Apple Newtons)*, 1 piece................... 16.0
  pastry *(Stella D'Oro Dietetic)*, 1 piece 13.0
apple filled *(Archway)*, 1 piece.................................... 20.0
apple filled *(Little Debbie Apple Delights)*, 1 piece............. 22.0
apple-oatmeal tart *(Pepperidge Farm Wholesome
  Choice)*, 1 piece 12.0
apple'n raisin *(Archway)*, 1 piece................................. 20.0

Cookie (cont.)

apple-raisin filled (Health Valley Fruit Centers),
  1 piece.. 16.0
apple or apricot filled (Health Valley Fruit Centers),
  1 piece.. 17.0
apricot filled (Archway), 1 piece 19.0
apricot-raspberry (Pepperidge Farm Fruit Cookies),
  2 pieces.. 15.0
apricot-raspberry (Pepperidge Farm Zurich), 1 piece........ 10.0
arrowroot biscuit (National), 1 piece.................................... 3.0
arrowroot biscuit (Peek Freans), 5 pieces 30.5
biscottini cashews (Stella D'Oro), 1 piece.......................... 13.5
blueberry filled (Archway), 1 piece 20.0
bourbon creme (Peek Freans), 3 pieces 28.9
bran crunch (Peek Freans), 4 pieces................................... 26.0
brownie chocolate nut (Pepperidge Farm), 2 pieces......... 11.0
butter flavor:
  (Peek Freans Petit Beurre), 6 pieces 32.0
  (Pepperidge Farm Chessmen), 1 piece 6.0
  fudge creme filled (Keebler E.L. Fudge), 1 piece 8.0
butter pecan (Dare), 1 piece.. 7.5
caramel, golden (Dare), 1 piece.. 9.0
caramel bar (Little Debbie), 1 piece 22.0
carob chip (Health Valley Healthy Chip), 1.17 oz. or
  3 pieces 18.0
carrot cake (Archway), 1 piece.. 19.0
carrot walnut (Pepperidge Farm Wholesome Choice),
  1 piece.. 11.0
(Carr's Hob Nobs), 1 piece.. 9.3
cherry filled (Archway), 1 piece 20.0
chocolate (see also "fudge," below):
  (Grandma's Grab), 8 pieces 19.0
  (Stella D'Oro Castelets), 1 piece....................................... 9.0
  (Stella D'Oro Margherite), 1 piece..................................... 10.0
  dark (Peek Freans), 3 pieces... 25.8
  fudge (Dare), 1 piece... 13.0
  milk (Peek Freans), 3 pieces 26.3

milk, fudge *(Dare)*, 1 piece 13.0
snaps *(Nabisco)*, 4 pieces 10.0
chocolate chip or chunk:
  (Almost Home Real), 1 piece 7.0
  (Archway Mini), 12 pieces 20.0
  (Archway Super Pak), 1 piece....................................... 20.0
  (Barbara's), 1 oz. 16.0
  (Chips Ahoy!), 1 piece 7.0
  (Chips Ahoy! Rockers), 1 piece.................................... 8.0
  (Dare), 1 piece 9.7
  (Dare Breaktime), 1 piece... 5.0
  (Drake's), 2 pieces 18.0
  (Famous Amos), 3 pieces.. 20.0
  (Grandma's), 2 pieces 50.0
  (Grandma's Rich'N Chewy), 3 pieces 20.0
  (Hostess), 5 pieces 33.0
  (Keebler Chips Deluxe), 1 piece.................................. 10.0
  (Keebler Chips Deluxe Bakery Crisp), 1 piece.................. 7.0
  (Master Choice), 1 piece 10.0
  (Mini Chips Ahoy!), 6 pieces 9.0
  (Pepperidge Farm Family Request), 2 pieces.................... 15.0
  (Pepperidge Farm Old Fashioned), 2 pieces.................... 12.0
  (SnackWell's), 6 pieces.. 11.0
  (Tom's), 2.25-oz. pkg.. 43.0
  bar *(Tastykake)*, 1 piece 28.0
  chewy *(Chips Ahoy!)*, 1 piece....................................... 8.0
  chocolate *(Barbara's)*, 1 oz. 17.0
  chocolate *(Drake's)*, 2 pieces 19.0
  pecan *(Keebler Pecan Chips Deluxe)*, 1 piece 8.0
  toffee *(Pepperidge Farm)*, 2 pieces................................ 12.0
  chocolate walnut *(Pepperidge Farm* Beacon Hill),
    1 piece 14.0
  chocolate walnut *(Pepperidge Farm* Soft Baked),
    1 piece 17.0
  chunk *(Pepperidge Farm* Nantucket), 1 piece.................. 15.0
  chunk *(Pepperidge Farm* Soft Baked), 1 piece 17.0
  chunk, macadamia *(Tastykake)*, 1 piece 42.0
  chunk, pecan *(Chips Ahoy!)*, 1 piece................................ 10.0

Cookie, chocolate chip or chunk *(cont.)*
   chunk, pecan *(Pepperidge Farm Chesapeake)*,
     1 piece 14.0
   chunky *(Chips Ahoy!)*, 1 piece 11.0
   coconut *(Keebler Chocolate Drop)*, 1 piece 10.0
   drop *(Archway)*, 1 piece 16.0
   Dutch, crunch or mint *(Master Choice Patisserie)*,
     1 piece 10.0
   fudge *(Almost Home)*, 1 piece 9.0
   fudge *(Grandma's)*, 2 pieces 54.0
   fudge, white, chunk *(Chips Ahoy!)*, 1 piece 5.0
   Heath toffee chunk *(Chips Ahoy!)*, 1 piece 10.0
   milk *(Dare Jersey Milk Chip)*, 1 piece 8.0
   milk, macadamia *(Pepperidge Farm Sausalito)*,
     1 piece 14.0
   milk, macadamia *(Pepperidge Farm Soft Baked)*,
     1 piece 16.0
   milk or regular *(Duncan Hines)*, 2 pieces 15.0
   pecan *(Famous Amos)*, 3 pieces 18.0
   snaps *(Nabisco)*, 3 pieces 11.0
   sprinkled *(Chips Ahoy!)*, 1 piece 8.0
   striped *(Chips Ahoy!)*, 1 piece 10.0
   toffee *(Archway)*, 1 piece 19.0
  chocolate sandwich:
   (Famous Amos), 3 pieces 21.0
   (Little Debbie), 1 piece 35.0
   (Mini Oreo), 5 pieces 10.0
   (Oreo), 1 piece 8.0
   (Oreo Double Stuf), 1 piece 9.0
   creme *(Tom's)*, 1.6-oz. pkg. 32.0
   fudge covered *(Oreo)*, 1 piece 13.0
   peanut butter creme *(Dunkaroos)*, 1 tray 15.0
   vanilla creme filled *(Keebler E.L. Fudge)*, 1 piece 8.0
   white fudge covered *(Oreo)*, 1 piece 14.0
  chocolate filled sandwich:
   (Nabisco Pure Chocolate Middles), 1 piece 9.0
   (Pepperidge Farm Brussels), 2 pieces 13.0

(Pepperidge Farm Lido), 1 piece 10.0
(Pepperidge Farm Milano), 2 pieces 15.0
mint *(Pepperidge Farm* Brussels Mint), 2 pieces 17.0
mint or orange *(Pepperidge Farm* Milano), 2 pieces...... 17.0
chocolate peanut bar *(Ideal)*, 1 piece................................. 10.0
cinnamon:
   crisp *(Tom's)*, 2.5-oz. pkg...................................... 49.0
   snap *(Archway)*, 6 pieces 20.0
   sugar *(Pepperidge Farm* Family Request), 2 pieces 12.0
cocoa, Dutch *(Archway)*, 1 piece.................................... 19.0
coconut:
   (Dare Breaktime), 1 piece..................................... 5.0
   (Drake's), 2 pieces 19.0
   (Stella D'Oro Dietetic), 1 piece............................... 6.0
   creme *(Dare)*, 1 piece 12.0
   macaroon *(Archway)*, 1 piece.................................. 19.0
   macaroon *(Drake's)*, 1 piece 17.0
   macaroon *(Stella D'Oro)*, 1 piece.............................. 7.0
coffee creme *(Peek Freans)*, 3 pieces 26.8
cranberry honey *(Pepperidge Farm* Wholesome
   Choice), 1 piece 11.0
creme sandwich, see specific listings
Danish *(Imported Danish Cookies)*, 2 pieces 9.0
(Dare Harvest from the Rain Forest), 1 piece 8.0
date filled *(Health Valley Fruit Centers)*, 1 piece 16.0
date walnut *(Pepperidge Farm* Wholesome Choice),
   1 piece.. 10.0
devil's food cakes *(Nabisco)*, 1 piece 15.0
devil's food cakes *(SnackWell's)*, 1 piece 12.0
egg biscuit:
   (Stella D'Oro Dietetic), 1 piece.............................. 6.5
   (Stella D'Oro Jumbo), 1 piece................................. 9.0
   Roman *(Stella D'Oro)*, 1 piece 20.0
   sugared *(Stella D'Oro)*, 1 piece............................... 14.0
fig bar:
   (Drake's), 1 piece.. 50.0
   (Fig Newtons), 1 piece 11.0

Cookie, fig bar *(cont.)*
   (Fig Newtons Fat Free), 1 piece................................... 15.0
   (Little Debbie Figaroo), 1.5 oz............................... 31.0
   (Tom's), 2-oz. pkg.. 43.0
  fortune *(La Choy),* 1 piece 4.0
  French creme *(Dare),* 1 piece 8.4
  fruit (see also specific fruits):
   all varieties *(Health Valley* Fat Free Jumbo Fruit
    Cookies), 1 piece... 17.0
   chunks, all varieties *(Health Valley* Fat Free),
    3 pieces... 19.0
   creme *(Peek Freans),* 3 pieces............................. 27.6
   filled, all varieties *(Baker's Own),* 1 piece 12.0
   filled, all varieties *(Health Valley Mini Fruit Centers*
    Fat Free), 3 pieces.. 17.0
   slices *(Stella D'Oro),* 1 piece.............................. 9.0
   tropical, filled *(Health Valley Fruit Centers),* 1 piece 17.0
  fruit cake *(Archway),* 3 pieces 20.0
  fruit and honey bar *(Archway),* 1 piece 18.0
  fruit and nut *(Barbara's),* 1 oz................................ 18.0
  fudge (see also "chocolate," above):
   (Stella D'Oro Swiss), 1 piece 9.0
   bar *(Tastykake),* 1 piece....................................... 35.0
   bar, with caramel and peanut *(Heyday),* 1 piece............ 13.0
   deep night *(Stella D'Oro),* 1 piece...................... 8.0
   fudge creme filled *(Keebler E.L. Fudge),* 1 piece 7.0
   mint *(Keebler Grasshopper),* 2 pieces 10.0
   nut *(Tom's),* 2.25-oz. pkg. 39.0
   nut bar *(Archway),* 1 piece.................................... 17.0
   wafer *(Nabisco Famous Wafers),* ½ oz.................. 11.0
  garden creme *(Peek Freans),* 3 pieces................. 26.9
  ginger:
   (Little Debbie), 1 piece 14.0
   (Pepperidge Farm Gingerman), 2 pieces.......................... 10.0
   crisp *(Peek Freans),* 5 pieces.............................. 31.7
  gingersnaps:
   (Archway), 6 pieces 23.0
   (Nabisco Old Fashioned), 2 pieces...................... 11.0

(Sunshine), 5 pieces 16.0
golden bar *(Stella D'Oro)*, 1 piece 16.0
graham cracker:
  (Carr's Home Wheat), 1 piece 10.0
  (Nabisco), 2 pieces 11.0
  (Regal), 2 pieces 19.0
  carob chip, ginger or orange *(Mitchelhill)*, 1 piece 8.0
  chocolate, see "graham cracker, chocolate,"
    below
  cinnamon *(SnackWell's)*, 9 pieces 12.0
  cinnamon *(Snoopy's)*, 11 pieces 11.0
  cinnamon *(Sunshine)*, 4 scored sections 11.0
  cinnamon *(Honey Maid)*, 2 pieces 12.0
  cinnamon *(Teddy Grahams)*, 11 pieces 11.0
  honey *(Grahamy Bears)*, 9 pieces 21.0
  honey *(Honey Maid)*, 2 pieces 11.0
  honey *(Mitchelhill)*, 1 piece 9.0
  honey *(Snoopy's)*, 11 pieces 11.0
  honey *(Sunshine)*, 4 scored sections 10.0
  honey or vanilla *(Teddy Grahams)*, 11 pieces 11.0
  muesli *(Mitchelhill)*, 1 piece 9.0
  vanilla frosted *(Dunkaroos)*, 1 tray 21.0
  wheat *(Carr's* Home Graham), 1 piece 10.9
  wholemeal *(Mitchelhill)*, 1 piece 8.0
graham cracker, chocolate:
  (Nabisco), 1 piece 7.0
  (Teddy Grahams), 11 pieces 10.0
  (Snoopy's), 11 pieces 10.0
  dark *(Carr's* Home Wheat), 1 piece 8.2
  milk *(Carr's* Home Wheat), 1 piece 8.3
  frosted *(Dunkaroos)*, 1 tray 19.0
  with fudge *(Cookies'N Fudge)*, 1 piece 6.0
  fudge covered *(Keebler* Deluxe), 2 pieces 12.0
hazelnut *(Pepperidge Farm)*, 2 pieces 15.0
hazelnut crunch *(Master Choice)*, 1 piece 9.0
heart *(Little Debbie)*, 1 piece 12.0
kichel *(Stella D'Oro* Dietetic), 1 piece 7

Cookie *(cont.)*
lemon:
  butter finger *(Master Choice)*, 1 piece 7.0
  creme *(Dare)*, 1 piece 13.0
  creme sandwich *(Tom's)*, 1 pkg. 32.0
  frosty *(Archway)*, 1 piece 19.0
  nut crunch *(Pepperidge Farm)*, 2 pieces 13.0
  snaps *(Archway)*, 6 pieces 19.0
maple leaf creme *(Dare)*, 1 piece 15.0
maple walnut fudge *(Dare)*, 1 piece 12.0
marshmallow cake:
  (Mallomars), 1 piece 9.0
  (Nabisco Puffs), 1 piece 14.0
  (Nabisco Twirls), 1 piece 20.0
  (Pinwheels), 1 piece 20.0
  all flavors *(Dare Belmont Mallow)*, 1 piece 11.0
mint *(Dare Midnight Mint)*, 1 piece 9.0
mint *(Mystic Mint)*, 1 piece 11.0
molasses:
  (Archway/Archway Old Fashioned), 1 piece 20.0
  (Grandma's Old Time), 2 pieces 58.0
  crisps *(Pepperidge Farm)*, 2 pieces 8.0
  iced *(Archway)*, 1 piece 19.0
New Orleans cake *(Archway)*, 1 piece 18.0
nougat, nutty *(Archway)*, 3 pieces 18.0
oat bran raisin *(Awrey's)*, 1 piece 14.0
oatmeal:
  (Archway), 1 piece 20.0
  (Archway Mini), 12 pieces 19.0
  (Baker's Bonus), 1 piece 12.0
  (Dare Breaktime), 1 piece 5.0
  (Drake's), 2 pieces 19.0
  (Peek Freans Traditional), 4 pieces 30.3
  (Pepperidge Farm Family Request), 2 pieces 13.0
  (Sunshine), 2 pieces 16.0
  apple spice *(Grandma's)*, 2 pieces 51.0

chocolate *(Pepperidge Farm* Dakota), 1 piece 15.0
creme *(Drake's)*, 1 piece 38.0
creme cakes *(Tom's)*, 1.8-oz. pkg. 33.0
date filled *(Archway)*, 1 piece 19.0
golden *(Archway Ruth's)*, 1 piece 19.0
iced *(Archway)*, 1 piece 19.0
Irish *(Pepperidge Farm)*, 2 pieces 13.0
oatmeal raisin:
  (Almost Home), 1 piece 10.0
  (Archway), 1 piece 19.0
  (Barbara's), 1 oz. 19.0
  (Dare), 1 piece 7.9
  (Duncan Hines), 2 pieces 15.0
  (Pepperidge Farm Old Fashioned), 2 pieces 15.0
  (Pepperidge Farm Santa Fe), 1 piece 16.0
  (Pepperidge Farm Wholesome Choice), 1 piece 11.0
  (SnackWell's), 1 piece 10.0
  bar *(Tastykake)*, 1 piece 32.0
  bran *(Archway)*, 1 piece 19.0
  regular or chocolate coated raisins *(Keebler Raisin*
    Ruckus), 1 piece 10.0
  cinnamon *(Famous Amos)*, 3 pieces 19.0
orange:
  butter fingers *(Master Choice)*, 1 piece 7.0
  frosty *(Archway)*, 1 piece 19.0
  chocolate tea *(Peek Freans)*, 5 pieces 28.0
peach-apricot pastry *(Stella D'Oro)*, 1 piece 13.0
peanut butter:
  (Archway), 1 piece 16.0
  (Dare Peanut Butter Delites), 1 piece 8.0
  (Grandma's), 2 pieces 43.0
  (Grandma's Grab), 8 pieces 19.0
  (Pepperidge Farm Family Request), 2 pieces 10.0
  bar *(Frito-Lay's)*, 1.75 oz. 30.0
  'n chips *(Archway)*, 1 piece 16.0
  chip *(Dare)*, 1 piece 7.3
  chocolate chip *(Pepperidge Farm* Cheyenne),
    1 piece 13.0

Cookie, peanut butter *(cont.)*
    nougat *(Archway)*, 3 pieces.................................. 18.0
    sandwich *(Nutter Butter)*, 1 piece 9.0
    sandwich *(Nutter Butter Bites)*, ½ oz. 9.0
    wafer *(Drake's)*, 1 piece.................................... 43.0
peanut creme patties *(Nutter Butter)*, 2 pieces.................... 8.0
pecan:
    (Pecan Supremes), 1 piece................................ 9.0
    crunch *(Archway)*, 1 piece................................. 17.0
    ice box *(Archway)*, 1 piece................................ 18.0
    nougat, malted *(Archway)*, 3 pieces 17.0
pineapple filled *(Archway)*, 1 piece............................... 16.0
prune pastry *(Stella D'Oro* Dietetic), 1 piece.................. 13.0
raisin:
    bran *(Pepperidge Farm)*, 2 piece 13.0
    oatmeal *(Archway)*, 1 piece................................ 19.0
    oatmeal *(Dare Sun-Maid* Raisin Oatmeal), 1 piece 7.5
    soft *(Grandma's)*, 2 pieces.................................. 54.0
raspberry filled:
    (Archway), 1 piece.. 18.0
    (Health Valley Fruit Centers), 1 piece................. 17.0
    (Health Valley Fruit Centers 2-pack), 1 piece 19.0
    (Pepperidge Farm Liner), 1 piece...................... 20.0
    (Raspberry Newtons), 1 piece............................ 15.0
    regular or chocolate *(Pepperidge Farm* Chantilly),
      1 piece 14.0
raspberry tart *(Pepperidge Farm* Wholesome
  Choice), 1 piece 11.0
rocky road *(Archway)*, 1 piece.................................... 18.0
sesame *(Stella D'Oro Regina)*, 1 piece..................... 6.0
shortbread:
(Lorna Doone), 2 pieces... 9.0
(Pepperidge Farm), 2 pieces..................................... 17.0
butter *(Dare)*, 1 piece 7.0
with chocolate drop *(Keebler Sweet Spots)*, 2 pieces 8.0
fudge covered, with toffee *(Keebler Toffee Toppers)*,
  2 pieces 10.0
fudge striped *(Keebler)*, 1 piece 7.0

fudge striped *(Cookies'N Fudge)*, 1 piece.................... 7.0
fudge-caramel covered *(Keebler Fudge'n Caramel)*,
  1 piece.. 8.0
pecan *(Pepperidge Farm)*, 1 piece 7.0
toffee chip *(Keebler Toffee Sandies)*, 1 piece 8.0
shortcake *(Peek Freans)*, 3 pieces 26.3
spice drops *(Stella D'Oro Pfeffernusse)*, 1 piece 7.0
(Stella D'Oro Angel Bars/Wings), 1 piece............................ 7.0
(Stella D'Oro Angelica Goodies), 1 piece 16.0
(Stella D'Oro Como Delights), 1 piece 18.0
(Stella D'Oro Love Cookies), 1 piece................................ 13.0
strawberry:
  (Pepperidge Farm Fruit Cookies), 2 pieces 15.0
  bar *(Strawberry Newtons)*, 1 piece 15.0
  filled *(Archway)*, 1 piece 18.0
sugar:
  (Almost Home Old Fashioned), 1 piece...................... 10.0
  (Archway)... 19.0
  (Dare), 1 piece 6.0
  (Pepperidge Farm), 2 pieces....................................... 13.0
  drop, soft *(Archway)*, 1 piece....................................... 18.0
  wafer *(Biscos)*, 4 pieces 10.0
  wafer, vanilla *(Tastykake)*, 1 piece................................ 4.0
sweetmeal *(Peek Freans)*, 4 pieces 27.7
tea biscuit:
  (Dare Social Tea), 1 piece 4.1
  (Social Tea), 3 pieces 11.0
  rich *(Peek Freans)*, 4 pieces....................................... 29.6
vanilla:
  (Grandma's Grab), 8 pieces 20.0
  (Pepperidge Farm Bordeaux), 2 pieces 11.0
  (Stella D'Oro Castelets), 1 piece 10.0
  (Stella D'Oro Margherite), 1 piece............................... 11.0
  chocolate laced *(Pepperidge Farm Pirouettes)*,
    2 pieces.. 8.0
  chocolate nut coated *(Pepperidge Farm Geneva)*,
    2 pieces.. 14.0
  creme sandwich *(Cameo)*, 1 piece 10.0

Cookie, vanilla *(cont.)*

creme sandwich *(Tom's)*, 1.6-oz. pkg. 32.0

creme sandwich, French *(Peek Freans)*, 3 pieces 24.9

wafer *(Nilla Wafers)*, ½ oz. 11.0

wafer *(Tom's)*, 2.5-oz. pkg. 52.0

wafer (see also specific cookie listings):

brown edge *(Nabisco)*, ½ oz. 10.0

creme, fudge covered *(Keebler Fudge Sticks)*,
2 pieces 13.0

fudge striped *(Cookies'N Fudge)*, 1 piece 8.0

waffle cremes *(Biscos)*, 1 piece 6.0

wedding cake *(Archway)*, 3 pieces 20.0

wheat *(Carr's Wheatolo)*, 1 piece 10.0

wheatmeal, large *(Carr's)*, 1 piece 9.0

wheatmeal, small *(Carr's)*, 1 piece 5.5

windmill *(Archway Old Fashioned)*, 1 piece 20.0

Cookie, frozen:

chocolate chip, double *(Nestlé Toll House Ready To
Bake)*, 1.2 oz. 20.0

chocolate chip, with nuts *(Nestlé Toll House Ready
To Bake)*, 1.2 oz. 19.0

oatmeal raisin *(Nestlé Toll House Ready To Bake)*,
1.2 oz. 19.0

Cookie, mix, see "Dessert bar mix"

Cookie crumbs, see "Pie crust"

Cookie dough, refrigerated*:

candy *(Pillsbury Oven Lovin')*, 1 piece 10.0

chocolate chip:

(Pillsbury Oven Lovin'), 1 piece 9.0

(Pillsbury's Best), 1 piece 9.0

chocolate *(Pillsbury's Best)*, 1 piece 9.0

oatmeal raisin *(Pillsbury's Best)*, 1 piece 10.0

peanut butter *(Pillsbury's Best)*, 1 piece 9.0

Reese's Pieces (Pillsbury Oven Lovin'), 1 piece 9.0

sugar *(Pillsbury's Best)*, 1 piece 9.0

Coquito nut, shelled *(Frieda's)*, 1 oz. 5.0

Coriander:
fresh, ¼ cup... .1
dried, leaf, 1 tsp.. .3
seeds, 1 tsp. 1.0

Corn:
fresh, kernels, boiled, drained, ½ cup 20.6
canned, kernels:
   drained, ½ cup.. 15.2
   (Comstock), ½ cup 21.0
   (Green Giant Delicorn) 19.0
   (Green Giant Niblets), ½ cup 20.0
   (Green Giant Niblets No Salt No Sugar), ½ cup 18.0
   (Green Giant Sweet Select), ½ cup............................. 15.0
   golden *(Stokely)*, ½ cup 16.0
   golden, sweet *(Green Giant)*, ½ cup 18.0
   golden, sweet *(Green Giant 50% Less Salt)*,
     ½ cup.. 16.0
   white *(Green Giant)*, ½ cup....................................... 20.0
   with peppers *(Green Giant Mexicorn)*, ½ cup 18.0
   cream-style *(Green Giant)*, ½ cup 24.0
   cream-style *(Stokely)*, ½ cup 23.0
freeze-dried* *(Mountain House)*, ½ cup 18.0
frozen, on cob:
   (Green Giant Nibblers), 2 ears 27.0
   (Green Giant Nibblers One Serving), 2 half ears 26.0
   (Green Giant Niblet Ears), 1 ear 27.0
   (Green Giant Sweet Select), 1 ear 19.0
   (Green Giant Sweet Select Half Ears), 2 ears 19.0
   (Ore-Ida), 1 ear 40.0
   miniature *(Ore-Ida Mini-Gold)*, 1 ear 20.0
frozen, kernels:
   (Green Giant Harvest Fresh Niblets), ½ cup 17.0
   (Green Giant Niblets), ½ cup 19.0
   (Green Giant Sweet Select), ½ cup............................. 13.0
   cream-style *(Green Giant)*, ½ cup 25.0
   cut *(Frosty Acres)*, 3.3 oz....................................... 20.0
   white *(Seabrook)*, 3.3 oz.. 19.0
   white shoepeg *(Green Giant Harvest Fresh)*, ½ cup...... 19.0

Corn, frozen, kernels *(cont.)*
   white shoepeg *(Green Giant* Select), ½ cup 19.0
   in butter sauce *(Green Giant Niblets),* ½ cup 19.0
   in butter sauce *(Green Giant Niblets* One Serving),
     4.5 oz. 23.0
   in butter sauce, white shoepeg *(Green Giant),*
     ½ cup... 20.0
Corn, whole-grain:
1 oz. 21.1
1 cup 123.3
blue *(Arrowhead Mills),* 2 oz. 41.0
yellow *(Arrowhead Mills),* 2 oz. 43.0
Corn bran, crude:
1 oz. 24.3
1 cup 65.1
Corn chips and similar snacks:
(Barbara's Blue Corn/Pinta Chips/Potillas), 1 oz. 18.0
(Bugles), 1 oz. 18.0
(Fritos Original/Dip Size/*Fritos Crisp'N Thin),* 1 oz. 16.0
(Santitas Cantina Style/Chips/Strips), 1 oz. 19.0
(Tom's), 1¾-oz. pkg. 29.0
barbecue flavor *(Fritos Rowdy Rustlers Bar-B-Q),*
   1 oz. 17.0
barbecue flavor *(Tom's),* 1⅝-oz. pkg. 26.0
caramel corn puffs, apple cinnamon or peanut flavor
   (Health Valley), 1 oz. 21.0
cheese:
   (Cheddar Valley), 1 oz. 16.0
   (Chee•tos Balls/Puffs), 1 oz. 16.0
   (Chee•tos Crunchy/Curls), 1 oz. 17.0
   (Chee•tos Light), 1 oz. 19.0
   (Chee•tos Paws), 1 oz. 15.0
   (Health Valley Cheese Puffs), 1 oz. 21.0
   (Tom's Cheese Crunchies), 1 oz. 23.0
   (Tom's Cheese Puffs), ⅞-oz. pkg. 20.0
   chili, zesty or green onion *(Health Valley* Cheese
     Puffs), 1 oz. 21.0
   hot *(Flamin' Hot),* 1 oz. 16.0

nacho *(Bugles)*, 1 oz.. 17.0
nacho *(Fritos* Non-Stop), 1 oz.. 16.0
nacho, rings *(Tom's)*, ⅞ oz.. 10.0
puffs *(No Fries)*, 1 oz... 22.0
chili cheese *(Fritos)*, 1 oz. 15.0
fajita flavor *(Santitas* Cantina Style), 1 oz.................... 18.0
nuggets, toasted *(Frito-Lay's)*, 1.38 oz......................... 29.0
ranch:
    (Bugles), 1 oz.. 16.0
    (Fritos Wild'N Mild), 1 oz...................................... 16.0
    (No Fries Ranch-O's), 1 oz.................................... 22.0
roasted, fresh *(Pringles)*, 1 oz. 17.0
tortilla, see "Tortilla chips"
Corn combinations, packaged:
with carrots *(Del Monte Vegetable Classics)*, ½ cup 12.0
with green beans, carrots, and pasta *(Green Giant
    Pantry Express)*, ½ cup..................................... 17.0
Corn flake crumbs *(Kellogg's)*, 1 oz. 24.0
Corn flour:
whole-grain, 1 oz. 21.8
whole-grain, 1 cup 89.9
masa, 1 oz. 21.6
masa, 1 cup 87.0
Corn fritter, frozen *(Mrs. Paul's)*, 4 oz.......................... 35.0
Corn grits:
dry:
    instant *(Quaker* Original), 1 oz............................... 22.0
    instant, quick, dry *(Albers* Hominy), ¼ cup............... 33.0
    white *(Arrowhead Mills)*, 2 oz................................. 43.0
    yellow *(Arrowhead Mills)*, 2 oz. 44.0
cooked, 1 cup 31.4
Corn soufflé, frozen *(Stouffer's)*, 6 oz. 27.0
Corn syrup, dark or light *(Karo)*, 1 tbsp. 15.0
Cornbread, see "Bread, sweet, mix"
Cornish game hen, without added ingredients..................... 0
Cornish game hen, roasted, refrigerated:
dark or white meat *(Perdue)*, 1 oz.. 0

Cornish game hen, roasted *(cont.)*
dark or white meat *(Perdue Done It!)*, 1 oz.........................,..... <1.0
Cornish game hen, frozen:
with skin *(Tyson)*, 3.5 oz. 1.0
Cornmeal (see also "Corn flour" and "Polenta"):
blue *(Arrowhead Mills)*, 2 oz. 41.0
white or yellow *(Albers)*, 1 oz. 22.0
white or yellow *(Quaker)*, 1 oz. 22.0
yellow or hi-lysine *(Arrowhead Mills)*, 2 oz...................... 43.0
Cornmeal mix, white *(Aunt Jemima)*, 1 oz......................... 18.0
Cornstarch *(Argo/Kingsford)*, 1 tbsp. 7.0
Cottonseed kernels, roasted, 1 tbsp................................. 2.2
Cottonseed meal, partially defatted, 1 oz. 10.9
Cough drop, see "Candy"
Country coating mix, mild *(Shake'n Bake)*, ¼ pouch 10.0
Country gravy mix*:
regular or sausage *(McCormick/Schilling)*, ¼ cup 5.0
vegetarian *(LaLoma Gravy Quik)*, 2 tbsp. 2.0
Couscous:
dry, 1 oz. 22.0
cooked, ½ cup.. 20.9
Couscous mix*:
(Fantastic Foods), ½ cup.. 21.0
almond chicken *(Casbah Couscous Cup)*, 6 oz................ 22.0
asparagus au gratin *(Casbah Couscous Cup)*, 6 oz. 21.0
cheddar broccoli *(Casbah Couscous Cup)*, 6 oz. 22.0
lentil curry *(Marakesh Express)*, ½ cup 25.0
mushroom tofu *(Casbah Couscous Cup)*, 6 oz................... 24.0
pilaf, savory *(Quick Pilaf)*, ½ cup... 24.0
pilaf, spicy, raisins and almonds *(Knorr Pilafs)*,
   1 serving... 29.4
shrimp paella *(Casbah Couscous Cup)*, 6 oz..................... 21.0
tomato Parmesan *(Casbah Couscous Cup)*, 6 oz.............. 22.0
whole wheat *(Fantastic Foods)*, ½ cup 21.0
Cowpeas:
fresh:
   raw, trimmed, ½ cup.. 13.6
   boiled, drained, ½ cup.. 16.7

leafy tips, raw, chopped, ½ cup...9
leafy tips, boiled, drained, 4 oz. 3.2
pods, with seeds, raw, trimmed, ½ cup 4.5
pods, with seeds, boiled, drained, ½ cup....................... 3.3
canned:
  (Allens/East Texas Fair), ½ cup................................. 18.0
  with jalapeños *(Home-Folks)*, ½ cup 10.0
  with snaps *(Allens/East Texas Fair)*, ½ cup 20.0
frozen, boiled, drained, ½ cup 20.2
frozen *(Frosty Acres)*, 3.3 oz.. 23.0
Cowpeas, mature:
dry, boiled, ½ cup 17.9
canned, ½ cup:
  with liquid, ½ cup 16.4
  (Allens/East Texas Fair), ½ cup................................. 20.0
  (Green Giant/Joan of Arc), ½ cup 18.0
  with bacon *(Allens/Sunshine)*, ½ cup 18.0
  with pork, ½ cup.. 19.8
Cowpeas, catjang, see "Catjang"
Crab, meat only:
Alaska king, raw, 4 oz. 7
Alaska king, boiled, poached, or steamed, 4 oz. 0
blue, raw, 4 oz. 1
blue, boiled, poached, or steamed, 4 oz. 0
dungeness, raw, 4 oz. 8
dungeness, boiled, poached, or steamed, 4 oz. 1.1
queen, raw, or boiled, 4 oz. 0
Crab, canned, blue, 4 oz... 0
"Crab," imitation:
made from surimi, 1 oz.. 3.0
(Louis Kemp Crab De-Lights), 2 oz. 5.0
Crab cake, deviled, frozen:
(Mrs. Paul's), 3 oz. 18.0
miniature *(Mrs. Paul's)*, 3.5 oz. 25.0
Crab cake seasoning mix *(Old Bay Crab Cake*
  Classic), 1 pkg.. 18.0
Crabapple:
fresh, unpeeled, 1 oz.. 5.7

Crabapple *(cont.)*
fresh, unpeeled, sliced, ½ cup 11.0
fresh *(Frieda's)*, 1 oz. 5.0
Cracker:
all varieties *(Barbara's Wheatines)*, ½ oz. 9.0
all varieties *(McCrakens Cracker Crisp)*, 1 oz. 18.0
all varieties, except pretzel *(Pepperidge Farm
   Goldfish)*, ½ oz. 9.0
animal crackers, see "Cookies"
bacon flavor *(Nabisco)*, ½ oz. 9.0
with bacon and cheese *(Handi-Snacks)*, 1 pkg. 8.0
butter flavor:
   (Carr's Butterpuff), 1 piece 6.3
   (Escort), 3 pieces 9.0
   (Keebler Club/Keebler Club Low Salt), 4 pieces 9.0
   (Keebler Toasteds Complements), 4 pieces 8.0
   *(Keebler Town House/Keebler Town House Low
      Salt)*, 4 pieces 8.0
   (Ritz/Ritz Bits), ½ oz. 9.0
   dairy *(American Classic)*, 4 pieces 9.0
   thins *(Pepperidge Farm)*, 4 pieces 10.0
cheddar:
   (Carr's), 1 piece 1.9
   (Cheddar Wedges), ½ oz. 9.0
   (Combos), 1.8 oz. 34.0
   (Frito-Lay Cracker Snacks), ½ oz. 8.0
   (Munch'ems), ½ oz. 9.0
   (Snorkels), ½ oz. 9.0
   thins *(Better Cheddars/Better Cheddars Low Salt)*,
      ½ oz. 8.0
cheese:
   (Cheese Nips), ½ oz. 9.0
   (Cheez-it/Cheez-it Low Salt), ½ oz., 12 pieces 7.0
   (Hain), ½ oz., 6 pieces 9.0
   (Nips), ½ oz. 9.0
   (Ritz Bits), ½ oz. 8.0
   (SnackWell's), ½ oz. 11.0

(Tid Bits), ½ oz. 8.0
nacho *(Doritos Nacho Cheese)*, 1 oz. 18.0
nacho *(Munch'ems)*, ½ oz. 8.0
Swiss *(Nabisco Swiss Cheese)*, ½ oz. 9.0
three *(Pepperidge Farm Snack Sticks)*, 8 pieces 19.0
cheese sandwich:
    (Tom's Cheese Crisp), 1¼ oz. 18.0
    (Tom's Cheezer), 1¼ oz. 21.0
    cheese filled *(Ritz Bits Real Cheese)*, ½ oz. 7.0
    cheese or peanut butter filled *(Frito-Lay's)*, 1.5 oz. 24.0
    nacho or pizza *(Ritz Bits)*, ½ oz. 8.0
    and peanut butter *(Handi-Snacks)*, 1 pkg. 11.0
    and peanut butter *(Tom's Eat-A-Snax)*, 1.4 oz. 22.0
    and cheese *(Handi-Snacks)*, 1 pkg. 9.0
(Chicken In A Biskit), ½ oz. 8.0
chips *(Zings! Original)*, ½ oz. 10.0
chips, cheddar or ranch *(Zings!)*, ½ oz. 9.0
club *(Red Oval Farms)*, 6 pieces 16.7
crispbread (see also specific cracker listings):
    (Wasa Breakfast), 1 piece 8.0
    (Wasa Extra Crisp/Fiber Plus), 1 piece 5.0
    cinnamon sugar wheat *(Pepperidge Farm)*, ½ oz. 11.0
    dark, regular, or with caraway *(Finn Crisp)*,
      2 pieces 9.0
    high fiber *(Ryvita Crisp Bread)*, 1 piece 4.0
    high fiber *(Ryvita Snackbread)*, 1 piece 3.0
croissant *(Carr's)*, 1 piece 3.2
(Dare Breton/Dare Breton 50% Less Salt), 1 piece 2.6
(Dare Cabaret), 1 piece 3.0
(Dare Vivant), 1 piece 2.8
flatbread:
    (J.J. Flats Flavorall), 1 piece 10.0
    all varieties, except poppy and sesame *(J.J. Flats)*,
      1 piece 11.0
    garlic *(New York)*, 1 piece 12.0
    poppy or sesame *(J.J. Flats)*, 1 piece 10.0
garlic *(Manischewitz Tams)*, 10 pieces 19.0
graham crackers, see "Cookies"

Cracker *(cont.)*

grain, mixed *(Harvest Crisps 5 Grain)*, ½ oz. 10.0
grain, multi *(Pepperidge Farm* Wholesome), 4 pieces 12.0
Italian, zesty *(Frito-Lay* Cracker Snacks), ½ oz. 9.0
(Manischewitz Tam Tams), 10 pieces 17.0
(Manischewitz Tam Tams No Salt), 10 pieces 18.0
matzo:
   (Manischewitz Daily Unsalted), 1 board 24.0
   (Manischewitz Miniatures), 10 pieces 20.0
   American *(Manischewitz)*, 1 board 22.0
   plain or egg *(Manischewitz* Passover), 1 board 27.0
   egg *(Manischewitz* Passover Crackers), 10 pieces 20.0
   egg'n onion *(Manischewitz)*, 1 board 23.0
   tea, thin *(Manischewitz)*, 1 board 22.0
   thin *(Manischewitz)*, 1 board 21.0
   thin, dietetic *(Manischewitz)*, 1 board 19.0
   whole wheat with bran *(Manischewitz)*, 1 board 21.0
melba toast:
   (Devonsheer Rounds), ½ oz. 11.0
   all varieties, except sesame *(Old London* Snacks),
     ½ oz. 9.0
   garlic *(Devonsheer* Rounds), ½ oz. 10.0
   honey bran *(Devonsheer* Rounds), ½ oz. 12.0
   oat bran or onion *(Devonsheer* Rounds), ½ oz. 11.0
   sesame *(Devonsheer* Rounds), ½ oz. 9.0
   sesame *(Old London* Snacks), ½ oz. 8.0
   sesame, plain or unsalted *(Old London* Toast),
     ½ oz. 9.0
   white, wheat, or whole grain *(Old London* Toast),
     ½ oz. 10.0
milk *(Royal Lunch)*, ½ oz. 10.0
oat *(Harvest Crisps)*, ½ oz. 10.0
oat *(Oat Thins)*, ½ oz. 10.0
oat bran *(Oat Bran Krisp)*, ½ oz. 9.0
onion *(Hain/Hain* No Salt Added), 6 pieces 9.0
onion *(Manischewitz Tams)*, 10 pieces 18.0
oyster, see "soup and oyster," below

peanut butter:
   (Combos), 1.8 oz. 30.0
   (Tom's Peanut Butter Malt), 1¼ oz. 20.0
   (Tom's Peanut Butter Squares), 1¾ oz. 31.0
   (Tom's Peanut Butter Toast), 1¼ oz. 19.0
   sandwich *(Little Debbie* Toasty), 4 pieces 15.0
   sandwich *(Ritz Bits)*, ½ oz. 8.0
pizza flavor *(Snorkels)*, ½ oz. 10.0
poppy, toasted *(American Classic)*, ½ oz. 9.0
poppy and sesame seed *(Carr's)*, 1 piece 2.1
pretzel *(Pepperidge Farm* Goldfish), ½ oz. 10.0
pretzel *(Pepperidge Farm* Snack Sticks), 8 pieces 23.0
pumpernickel *(Pepperidge Farm* Snack Sticks),
   8 pieces 20.0
ranch *(Munch'ems)*, ½ oz. 17.0
ranch *(Snorkels)*, ½ oz. 10.0
rich *(Hain/Hain* No Salt Added), 4 pieces 9.0
rye:
   (Hain/Hain No Salt Added), 6 pieces 10.0
   (Rykrisp), ½ oz. 11.0
   (Triscuit Deli Style), ½ oz. 10.0
   dark or light *(Ryvita* Crisp Bread), 1 piece 6.0
   light *(Wasa* Crispbread), 1 piece 5.0
   seasoned *(Rykrisp)*, ½ oz. 11.0
   sesame *(Rykrisp)*, ½ oz. 10.0
   sesame, toasted *(Ryvita* Crisp Bread), 1 piece 5.0
   stoned *(Red Oval Farms)*, 7 pieces...................... 18.0
saltine:
   (Premium/Premium Low Salt/Unsalted Tops),
   ½ oz. 10.0
   (Premium Bits), ½ oz. 9.0
   (Premium Fat Free), ½ oz. 12.0
   (Sunshine Krispy/Sunshine Crispy Unsalted Tops),
   ½ oz., 5 pieces... 11.0
   multi grain *(Premium)*, ½ oz. 10.0
sandwich, see specific cracker listings
seasoned *(Munch'ems* Original), ½ oz. 9.0

Cracker *(cont.)*
sesame:
  (Dare Breton), 1 piece 2.5
  (Hain/Hain No Salt Added), 6 pieces 9.0
  (Keebler Toasteds Complements), 4 pieces 8.0
  (Pepperidge Farm), 4 pieces 12.0
  (Pepperidge Farm Snack Sticks), 8 pieces 19.0
  golden *(American Classic)*, ½ oz. 9.0
  thins *(Sesmark Original)*, 4 pieces.................................... 8.0
sesame and cheese *(Twigs Snack Sticks)*, ½ oz................ 8.0
sesame and onion *(Red Oval Farms)*, 6 pieces 16.7
soda or water:
  (Carr's Table Water, Bite Size), 1 piece 2.7
  (Carr's Table Water, King Size), 1 piece 5.9
  (Carr's Table Water Oblong), 1 piece 3.1
  (Crown Pilot), ½ oz. 11.0
  (Pepperidge Farm English Water Biscuit), 4 pieces 13.0
  with cracked pepper or sesame seeds *(Carr's*
    Table Water)*, 1 piece 2.6
soup and oyster:
  (Carr's Scalloped Round), 1 piece.................................... 2.5
  (Oysterettes), ½ oz. 10.0
  (Premium), ½ oz. 10.0
  (Sunshine), ½ oz., 16 pieces.. 11.0
sour cream and onion *(Munch'ems)*, ½ oz. 9.0
sourdough *(Hain/Hain Low Salt)*, 6 pieces........................ 9.0
toast *(Uneeda Biscuits Unsalted Tops)*, ½ oz.................... 10.0
vegetable:
  (Garden Crisps), ½ oz. 11.0
  (Hain/Hain No Salt Added), 6 pieces 9.0
  (Vegetable Thins), ½ oz... 8.0
  garden *(Pepperidge Farm Wholesome)*, 5 pieces 10.0
wheat:
  (Keebler Toasteds Complements), ½ oz., 4 pieces.......... 8.0
  (Manischewitz Tams), 10 pieces....................................... 18.0
  (Ryvita Original Snackbread), 1 piece 4.0
  (SnackWell's), ½ oz. 12.0

(Sociables), 1/2 oz. 9.0
(Sunshine Wheats), 8 pieces 9.0
(Triscuit/Triscuit Low Salt), 1/2 oz. 10.0
(Waverly/Waverly Low Salt), 1/2 oz. 10.0
(Wheat Thins/Wheat Thins Low Salt), 1/2 oz. 9.0
(Wheatsworth Stone Ground), 1/2 oz. 9.0
cracked *(Nabisco American Classic)*, 1/2 oz. 8.0
cracked *(Pepperidge Farm)*, 3 pieces 14.0
grain *(Carr's)*, 1 piece 6.1
hearty *(Pepperidge Farm)*, 4 pieces 13.0
multi-grain *(Wheat Thins)*, 1/2 oz. 10.0
nutty *(Wheat Thins)*, 1/2 oz. 9.0
thins, stoned *(Red Oval Farms)*, 7 pieces 18.0
thins, stoned *(Red Oval Farms* Low Salt), 7 pieces 18.4
toasted, with onion *(Pepperidge Farm)*, 4 pieces 12.0
wheat, whole:
  (Carr's Star), 1 piece 2.5
  (Carr's Wheatmeal), 1 piece 5.5
  (Keebler Club), 4 pieces 9.0
  (Keebler Town House), 4 pieces 8.0
  (Keebler Wheatables/Keebler Wheatables Low
    Salt), 1/2 oz. 8.0
  (Manischewitz), 10 pieces 18.0
  (Ritz), 1/2 oz. 10.0
wheat'n bran *(Triscuit)*, 1/2 oz. 10.0
wheat sandwich:
  cheese *(Tom's Wheat'N Cheese)*, 1.4 oz. 22.0
  cheese, cheddar *(Little Debbie)*, 4 pieces 17.0
  peanut butter *(Tom's Wheat'N Peanut Butter)*,
    1.4 oz. 22.0
zwieback toast *(Nabisco)*, 2 pieces 10.0
Cracker crumbs and meal:
(Golden Dipt), 1 oz. 22.0
matzo *(Manischewitz Farfel)*, 1 cup 60.0
matzo meal *(Manischewitz* Daily), 1 cup 109.0
meal *(Nabisco)*, 1/4 cup 23.0
saltine, fat free *(Premium)*, 2 tbsp. 11.0

Cranberry, fresh, raw:
whole, ½ cup 6.0
chopped, ½ cup 7.0
Cranberry beans:
boiled, ½ cup 21.5
canned, with liquid, ½ cup 19.7
Cranberry fruit concentrate (Hain), 2 tbsp. 12.0
Cranberry juice:
(R.W. Knudsen Just Cranberry), 8 fl. oz. 10.0
(Master Choice), 6 fl. oz. 25.0
(Smucker's Naturally 100%), 8 fl. oz. 30.0
cocktail, 6 fl. oz.:
   (Ocean Spray), 6 oz. 25.0
   (Sunkist), 6 oz. 28.2
   frozen* (Welch's), 6 oz. 26.0
   frozen* (Welch's No Sugar Added), 6 oz. 10.0
sparkling (Santa Cruz Natural), 8 fl. oz. 22.0
Cranberry juice drink, blend (Ocean Spray
   CranTastic), 6 fl. oz. 26.0
Cranberry nectar:
(R.W. Knudsen), 8 fl. oz. 28.0
(Santa Cruz Natural), 8 fl. oz. 28.0
Cranberry sauce, canned:
(R.W. Knudsen), 1 oz. 8.0
whole or jellied, ½ cup 53.7
whole (Ocean Spray), 2 oz. 21.0
jellied (Ocean Spray), 2 oz. 22.0
Cranberry sauce blends, for chicken:
with orange or raspberry (Ocean Spray Cran•Fruit),
   2 oz. 23.0
with strawberry (Ocean Spray Cran•Fruit), 2 oz. 22.0
Cranberry-apple drink (Ocean Spray CranApple),
   6 fl. oz. 31.0
Cranberry-apple juice cocktail:
canned (Minute Maid), 6 fl. oz. 30.0
frozen* (Welch's), 6 fl. oz. 30.0
Cranberry-apricot juice drink (Ocean Spray
   Cranicot), 6 fl. oz. 29.0

Cranberry-blueberry juice:
(Ocean Spray Cran•Blueberry), 6 fl. oz. 31.0
(R.W. Knudsen), 8 fl. oz. 36.0
cocktail, frozen* *(Welch's),* 6 fl. oz. 27.0
Cranberry-cherry juice cocktail, frozen* *(Welch's),*
   6 fl. oz. 28.0
Cranberry-grape drink *(Ocean Spray Cran•Grape),*
   6 fl. oz. 31.0
Cranberry-grape juice cocktail, frozen* *(Welch's),*
   6 fl. oz. 27.0
Cranberry-orange juice cocktail, frozen* *(Welch's),*
   6 fl. oz. 28.0
Cranberry-orange relish, canned, ½ cup 63.8
Cranberry-raspberry drink *(Ocean Spray*
   Cran•Raspberry), 6 fl. oz. 27.0
Cranberry-raspberry juice:
(R.W. Knudsen), 8 fl. oz. 25.0
cocktail, frozen* *(Welch's),* 6 fl. oz. 28.0
cocktail, frozen* *(Welch's* No Sugar Added), 6 fl. oz. 10.0
Cranberry-raspberry-strawberry juice drink
   (Tropicana Twister), 6 fl. oz. 27.0
Cranberry-strawberry drink *(Ocean Spray*
   Cran•Strawberry), 6 fl. oz. 27.0
Crayfish, without added ingredients.................................... 0
Cream (see also "Creamer, nondairy"):
half and half, 1 cup.. 10.4
half and half, 1 tbsp. 6
light, coffee or table, 1 cup 8.8
light, coffee or table, 1 tbsp. 6
medium (25% fat), 1 cup 8.3
medium (25% fat), 1 tbsp. 5
sour, see "Cream, sour"
whipping[1]:
   light, 1 cup.. 7.1
   light or heavy, 1 tbsp. 4
   heavy, 1 cup.. 6.6

---

[1] *Unwhipped; volume approximately doubled when whipped.*

Cream *(cont.)*
whipped topping:
   frozen *(Kraft Real Cream)*, ¼ cup 2.0
   frozen *(La Creme)*, 1 tbsp. 1.0
   nondairy, see "Cream topping, nondairy"
   pressurized, 1 tbsp.. .4
Cream, sour:
1 cup 9.8
1 tbsp. 5
(Bison), 1 oz. 2.0
(Breakstone's/Sealtest), 1 tbsp. 1.0
(Friendship), 1 oz. or 2 tbsp. 1.0
(Knudsen Hampshire), 1 oz................................. 1.0
half and half, 1 tbsp... .6
half and half *(Breakstone's Light Choice/Sealtest*
   Light), 1 tbsp. 1.0
light:
   (Borden Lite-Line/Viva Lite), 2 tbsp. 2.0
   (Friendship), 2 tbsp.. 2.0
   (Knudsen Light'n Lively), 2 tbsp........................ 2.0
   (Land O'Lakes), 2 tbsp. 4.0
   with chives *(Land O'Lakes)*, 2 tbsp................... 4.0
no fat *(Land O'Lakes)*, 2 tbsp. 5.0
Cream, sour, nondairy:
1 oz. 1.9
(Friendship Sour Treat), 1 oz............................... 2.0
imitation *(Pet/Dairymate)*, 1 tbsp. .... <1.0
Creme de menthe, 72 proof, 1 fl. oz. 14.0
Cream gravy, canned *(Franco-American)*, 2 oz. 4.0
Cream puff, Bavarian, frozen *(Rich's)*, 1 piece 17.0
Cream of tartar *(Tone's)*, 1 tsp................................. .6
Cream topping, dairy, see "Cream"
Cream topping, nondairy:
frozen:
   1 cup.. 17.3
   (Kraft Whipped Topping), ¼ cup....................... 2.0
   (Pet Whip), 1 tbsp. 1.0

(Richwhip), 1 tbsp. 1.0
all varieties *(Cool Whip)*, 1 tbsp. 1.0
mix*:
   1 cup.. 13.2
   (D-Zerta), 1 tbsp. 0
   (Dream Whip), 1 tbsp. 1.0
pressurized *(Rich's)*, ¼ oz. 1.0
Creamer, nondairy:
(N.Rich), 1 tsp. 1.0
(Rich's Coffee Rich), 1 tbsp. 2.0
(Rich's Coffee Rich Light), 1 tbsp. 1.0
(Rich's Farm Rich), 1 tbsp. 1.0
(Rich's Farm Rich Light), 1 tbsp. .... <1.0
liquid:
   (Coffee-mate), 1 tbsp. 2.0
   (Coffee-mate Lite), 1 tbsp. 1.0
   all flavors *(Carnation)*, 1 tbsp. 5.0
   all flavors *(International Delight)*, 1 tbsp. 7.0
powder *(Coffee-mate)*, 1 tsp.. 1.0
powder *(Coffee-mate Lite)*, 1 tsp. 2.0
Creole sauce, Cajun *(Enrico's Light)*, 4 oz........................ 9.0
Crepe, fresh *(Frieda's)*, 1 piece 7.0
Cress, garden:
raw, ½ cup 1.4
boiled, drained, ½ cup 2.6
Cress, water, see "Watercress"
Croaker, without added ingredients 0
Croissant:
butter *(Awrey's)*, 3-oz. piece.. 32.0
margarine *(Awrey's)*, 2.5-oz. piece 26.0
wheat *(Awrey's)*, 1 piece... 24.0
frozen, butter *(Sara Lee Original)*, 1 piece 19.0
Crookneck squash:
fresh, raw, ends trimmed, sliced. ½ cup 2.6
fresh, boiled, drained, sliced, ½ cup................................. 3.9
canned, drained, cut, ½ cup 3.2
canned, yellow *(Allens/Sunshine)*, ½ cup 3.0
frozen, boiled, sliced, ½ cup... 5.3

Croquettes, vegetarian, frozen *(Worthington
Golden),* 5 pieces 20.0
Croutons:
Caesar *(Pepperidge Farm* Homestyle), ½ oz. 8.0
Caesar salad *(Brownberry),* ½ oz. 7.0
cheddar or cheese and garlic *(Brownberry),* ½ oz. 8.0
cheddar and Romano *(Pepperidge Farm),* ½ oz. 10.0
cheese and garlic or onion and garlic *(Arnold*
Crispy), ½ oz. 9.0
cheese and garlic or onion and garlic *(Pepperidge*
Farm), ½ oz. 9.0
fine herb *(Arnold* Crispy), ½ oz. 10.0
Italian *(Arnold* Crispy), ½ oz. 8.0
Italian *(Pepperidge Farm* Homestyle), ½ oz. 9.0
olive oil and garlic *(Pepperidge Farm),* ½ oz. 10.0
onion and garlic, ranch, or toasted *(Brownberry),*
½ oz. 9.0
ranch *(Pepperidge Farm),* ½ oz. 9.0
seasoned:
(Arnold/Brownberry), ½ oz. 8.0
(Pepperidge Farm), ½ oz. 9.0
wheat *(Brownberry),* ½ oz. 9.0
sourdough cheese *(Pepperidge Farm* Homestyle),
½ oz. 9.0
Cucumber, unpeeled:
1 medium, 8¼" long 8.3
sliced, ½ cup 1.4
hot house *(Frieda),* 1 oz. 8
Cucumber dip:
creamy *(Kraft* Premium), 2 tbsp. 2.0
and onion *(Breakstone's/Sealtest),* 2 tbsp. 2.0
Cumin seeds, 1 tsp. 9
Cupcake, see "Cake, snack"
Cupuassu punch *(R. W. Knudsen* Rain Forest),
8 fl. oz. 25.0
Currant, trimmed, ½ cup:
black, European, ½ cup 8.6

red or white, ½ cup 7.7
zante, dried, ½ cup 53.3
Curry powder:
1 tbsp. 3.7
1 tsp. 1.2
Curry sauce mix, 1.25-oz. packet.................................... 17.9
Cusk, without added ingredients 0
Custard, see "Pudding mix"
Custard apple, trimmed, 1 oz. 7.1
Cutlets, vegetarian:
canned:
    (LaLoma Dinner Cuts), 2 pieces............................... 2.0
    (Worthington), 2 pieces 4.0
    multigrain *(Worthington),* 2 pieces 5.0
frozen, breaded *(Morningstar Farms),* 1 piece 12.0
Cuttlefish, meat only:
raw, 4 oz. 9
boiled or steamed, 4 oz.. 1.9

D

Food and Measure	Carbohydrate Grams

Daikon, see "Radish, Oriental"
Daiquiri mixer:
bottled:
   (Holland House), 3 fl. oz.. 27.0
   raspberry *(Holland House),* 3 fl. oz. 21.0
   strawberry *(Holland House),* 3 fl. oz. 24.0
instant *(Holland House),* .56 oz. dry 16.0
frozen*, with rum:
   banana *(Bacardi),* 7 fl. oz. 35.0
   lime or peach *(Bacardi),* 7 fl. oz. 33.0
   strawberry *(Bacardi),* 7 fl. oz. 34.0
Dairy Queen/Brazier, 1 serving:
burgers and sandwiches:
   BBQ beef 34.0
   chicken fillet, breaded 37.0
   chicken fillet, breaded, with cheese 38.0
   chicken fillet, grilled 33.0
   DQ Homestyle Ultimate burger 30.0
   fish fillet 39.0
   fish fillet, with cheese 40.0
   hamburger, single or double 29.0
   cheeseburger, single 30.0
   cheeseburger, double.. 31.0
   hot dog 23.0
   hot dog, with cheese 24.0
   hot dog, with chili... 26.0
   hot dog, 1/4# *Super Dog* 41.0

side dishes:
  french fries, large... 52.0
  french fries, regular 40.0
  french fries, small 29.0
  onion rings, regular.. 29.0
salad, garden, without dressing 7.0
salad, side, without dressing 4.0
salad dressing, French, reduced calorie, 2 oz. 11.0
salad dressing, Thousand Island, 2 oz.................... 10.0
desserts and shakes, regular size:
  banana split 93.0
  Blizzard, Heath.. 114.0
  Blizzard, strawberry 92.0
  Breeze, Heath 113.0
  Breeze, strawberry.. 90.0
  Buster Bar.. 40.0
  cone, chocolate or vanilla 36.0
  cone, chocolate dip... 40.0
  Dilly Bar 21.0
  DQ cake slice, undecorated.............................. 50.0
  DQ Sandwich.. 24.0
  Hot Fudge Brownie Delight 102.0
  malt, vanilla... 106.0
  Mr. Misty 63.0
  Nutty Double Fudge 85.0
  Peanut Buster Parfait 94.0
  QC Big Scoop, chocolate 40.0
  QC Big Scoop, vanilla 39.0
  shake, chocolate 94.0
  shake, vanilla 88.0
  Strawberry Waffle Cone Sundae.......................... 56.0
  sundae, chocolate 54.0
  yogurt, cone 38.0
  yogurt, cup 35.0
  yogurt, strawberry sundae 43.0
Dandelion greens:
raw, chopped, 1 oz. or ½ cup 2.6
boiled, drained, chopped, ½ cup............................. 3.3

Danish:
packaged:
  all varieties, miniature *(Awrey's)*, 1 piece........................ 21.0
  apple, round *(Awrey's)*, 1 piece 50.0
  apple, square *(Awrey's)*, 1 piece.................................... 34.0
  cheese, round *(Awrey's)*, 1 piece................................... 52.0
  cheese, square *(Awrey's)*, 1 piece 25.0
  cinnamon raisin, square *(Awrey's)*, 1 piece.................... 41.0
  cinnamon walnut, round *(Awrey's)*, 1 piece................... 31.0
  raspberry, square *(Awrey's)*, 1 piece 45.0
  strawberry, round *(Awrey's)*, 1 piece 53.0
Danish, frozen or refrigerated:
apple or cinnamon raisin *(Pepperidge Farm)*, 1 piece 35.0
cheese *(Pepperidge Farm)*, 1 piece.................................... 25.0
cinnamon raisin, iced *(Pillsbury)*, 1 piece........................... 20.0
orange, iced *(Pillsbury)*, 1 piece 19.0
raspberry *(Pepperidge Farm)*, 1 piece................................ 31.0
Dasheen, see "Taro"
Date, pitted:
(Bordo), 2 oz. 47.2
(Dole), ½ cup 62.0
(Dromedary), 1 oz. or 5 dates................................... 23.0
chopped *(Dole)*, ½ cup... 56.0
chopped *(Dromedary)*, ¼ cup 31.0
diced *(Bordo)*, 2 oz. 47.5
domestic, natural, dry, 10 dates, 2.9 oz. 61.0
Date bar, see "Dessert bar, mix"
Denny's, 1 serving:
breakfast:
  bacon, 1 slice 5
  bagel.. 47.0
  biscuit 35.0
  blueberry muffin.. 42.0
  cinnamon roll 73.0
  country gravy, 1 oz. 14.0
  eggs... 0
  eggs Benedict 20.2
  English muffin... 25.8

French toast, 2 slices 46.0
ham slice 9
hash browns, 4 oz. 32.1
omelette:
  chili cheese 17.0
  Denver 4.0
  ham'n cheddar 7.0
  Mexican 14.0
  ultimate 7.7
pancakes 26.0
sausage, 1 link 0
waffles 35.0
sandwiches and burgers:
  BLT 42.0
  bacon Swiss burger, without lettuce and tomato 38.0
  cheese, grilled 29.0
  chicken, grilled, without lettuce and tomato 40.0
  club sandwich 40.0
  Dennyburger 36.7
  patty melt 27.0
  roast beef deluxe 44.0
  San Fran burger, without lettuce, tomato, and
    guacamole 51.0
  Superbird 81.0
  veggie cheese 29.0
  works burger, without lettuce and tomato 48.0
finger food:
  chicken strips, 4 pieces 21.0
  mozzarella strips, 1 piece 7.3
entree (entree only):
  catfish, seasoned 1.0
  chicken, fried, 4 pieces 7.5
  chicken, grilled 2.5
  chicken fried steak, without gravy 16.0
  fried shrimp, 1 piece 7.3
  hamburger steak 8.6
  liver with bacon and onions, 2 slices 10.0
  New York steak 0

Denny's, entree (entree only) *(cont.)*
 roast beef.. 41.0
 spaghetti with meatballs 119.0
 stir-fry.. 5.0
 top sirloin steak.. .7
 turkey, without gravy, 6 slices............................. 40.0
side dishes:
 carrots, 3 oz. 3.8
 chili, 4 oz. 15.0
 coleslaw, 1 cup 8.5
 corn, 3 oz. 15.0
 french fries, 4 oz. 38.0
 green beans, 3 oz. 2.6
 onion rings, 1 piece... 9.0
 peas, 3 oz.. 7.0
 potato, baked 21.0
 potato, mashed, 4 oz. 15.0
 rice pilaf, 1/3 cup 15.5
 stuffing, 1/2 cup 20.0
soups, 1 bowl:
 beef barley.. 10.9
 cheese 19.0
 chicken noodle 14.8
 clam chowder... 21.0
 potato 38.0
 split pea.. 33.0
salad:
 chef.. 12.9
 chicken, without shell... 4.0
 taco, without shell 35.0
 tuna.. 13.2
salad condiments:
 cheese, American, 1 slice 5
 cheese, cheddar, 1 oz... 0
 cheese, jack, 1 slice.. .2
 cheese, Swiss, 1 slice.. .3
 guacamole, 1 oz... 2.3

ranch dressing, 1 tbsp. 6
tortilla shell, fried 37.0
Dessert bar mix:
caramel oatmeal *(Betty Crocker* Supreme), 1 bar* 15.0
chocolate peanut butter *(Betty Crocker* Supreme),
  1 bar* 14.0
chocolate and toffee *(Betty Crocker* Supreme), 1 bar*...... 17.0
date *(Betty Crocker* Classic), 1/32 pkg. 9.0
Sunkist lemon *(Betty Crocker* Supreme), 1 bar* 17.0
Diable sauce *(Escoffier),* 1 tbsp. 4.0
Dill dip:
(Nasoya Vegi-Dip), 1 oz.. 4.0
mix*, garden *(Knorr),* 1 tbsp. 1.0
Dill seasoning *(McCormick/Shilling Parsley Patch*
  It's a Dilly), 1/2 tsp. 1.0
Dill seeds:
1 tsp. 1.2
sprouted, raw *(Shaw's),* 2 oz. .... <1.0
Dill weed:
fresh, 5 sprigs 1
fresh, 1/2 cup loosely packed 3
dried, 1 tsp... .6
Dock, boiled, drained, 4 oz.. 3.3
Dolphin fish, without added ingredients 0
Donut:
plain:
  (Awrey's), 1 piece 48.0
  (Hostess Breakfast Bake Shop Pantry), 1 piece.............. 21.0
  (Tastykake Assorted), 1 piece................................... 22.0
cinnamon:
  (Hostess Breakfast Bake Shop Donette Gems),
    1 piece 7.0
  (Hostess Breakfast Bake Shop Pantry), 1 piece.............. 24.0
  (Tastykake Assorted), 1 piece................................... 25.0
  (Tastykake Mini), 1 piece 6.0
  apple filled *(Hostess Breakfast Bake Shop Donette*
    Gems), 1 piece.. 10.0
crumb *(Hostess Breakfast Bake Shop),* 1 piece................. 16.0

Donut *(cont.)*
crumb *(Hostess Breakfast Bake Shop Donette
    Gems)*, 1 piece 8.0
crunch *(Awrey's)*, 1 piece 65.0
frosted:
    (Hostess Breakfast Bake Shop), 1.5 oz. 20.0
    (Hostess Breakfast Bake Shop Donette Gems),
        1 piece 8.0
    (Hostess Breakfast Bake Shop O's), 1 piece 32.0
    rich *(Tastykake)*, 1 piece 28.0
    rich *(Tastykake Mini)*, 1 piece 8.0
    strawberry filled *(Hostess Breakfast Bake Shop
        Donette Gems)*, 1 piece 10.0
glazed *(Hostess Breakfast Bake Shop Old
    Fashioned)*, 1 piece 33.0
glazed, whirl *(Hostess Breakfast Bake Shop)*, 1 piece 27.0
honey wheat:
    (Hostess Breakfast Bake Shop), 1 piece 32.0
    (Tastykake), 1 piece 32.0
    (Tastykake Mini), 1 piece 7.0
(Hostess Breakfast Bake Shop O's), 1 piece 34.0
(Hostess Breakfast Bake Shop Old Fashioned),
    1 piece 21.0
orange glazed *(Tastykake)*, 1 piece 32.0
powdered sugar:
    (Awrey's), 1 piece 68.0
    (Hostess Breakfast Bake Shop Assorted), 1 piece 24.0
    (Hostess Breakfast Bake Shop Donette Gems),
        1 piece 7.0
    (Tastykake Assorted), 1 piece 24.0
    (Tastykake Mini), 1 piece 7.0
    strawberry filled *(Hostess Breakfast Bake Shop
        Donette Gems)*, 1 piece 10.0
frozen, glazed *(Rich's Ever Fresh)*, 1 piece 14.0
frozen, sugar and spice *(Rich's Ever Fresh Mini)*,
    3 pieces 24.0
Doughnut, see "Donut"
Drum, without added ingredients 0

Duck, without added ingredients 0
Duck sauce, see "Sweet and sour sauce"
Dunkin' Donuts:
apple filled, cinnamon sugar, 1 piece 33.0
Bavarian filled, chocolate frosting, 1 piece 32.0
blueberry filled, 1 piece 29.0
buttermilk ring, glazed, 1 piece 37.0
cake ring, plain, 1 piece 25.0
chocolate ring, glazed, 1 piece 34.0
coffee roll, glazed, 1 piece 37.0
cookie:
   chocolate chunk, 1 piece 25.0
   chocolate chunk, nuts, 1 piece 23.0
   oatmeal pecan raisin, 1 piece 28.0
croissant, plain, 1 piece 27.0
croissant, almond or chocolate, 1 piece 38.0
French cruller, glazed, 1 piece 16.0
jelly filled, 1 piece 31.0
lemon filled, 1 piece 33.0
muffin:
   apple 'n spice, 1 piece 52.0
   banana nut, 1 piece 49.0
   blueberry, 1 piece 46.0
   bran with raisins or corn, 1 piece 51.0
   cranberry nut, 1 piece 44.0
   oat bran muffin, 1 piece 50.0
whole wheat ring, glazed, 1 piece 39.0
yeast ring, chocolate frosted, 1 piece 25.0
yeast ring, glazed, 1 piece 26.0
Dutch brand loaf *(Kahn's),* 1 slice 1.0

E

Food and Measure | Carbohydrate Grams

Eclair, chocolate, frozen:
(*Rich's*), 1 piece 25.0
(*Weight Watchers Sweet Celebrations*), 1 piece 26.0
Eel, fresh or smoked, without added ingredients 0
Egg, chicken:
raw, whole, 1 large 6
raw, white or yolk only, 1 large 3
cooked, hard-boiled, chopped, 1 cup 1.5
dried, whole, 1 oz. 1.4
dried, yolk, 1 oz. 1
Egg, substitute or imitation:
frozen:
(*Fleischmann's Egg Beaters*), 1/4 cup 1.0
(*Healthy Choice*), 1/4 cup 1.0
(*Morningstar Farms Better'n Eggs*), 1/4 cup 1.0
(*Morningstar Farms Scramblers*), 1/4 cup 2.0
with cheez (*Fleischmann's Egg Beaters*), 1/2 cup 3.0
mix*, with tofu (*Tofu Scrambler*), 1/2 cup 9.0
refrigerated, 2 oz.,
(*Morningstar Farms Better'n Eggs*), 1/4 cup 1.0
(*Second Nature/Second Nature No Fat*), 2 oz. 3.0
with garden vegetables (*Second Nature/Second
Nature No Fat*), 2 oz. 4.0
Egg, duck, 1 egg 1.0
Egg, goose, 1 egg 1.9
Egg, pickled (*Penrose*), 1 egg 1.0
Egg, quail, 1 egg .... <.1
Egg, turkey, 1 egg 9

Egg breakfast, freeze-dried:
with bacon *(Mountain House)*, ½ pkg. 6.0
omelet, cheese *(Mountain House)*, ½ pkg. 8.0
Egg breakfast, frozen:
omelet, ham and cheese *(Weight Watchers Handy)*,
   4 oz. 18.0
scrambled eggs:
  with bacon, home fries *(Swanson Great Starts)*,
    5.25 oz. 16.0
  with Canadian bacon, cheese, jalapeños, home
    fries *(Swanson Fiesta)*, 6.5 oz. 18.0
  with home fries *(Swanson Budget)*, 4.35 oz. 15.0
  with pancakes, silver dollar *(Swanson Budget)*,
    4.25 oz. 20.0
  with sausages, hash browns *(Swanson Great
    Starts)*, 6.25 oz. 19.0
"Egg" breakfast, vegetarian, frozen:
with cheese and home fries *(Morningstar Farms
   Scramblers)*, 5 oz. 20.0
with hash browns and links *(Morningstar Farms
   Scramblers)*, 5 oz. 20.0
with links and muffins *(Morningstar Farms
   Scramblers)*, 4 oz. 22.0
Egg breakfast biscuit, frozen:
cheese and bacon *(Swanson Great Starts)*, 4.2 oz. 36.0
sausage and *(Hormel Quick Meal)*, 4.5 oz. 30.0
sausage and cheese *(Swanson Great Starts)*, 5.5 oz. 35.0
Egg breakfast muffin, frozen:
Canadian bacon, cheese:
  (Hormel Quick Meal), 4.5 oz. 29.0
  (Swanson Great Starts), 4.1 oz. 25.0
  green chili pepper *(Swanson Fiesta)*, 4.75 oz. 26.0
English *(Healthy Choice)*, 4.25 oz. 30.0
English *(Weight Watchers)*, 4 oz. 29.0
omelet:
  classic *(Weight Watchers)*, 3.84 oz. 22.0

Egg breakfast muffin, omelet *(cont.)*

garden *(Weight Watchers)*, 3.6 oz. 28.0

turkey sausage *(Healthy Choice)*, 4.75 oz. 30.0

western *(Healthy Choice)*, 4.75 oz. 29.0

sausage and cheese *(Hormel Quick Meal)*, 5.1 oz. 5.0

"Egg" breakfast sandwich, vegetarian, frozen:

with cheese *(Morningstar Farms Scramblers)*, 3.5 oz. 29.0

with pattie *(Morningstar Farms Scramblers)*, 4.5 oz. 29.0

with pattie and cheese *(Morningstar Farms
Scramblers)*, 5 oz. 33.0

Egg foo young, mix* *(La Choy Dinner Classics)*,
2 patties and 3 oz. sauce 20.0

Egg roll, frozen:

chicken:

(Chun King), 3.6 oz. 32.0

(La Choy Snack), 1.45 oz. 12.0

almond *(La Choy)*, 3 oz. 19.0

sweet and sour *(La Choy)*, 3 oz. 24.0

lobster *(La Choy Snack)*, 1.45 oz. 12.0

meat and shrimp *(Chun King)*, 3.6 oz. 31.0

meat and shrimp *(La Choy Snack)*, 1.45 oz. 11.0

pork *(Chun King Restaurant Style)*, 3 oz. 23.0

pork *(La Choy Restaurant Style)*, 3 oz. 20.0

shrimp:

(Chun King), 3.6 oz. 31.0

(La Choy Restaurant Style), 3 oz. 19.0

(La Choy Snack), 1.45 oz. 12.0

vegetarian *(Worthington)*, 3 oz. 20.0

Egg roll wrapper:

(Azumaya), 1 oz. 15.9

(Frieda's), 1 piece 1.0

(Nasoya), 1 piece 20.0

Eggless salad dip *(Nasoya Vegi-Dressing)*, 1 oz. 4.0

Eggnog, canned *(Borden)*, ½ cup 16.0

Eggplant, fresh:

raw, trimmed, 1" pieces, ½ cup 2.5

boiled, drained, 1" cubes, ½ cup 3.2

Japanese, raw, unpeeled *(Frieda's)*, 1 oz. 1.6

Eggplant appetizer:
(Progresso Caponata), ¼ cup 4.0
baby, stuffed *(Krinos)*, 1.1 oz. 0
Eggplant entree, frozen:
parmigiana:
    (Celentano), 6.25 oz. 36.0
    (Celentano), 10 oz. 30.0
    (Mrs. Paul's), 5 oz. 18.0
rollettes *(Celentano)*, 11 oz. 32.0
El Pollo Loco, 1 serving:
steak or chicken fajita meal[1] 120.0
chicken, all cuts 0
burritos and tacos:
    chicken burrito 30.0
    chicken taco 18.0
    steak burrito 31.0
    steak taco 18.0
    vegetarian burrito 54.0
salads and side dishes:
    beans 16.0
    chicken salad 11.0
    cole slaw 7.0
    corn 20.0
    corn tortilla 13.0
    flour tortilla 15.0
    guacamole, 1 oz. 2.0
    potato salad 21.0
    salsa, 2 oz. 3.0
    side salad 10.0
salad dressing, 1 oz.:
    blue cheese, ranch, or Thousand Island 4.0
    French, deluxe 7.0
    Italian, low calorie 2.0
dessert:
    cheesecake 30.0
    churros 14.0

---

[1] *Includes guacamole, cheese, and sour cream.*

El Pollo Loco, dessert *(cont.)*
Orange or Piña Colada Bang.. 26.0
Elderberries, ½ cup.. 13.3
Enchanada entree, frozen:
beef and bean *(Lean Cuisine),* 9¼ oz. 32.0
chicken *(Lean Cuisine),* 9⅞ oz. 34.0
Enchilada dinner, frozen:
beef *(Healthy Choice),* 13.4 oz. 66.0
beef *(Patio),* 13.25 oz.. 59.0
cheese *(Patio),* 12 oz. 58.0
chicken *(Banquet Healthy Balance),* 11 oz....................... 58.0
chicken *(Healthy Choice),* 13.4 oz.................................. 58.0
Enchilada dinner mix:
(Tio Sancho Dinner Kit):
   sauce mix, 3 oz.. 62.0
   1 shell 10.8
Enchilada entree, frozen:
beef:
   (Banquet Meals), 11 oz. 57.0
   with chili sauce *(Banquet* Family), 7 oz. 28.0
   Ranchero *(Weight Watchers Ultimate 200),* 9.12 oz....... 18.0
cheese:
   (Banquet Meals), 11 oz. 56.0
   (Stouffer's), 9.75 oz. 33.0
   nacho *(Weight Watchers),* 8.87 oz. 33.0
chicken:
   (Banquet Meals), 11 oz. 54.0
   (Healthy Choice), 9.5 oz. 44.0
   (Stouffer's), 10 oz. 31.0
   Suiza *(Weight Watchers),* 9 oz. 25.0
Enchilada sauce:
(Gebhardt), 3 tbsp.. 3.0
mild *(Rosarita),* 2.5 oz. 3.0
green *(Old El Paso),* 2 tbsp. 3.0
hot *(Las Palmas),* ½ cup 3.0
hot or mild *(Old El Paso),* ¼ cup.................................... 4.0
hot or mild *(Ortega),* 1 oz. 3.0

Enchilada seasoning mix:
(Lawry's Seasoning Blends), 1 pkg. 29.9
(French's), 1/5 pkg. 4.0
(Old El Paso), 1/18 pkg. 1.0
Endive, chopped, 1/2 cup 8
Endive, Belgian, see "Chicory, witloof"
Energy shake, see "Protein shake mix"
Entree sauce (see also specific listings):
Alfredo *(Betty Crocker* Recipe Sauces), 4 oz. 8.0
barbecue *(Beef Tonight)*, 4 oz. 15.0
cacciatore *(Betty Crocker* Recipe Sauces), 3.9 oz. 9.0
cacciatore *(Chicken Tonight)*, 4 oz. 12.0
country French *(Chicken Tonight)*, 4 oz. 6.0
herbed, with wine *(Chicken Tonight)*, 4 oz. 13.0
honey mustard *(Chicken Tonight Light)*, 4 oz. 12.0
lasagna, skillet *(Beef Tonight)*, 4 oz. 9.0
Oriental *(Chicken Tonight)*, 4 oz. 14.0
parmigiana *(Betty Crocker* Recipe Sauces), 3.9 oz. 9.0
pepper steak *(Betty Crocker* Recipe Sauces), 3.8 oz. 8.0
primavera, Italian *(Chicken Tonight Light)*, 4 oz. 9.0
Spanish *(Chicken Tonight)*, 4 oz. 10.0
Stroganoff *(Beef Tonight)*, 4 oz. 6.0
Stroganoff *(Betty Crocker* Recipe Sauces), 3.8 oz. 6.0
sweet and sour *(Betty Crocker* Recipe Sauces),
    4.1 oz. 32.0
sweet and sour *(Chicken Tonight)*, 4 oz. 19.0
sweet and spicy *(Chicken Tonight Light)*, 4 oz. 10.0
teriyaki *(Betty Crocker* Recipe Sauces), 3.9 oz. 13.0
Eppaw, 1/2 cup 15.8
Escarole, see "Endive"
Etouffee dinner mix *(Luzianne)*, 1/4 pkg. 42.0

F

Food and Measure	Carbohydrate Grams

Fajita entree, frozen:
chicken *(Healthy Choice)*, 7 oz. 25.0
chicken *(Weight Watchers)*, 6.75 oz. 24.0
Fajita mix:
(Tio Sancho Dinner Kit):
  sauce, 1 oz. 1.8
  tortilla, 1 piece 24.0
(Tyson), 4 oz. 2.0
Fajita sauce *(Lawry's* Skillet Sauce), 1 oz. 1.8
Fajita seasoning mix:
(French's), 1/5 pkg. 3.0
(Lawry's Seasoning Blends), 1 pkg. 14.0
(McCormick/Schilling), 1/4 pkg. 5.0
Falafel mix:
(Casbah), 1 oz. dry 15.0
(Fantastic Falafel), 3 oz. 21.0
(Near East), 3 patties* 22.0
Farina, whole-grain (see also "Cereal"):
dry, 1 oz. 22.1
cooked, 1 cup 24.6
Fat, see specific listings
Fat, imitation *(Rokeach Nyafat)*, 1 tbsp. 0
Fava beans, see "Broad beans"
Feijoa, raw:
with skin, 1 medium, 2.3 oz. 5.3
pureed, 1/2 cup 12.9

(Frieda's), 1 oz... 4.0
Fennel, bulb, raw:
1 bulb, 8.3 oz.. 17.1
trimmed, 1 oz... 2.1
trimmed, sliced, ½ cup.. 6.3
Fennel seeds, 1 tsp. 1.1
Fenugreek seeds, 1 tsp. 2.2
Fettuccine Alfredo, frozen *(Stouffer's)*, 5 oz............... 22.0
Fettuccine Alfredo mix*:
(Hain Pasta & Sauce), ½ cup 21.0
(Kraft Pasta & Cheese), ½ cup 19.0
Fettuccine entree, frozen:
Alfredo:
   (Healthy Choice Quick Meal), 8 oz. 36.0
   (Lean Cuisine), 9 oz... 41.0
   (Stouffer's Lunch Express), 10 oz. 45.0
   (Weight Watchers), 8 oz. 28.0
   chicken *(Stouffer's Lunch Express)*, 9⅝ oz............... 29.0
with beef and broccoli *(Healthy Choice Extra
   Portion)*, 12 oz. 46.0
chicken:
   (Armour Classics), 11 oz. 28.0
   (Healthy Choice), 8.5 oz. 29.0
   (Lean Cuisine), 9 oz... 33.0
   (Weight Watchers), 8.25 oz. 25.0
   with vegetable medley *Stouffer's* Homestyle),
     9.5 oz. 28.0
primavera *(Green Giant/Green Giant Garden
   Gourmet Right for Lunch)*, 1 pkg.......................... 26.0
primavera *(Lean Cuisine)*, 10 oz. 35.0
Fettuccine entree mix, Alfredo *(Hain* Pasta &
   Sauce), ¼ pkg. 27.0
Fiber supplement *(FiberSonic)*, 1.35-oz. pouch 24.0
Figs:
fresh:
   1 large, 2.3 oz... 12.3
   1 medium, 1.8 oz. 9.6
   California, 4 figs, 2 oz. 38.8

Figs, fresh *(cont.)*
Calimyrna *(Frieda's)*, 1 oz... 5.8
canned in heavy syrup, ½ cup 29.7
dried, 10 figs, 6.6 oz. 122.2
dried, Calamata string *(Agora)*, ½ cup 58.0
Filberts:
dried:
1 oz. 4.4
chopped, 1 cup 17.6
blanched, 1 oz. 4.5
dry-roasted, salted or unsalted, 1 oz. 5.1
oil-roasted, salted or unsalted, 1 oz. 5.4
Fillo pastry, frozen:
(Apollo), 1 oz. 18.0
(Athens Foods), 1 oz. 18.0
Finnan haddie, without added ingredients 0
Fish, see specific listings
"Fish," vegetarian:
frozen *(Worthington* Fillets), 2 pieces 9.0
mix *(LaLoma* Ocean Platter), ¼ cup 5.0
Fish batter mix, see "Fish seasoning and coating
mix"
Fish cakes, see "Fish entree"
Fish dinner, frozen (see also specific fish listings):
'n chips *(Swanson)*, 10 oz. 59.0
lemon pepper *(Healthy Choice)*, 10.7 oz. 52.0
with mashed potatoes and carrots *(Morton)*, 9.25 oz. 44.0
sticks *(Swanson)*, 7.5 oz. 32.0
Fish entree, frozen (see also specific fish listings):
cakes *(Mrs. Paul's)*, 4 oz. 24.0
fillets:
divan *(Lean Cuisine)*, 10⅜ oz. 13.0
Florentine *(Lean Cuisine)*, 9⅝ oz. 13.0
with macaroni and cheese *(Stouffer's* Homestyle),
9 oz. 40.0
fillets, battered:
(Gorton's Crispy/Potato Crisp), 2 pieces 18.0

(Gorton's Crunchy/Crunchy Microwave Portions),
  2 pieces.. 19.0
(Gorton's Value Pack Portions), 1 piece 15.0
(Mrs. Paul's), 6 oz.. 35.0
(Mrs. Paul's Crunchy), 4.5 oz.. 26.0
(Van de Kamp's), 1 piece 13.0
minced *(Mrs. Paul's)*, 3 oz.. 14.0
fillets, breaded:
  (Healthy Choice), 2 pieces 16.0
  (Mrs. Paul's Crispy Crunchy), 4 oz. 23.0
  (Mrs. Paul's Healthy Treasures), 3 oz.............................. 14.0
  (Van Kamp's/Van de Kamp's Crisp & Healthy),
    2 pieces.. 18.0
  (Van de Kamp's Crispy Large Microwave), 1 piece........ 21.0
  (Van de Kamp's Crispy Microwave), 1 piece.................... 9.0
  (Van de Kamp's Snack Pack), 2 pieces............................ 13.0
fillets, in sauce *(Mrs. Paul's* Light), 4.1 oz............................ 5.0
'n chips *(Swanson)*, 5.5 oz. 39.0
nuggets, battered *(Van de Kamp's)*, 4 pieces....................... 8.0
oven baked *(Weight Watchers Ultimate 200)*, 6.64 oz....... 10.0
portions, minced, battered *(Mrs. Paul's)*, 3.5 oz. 21.0
sandwich, see "Fish sandwich"
sticks, battered:
  (Gorton's Crispy/Potato Crisp), 4 pieces...................... 16.0
  (Gorton's Crunchy), 4 pieces 15.0
  (Gorton's Crunchy Microwave), 6 pieces....................... 27.0
  (Gorton's Value Pack), 4 pieces.................................... 13.0
  (Van de Kamp's), 4 pieces 12.0
  minced *(Mrs. Paul's)*, 3.5 oz.. 20.0
sticks, breaded:
  (Frionor Bunch O'Crunch), 4 pieces 13.0
  (Healthy Choice), 8 pieces 14.0
  (Mrs. Paul's Crispy Crunchy), 2.7 oz. 16.0
  (Mrs. Paul's Healthy Treasures), 2.25 oz....................... 14.0
  (Mrs. Paul's Sea Pals), 3 oz. 18.0
  (Van de Kamp's), 4 pieces 15.0
  (Van de Kamp's Crisp & Healthy), 4 pieces................... 17.0
  (Van de Kamp's Crispy Microwave), 3 pieces 11.0

Fish entree, sticks, breaded *(cont.)*
  (Van de Kamp's Snack/Value Pack), 4 pieces 13.0
  minced *(Mrs. Paul's)*, 3 oz. 14.0
Fish sandwich, frozen, fillet *(Hormel Quick Meal)*,
  5.2 oz. 56.0
Fish seasoning and coating mix:
(Shake'n Bake), ¼ packet 14.0
batter, Cajun *(Tone's)*, 1 tsp. 2.6
batter, fish & chips *(Golden Dipt)*, 1¼ oz. 27.0
blackened Redfish or broiled *(Golden Dipt)*, ¼ tsp. 0
fish fry, regular or Cajun style *(Golden Dipt)*, ⅔ oz. 14.0
herb, Italian *(McCormick/Schilling* Bag'n Season),
  1 pkg. 21.0
lemon butter *(French's* Roasting Bag), ¼ pkg. 6.0
lemon and dill *(McCormick/Schilling* Bag'n Season),
  1 pkg. 15.0
seafood:
  (Old Bay), 1 tsp. 8
  (Tone's), 1 tsp. 9
  all purpose *(Golden Dipt)*, ¼ tsp. 0
  Chesapeake Bay *(McCormick/Schilling* Spice
    Blends), 1 tsp. 8
  frying *(Golden Dipt)*, ⅔ oz. 14.0
  lemon pepper *(Golden Dipt)*, ¼ tsp. 1.0
shrimp and crab, Cajun style *(Golden Dipt)*, ¼ tsp. 0
Flatfish, without added ingredients 0
Flavor enhancer *(Ac'cent)*, ½ tsp. 0
Flax seeds *(Arrowhead Mills)*, 1 oz. 11.0
Flounder, without added ingredients 0
Flounder entree, frozen:
battered *(Gorton's* Crispy), 2 pieces 16.0
battered *(Mrs. Paul's* Crunchy Batter), 2 pieces 23.0
breaded:
  (Mrs. Paul's Light), 1 piece 20.0
  (Van de Kamp's Light), 1 piece 21.0
  crunchy *(Gorton's* Select), 1 piece 17.0
Flour, see "Wheat flour" and specific listings

Frankfurter:
(Healthy Deli), 1 oz. 1.3
(Hillshire Farm Bun Size Wieners), 1 link 2.0
(Hormel Light & Lean), 1 link 2.0
(Hormel Wranglers), 1 link... 1.0
(Jesse Jones 1 lb.), 1 link 2.0
(Kahn's Bun Size/Jumbo), 1 link.. 2.0
(Oscar Mayer Healthy Favorites/Light Wieners), 1 link 2.0
(Oscar Mayer Little Wieners), 6 links 1.0
(Oscar Mayer Wieners), 1 link.. 1.0
beef:
   (Healthy Deli), 1 oz. 1.5
   (Hebrew National), 1 link .... <1.0
   (Hillshire Farm Bun Size Wieners), 1 link....................... 2.0
   (Hormel Wranglers), 1 link 1.0
   (Jesse Jones), 1 link 3.0
   (Kahn's), 1 link 2.0
   (Kahn's Bun Size/Jumbo), 1 link.................................... 3.0
   (King Kold), 2 oz. 1.0
   (Oscar Mayer), 1 link 1.0
   (Oscar Mayer Big & Juicy), 4-oz. link............................ 2.0
   (Oscar Mayer Big & Juicy Brooklyn), 1 link 0
   (Oscar Mayer Bun Length/Light), 1 link 1.0
   with cheddar *(Kahn's)*, 1 link....................................... 2.0
   hot *(Hillshire Farm* Links), 2 oz. 1.0
cheese (cheesefurter or cheese smokie):
   (Hillshire Farm Bun Size Wieners), 1 link...................... 2.0
   (Kahn's Wiener), 1 link... 1.0
   (Oscar Mayer), 1 link .... <1.0
chicken, see "Chicken frankfurter"
chili, frozen, with cheese *(Hormel Quick Meal)*,
   4.5 oz. 25.0
corn dog *(Jesse Jones)*, 1 piece 22.0
corn dog, frozen *(Hormel)*, 2.75 oz. 24.0
hot *(Hillshire Farm)*, 2 oz. 2.0
hot and spicy *(Oscar Mayer)*, 1 link................................. <1.0
natural casing *(Hillshire Farm* Wieners), 2 oz. 2.0
red hots *(Jesse Jones)*, 1 link.. 3.0

Frankfurter *(cont.)*
smoked *(Kahn's Big Red/Bun Size Smokey/Bun Size Beef Smokey)*, 1 link 2.0
turkey, see "Turkey frankfurter"
"Frankfurter," vegetarian:
canned:
   (LaLoma), 1 link 2.0
   (LaLoma Linketts), 2 links 2.0
   (LaLoma Sizzle Franks), 2 links 3.0
   (Worthington Veja-Links), 2 links 4.0
   (Worthington Super-Links), 1 link 3.0
frozen:
   (Morningstar Farms Deli Franks), 1 link 4.0
   (Worthington Leanies), 1 link 2.0
   corn battered *(LaLoma Corn Dogs)*, 1 link 15.0
Frankfurter wrap *(Weiner Wrap)*, 1 piece 10.0
French toast, frozen:
(Aunt Jemima Original), 2 pieces 36.0
(Downyflake), 1 piece 22.0
cinnamon *(Aunt Jemima)*, 2 pieces 36.0
mini *(Swanson Breakfast Blast)*, 3 oz. 30.0
sticks *(Qwick-Krisp)*, 4 pieces 52.0
sticks *(Swanson Breakfast Blast)*, 3.75 oz. 44.0
French toast breakfast, frozen:
(Aunt Jemima Homestyle), 5.9 oz. 53.0
cinnamon swirl, with sausage *(Swanson Great Starts)*, 5.5 oz. 38.0
with sausages *(Aunt Jemima Homestyle)*, 5.3 oz. 35.0
with sausages *(Swanson Great Starts)*, 5.5 oz. 36.0
vegetarian, cinnamon swirl, with patty *(Morningstar Farms)*, 6.5 oz. 37.0
Frog's legs, without added ingredients 0
Frosting, ready-to-use:
butter fudge *(Pillsbury Frosting Supreme)*, 1/12 can 22.0
butter pecan *(Betty Crocker Creamy Deluxe)*, 1/12 can 26.0
caramel pecan *(Pillsbury Frosting Supreme)*, 1/12 can 20.0
cherry *(Betty Crocker Creamy Deluxe)*, 1/12 can 27.0

chocolate:
  (Betty Crocker Creamy Deluxe), ¹/₁₂ can 24.0
  (Betty Crocker Creamy Deluxe Light), ¹/₁₂ can 28.0
  (Duncan Hines), ¹/₁₂ can 24.0
  double Dutch *(Pillsbury Frosting Supreme)*, ¹/₁₂ can 22.0
chocolate, milk:
  (Betty Crocker Creamy Deluxe), ¹/₁₂ can 25.0
  (Betty Crocker Creamy Deluxe Light), ¹/₁₂ can 29.0
  (Duncan Hines), ¹/₁₂ can 24.0
  regular or fudge swirl *(Pillsbury Frosting Supreme)*,
    ¹/₁₂ can 23.0
chocolate chip *(Betty Crocker Creamy Deluxe)*,
  ¹/₁₂ can 27.0
chocolate chip *(Pillsbury Frosting Supreme)*, ¹/₁₂ can 27.0
chocolate fudge:
  (Pillsbury Frosting Supreme), ¹/₁₂ can 22.0
  Funfetti (Pillsbury Frosting Supreme), ¹/₁₂ can 23.0
  dark Dutch *(Betty Crocker Creamy Deluxe)*, ¹/₁₂ can 22.0
  Dutch *(Duncan Hines)*, ¹/₁₂ can 24.0
  or milk *(Pillsbury Lovin' Lites)*, ¹/₁₂ can 28.0
coconut almond *(Pillsbury Frosting Supreme)*,
  ¹/₁₂ can 17.0
coconut pecan *(Betty Crocker Creamy Deluxe)*,
  ¹/₁₂ can 20.0
coconut pecan *(Pillsbury Frosting Supreme)*, ¹/₁₂ can 17.0
cream cheese:
  (Betty Crocker Creamy Deluxe), ¹/₁₂ can 26.0
  (Duncan Hines), ¹/₁₂ can 24.0
  (Pillsbury Frosting Supreme), ¹/₁₂ can 26.0
decorator, all varieties *(Pillsbury)*, 1 tbsp. 12.0
lemon:
  (Betty Crocker Creamy Deluxe), ¹/₁₂ can 28.0
  (Duncan Hines), ¹/₁₂ can 18.0
  (Pillsbury Frosting Supreme), ¹/₁₂ can 25.0
rainbow chip *(Betty Crocker Creamy Deluxe)*, ¹/₁₂ can 27.0
sour cream, chocolate *(Betty Crocker Creamy
  Deluxe)*, ¹/₁₂ can 23.0

Frosting, ready-to-use *(cont.)*
sour cream, white *(Betty Crocker Creamy Deluxe)*,
  1/12 can 27.0
strawberry *(Pillsbury Frosting Supreme)*, 1/12 can 25.0
vanilla:
  (Betty Crocker Creamy Deluxe), 1/12 can 27.0
  (Betty Crocker Creamy Deluxe), 1/12 can 30.0
  (Duncan Hines), 1/12 can 24.0
  (Pillsbury Frosting Supreme), 1/12 can 25.0
  (Pillsbury Lovin' Lites), 1/12 can 29.0
  with fudge swirl *(Pillsbury Frosting Supreme)*,
    1/12 can 25.0
  Funfetti, plain, pink, or sunshine *(Pillsbury Frosting
    Supreme)*, 1/12 can 25.0
Frosting mix*:
chocolate fudge *(Betty Crocker)*, 1/12 mix 30.0
coconut pecan *(Betty Crocker)*, 1/12 mix 19.0
vanilla, creamy *(Betty Crocker)*, 1/12 mix 32.0
white, fluffy *(Betty Crocker)*, 1/12 mix 16.0
Fructose:
(Estee), 1 tsp. 4.0
(Estee), 1 packet 3.0
Fruit, see specific listings
Fruit, mixed (see also "Fruit cocktail" and "Fruit
  salad"):
canned:
  in juice *(Del Monte Fruit Naturals)*, 1/2 cup 16.0
  in extra light syrup *(Del Monte Lite)*, 1/2 cup 16.0
  in heavy syrup *(Del Monte)*, 1/2 cup 24.0
  in heavy syrup, with berry flavor, chunky *(Libby's)*,
    1/2 cup 24.0
dried:
  (Del Monte), 2 oz. 34.0
  (Sun-Maid/Sunsweet), 2 oz. 39.0
  bits *(Sun-Maid/Sunsweet)*, 2 oz. 40.0
freeze-dried *(Mountain House Fruit Crisps)*, 1/4 cup 15.0
frozen *(Stilwell)*, 1 1/4 cup 14.0

frozen, in syrup *(Birds Eye)*, 5 oz. 31.0
Fruit bar, see "Snack bar"
Fruit bar, frozen (see also "Ice bar" and "Yogurt bar"):
all varieties *(Welch's* Fruit Juice Bar), 1.75 fl.-oz. bar 11.0
all varieties *(Welch's* Fruit Juice Bar No Sugar
   Added), 1.75 fl.-oz. bar 6.0
all varieties, except banana, coconut, strawberry
   cream, or strawberry-banana *(Frozfruit)*, 1 bar 16.0
banana *(Frozfruit)*, 1 bar 19.0
berry, wild *(Sunkist* Fruit & Juice Bar), 1 bar 24.6
coconut or strawberry cream *(Frozfruit)*, 1 bar 18.0
coconut *(Sunkist)*, 1 bar 12.8
lemonade *(Sunkist)*, 1 bar 17.6
orange *(Sunkist* Juice Bar), 1 bar 17.6
strawberry-banana *(Frozfruit)*, 1 bar 20.0
and cream, all flavors *(Welch's* No Sugar Added),
   1.75 fl. oz. 6.0
and cream, orange *(Sunkist)*, 1 bar 16.6
Fruit cocktail, canned:
(Hunt's), 4 oz. 23.0
(Stokely), ½ cup 24.0
in water, ½ cup 10.4
in water *(Libby's)*, ½ cup 10.0
in juice *(Del Monte* Fruit Naturals), ½ cup 15.0
in extra light syrup *(Del Monte* Lite Fruits), ½ cup 13.0
in light syrup, ½ cup 18.8
in heavy syrup *(Libby's)*, ½ cup 24.0
Fruit juice blends (see also specific fruit listings):
(Chiquita Calypso Breeze), 6 fl. oz. 24.0
(Chiquita Caribbean Splash/Tropical Squeeze),
   6 fl. oz. 23.0
(Chiquita Hawaiian Sunrise), 6 fl. oz. 26.0
cocktail, frozen* *(Welch's Orchard* Harvest Blend),
   6 fl. oz. 27.0
Fruit juice drink:
(Boku Seven Fruit Blend), 8 fl. oz. 29.0
mixed *(Tang Fruit Box)*, 8.45 fl. oz. 36.0

Fruit punch (see also specific fruit listings):
canned or bottled:
    (Juicy Juice), 6 fl. oz. 23.0
    (Mott's 100%), 6 fl. oz. 47.0
    rainbow *(Kool-Aid Koolers)*, 8.45 fl. oz. 36.0
    tropical *(Crush)*, 11.5 fl. oz. 47.0
    tropical *(Juicy Juice)*, 6 fl. oz. 26.0
    tropical *(R.W. Knudsen)*, 8 fl. oz. 33.0
    tropical *(Santa Cruz Natural)*, 8 fl. oz. 26.0
canned or chilled *(Minute Maid)*, 6 fl. oz. 22.0
chilled *(Tropicana)*, 6 fl. oz. 21.0
cocktail, frozen* *(Welch's Orchard* Harvest Punch),
    6 fl. oz. 28.0
Fruit punch drink:
canned:
    (Hi-C/Hi-C Hula Cooler), 6 fl. oz. 23.0
    (Hi-C Hula Punch), 6 fl. oz. 21.0
    (Shasta), 12 fl. oz. 49.0
    (Shasta Plus), 12 fl. oz. 42.0
    (Wyler's), 8 fl. oz. 32.0
    tropical *(Kool-Aid Kool Bursts)*, 6.75 oz. 28.0
    tropical *(Kool-Aid Koolers)*, 8.45 fl. oz. 35.0
    tropical *(Wyler's)*, 6 fl. oz. 21.0
frozen* *(Bright & Early)*, 6 fl. oz. 22.0
mix*:
    tropical *(Kool-Aid)*, 8 fl. oz. 25.0
    tropical *(Kool-Aid* Presweetened), 8 fl. oz. 18.0
    tropical *(Wyler's* Crystals), 8 fl. oz. 21.0
Fruit roll, see "Fruit snack"
Fruit salad, canned:
in heavy syrup, ½ cup 24.5
tropical, in heavy syrup, ½ cup 28.6
Fruit snack (see also specific fruit listings):
all varieties:
    (Barbara's Real Fruit), ½-oz. bar 11.0
    (Fruit by the Foot), 1 roll 17.0
    (Fruit Roll-Ups), ½ oz. 12.0
    (Gushers), 1 pouch 21.0

   (Sunkist Fun Fruits), .9-oz. pouch 22.0
roll, all varieties, except apple *(Sunkist)*, 1 piece 18.0
roll, apple *(Sunkist)*, 1 piece 19.0
Fruit spreads (see also "Jam and preserves"):
all varieties:
   (Knott's Berry Farm Light), 1 tsp. 2.0
   (Master Choice), 2 tsp. 5.0
   (Polaner All Fruit), 1 tsp. 4.0
   (Smucker's Extra Fruit), 1 tsp. 3.0
   (Smucker's Simply Fruit), 1 tsp. 4.0
   (Smucker's Light/Low Sugar/Slenderella), 1 tsp. 2.0
   (Welch's), 2 tsp. 9.0
   (Welch's Totally Fruit), 1 tsp. 4.0
strawberry *(Master Choice)*, 2 tsp. 5.0
Fruit syrup and topping:
all varieties:
   (Knott's Berry Farm Light), 2 tbsp. 12.0
   (Knott's Berry Farm Light Microwave), 2 tbsp. 11.0
   (Knott's Berry Farm Microwave), 2 tbsp. 28.0
   (Smucker's), 2 tbsp. 26.0
   except apricot *(Knott's Berry Farm)*, 2 tbsp. 30.0
apple *(R.W. Knudsen)*, 2 tbsp. 15.0
apricot *(Knott's Berry Farm)*, 2 tbsp. 25.0
blueberry *(R.W. Knudsen)*, 2 tbsp. 19.0
with maple *(R.W. Knudsen Fruit 'N Maple)*, 2 tbsp. 26.0
raspberry or strawberry *(R.W. Knudsen)*, 2 tbsp. 18.0
Fudge, see "Candy"
Fudge topping, see "Chocolate topping"

G

Food and Measure	Carbohydrate Grams

Garbanzo, see "Chickpea"
Garlic:
trimmed, 1 oz. 9.4
1 clove, approximately 1 oz. 1.0
crushed *(Frieda's)*, 1 oz. 8.7
crushed or minced *(Gilroy)*, 1 tsp. 2.0
Garlic and herb dip *(Nasoya Vegi-Dip)*, 1 oz. 4.0
Garlic pepper:
(McCormick/Schilling California Style), 1 tsp. 2.0
(Lawry's Spice Blends), 1 tsp. 2.0
Garlic powder:
(McCormick/Schilling California Style), 1 tsp. 2.0
with parsley *(Lawry's Spice Blends)*, 1 tsp. 2.3
Garlic puree *(Progresso)*, 1 tsp. .... <1.0
Garlic salt:
(Lawry's Spice Blends), 1 tsp. 8
(McCormick/Schilling California Style), 1 tsp. 1.0
Garlic seasoning:
(McCormick/Schilling Garlicsaltless), ½ tsp. 1.1
(McCormick/Schilling Season All), 1 tsp. 5
bread sprinkle *(McCormick/Schilling Spice Blends)*,
  1 tsp. 4
spread *(Lawry's)*, ½ tbsp. 1.0
spread, concentrate *(Lawry's)*, ½ tbsp. 2
Gefilte fish:
(Mothers Low Sodium), 1 piece 2.0
(Rokeach, 4 piece), 1 piece 3.0
(Rokeach, 8 piece), 1 piece 1.0

(Rokeach Low Sodium/Old Vienna), 1 piece..........................2.0
(Rokeach No Sugar), 1 piece....................................1.0
jelled broth *(Mothers* Old Fashioned), 1 piece....................1.0
jelled broth *(Rokeach)*, 1 piece.................................1.0
liquid broth *(Mothers* Old Fashioned), 1 piece....................1.0
sweet:
   (Rokeach Gold Label Old Vienna), 1 piece......................2.0
   (Rokeach Old Vienna), 1 piece................................4.0
   jelled broth *(Mothers* Old World), 1 piece........................2.0
whitefish, jelled broth *(Rokeach* No Sugar), 1 piece..............0
whitefish and pike, jelled broth:
   (Mothers, 4 piece), 1 piece 2.0
   (Rokeach), 1 piece..1.0
   (Rokeach Old Vienna), 1 piece................................3.0
Gelatin, unflavored *(Knox)*, 1 packet........................0
Gelatin bar, frozen, all varieties *(Jell-O Gelatin*
   Pops), 1 bar...8.0
Gelatin dessert:
(Jell-O Snacks), 3.5-oz. cup 18.0
mix*, all flavors:
   (D-Zerta), 1/2 cup..0
   (Jell-O), 1/2 cup...19.0
   (Jell-O 1-2-3), 2/3 cup.....................................27.0
Gelatin drink mix, orange flavor, with *Nutrasweet*
   (Knox), 1 packet 4.0
Ginger, root, trimmed:
1 oz. 4.3
sliced, 1/4 cup 3.6
Ginger, crystallized *(Frieda's)*, 1 oz. 24.7
Ginger, ground, 1 tsp. 1.3
Ginger, pickled, Japanese, 1 oz. 2.1
Ginkgo nut, shelled:
raw, 1 oz. 10.7
canned, drained, 1 oz. 6.3
dried, 1 oz. 20.6
Glaze:
blueberry *(Marie's)*, 2.35 oz. 22.0
creamy, for bananas *(Marie's)*, 2.2 oz. 18.0

Glaze *(cont.)*
peach or strawberry *(Marie's)*, 2.35 oz..................... 21.0
Goat, without added ingredients................................ 0
Godfather's Pizza:
original crust cheese:
   mini, 1/4 pie... 20.0
   small, 1/6 pie.. 32.0
   medium, 1/8 pie 35.0
   large, 1/10 pie 37.0
   jumbo, 1/10 pie 54.6
original crust combo:
   mini, 1/4 pie... 21.0
   small, 1/6 pie.. 34.0
   medium, 1/8 pie 37.0
   large, 1/10 pie 39.0
   jumbo, 1/10 pie 58.5
original crust pepperoni:
   mini, 1/4 pie... 19.9
   small, 1/6 pie.. 32.3
   medium, 1/8 pie 35.1
   large, 1/10 pie 37.3
   jumbo, 1/10 pie 54.9
golden crust cheese:
   small, 1/6 pie.. 25.7
   medium, 1/8 pie 26.9
   large, 1/10 pie 29.5
golden crust combo:
   small, 1/6 pie.. 29.0
   medium, 1/8 pie 30.0
   large, 1/10 pie 33.0
golden crust pepperoni:
   small, 1/6 pie.. 25.9
   medium, 1/8 pie 27.1
   large, 1/10 pie 29.7
Goose, without added ingredients........................... 0
Goose liver, see "Liver" and "Pate"
Gooseberry:
fresh, 1/2 cup... 7.6

fresh, green *(Frieda's)*, 1 oz. 2.7
canned, in light syrup, ½ cup 23.6
Gourd:
dishcloth, boiled, drained, 1" slices, ½ cup 12.8
white-flower, boiled, drained, 1" cubes, ½ cup 2.7
Grain dish mix*, 3-grain, with herbs *(Quick Pilaf)*,
  ½ cup 24.0
Granola, see "Cereal"
Granola and cereal bars (see also "Snack bars"):
all varieties:
  (Carnation Breakfast Bar), 1 bar 20.0
  (Health Valley Fat Free), 1 bar 33.0
  (Kellogg's Nutri-Grain), 1 bar 25.0
  (Sunbelt Fruit Boosters), 1 bar 28.0
  except peanut butter *(Barbara's Nature's Choice)*,
    .75-oz. bar 15.0
  except peanut butter *(Kudos)*, 1 bar 20.0
with almonds, chewy *(Sunbelt)*, 1 bar 18.0
apple berry *(Quaker Chewy)*, 1 bar 20.0
apple cinnamon or honey nut *(Nature Valley Granola
  Bites)*, 1 pouch 25.0
butter almond *(Kudos)*, 1 bar 20.0
chocolate chip:
  (Quaker Chewy), 1 bar 20.0
  chewy *(Sunbelt)*, 1.25 oz. 23.0
  fudge dipped, chewy *(Sunbelt)*, 1 bar 26.0
cinnamon *(Nature Valley)*, 1 bar 17.0
cinnamon & oats *(Barbara's)*, 2-oz. bar 31.0
with coconut, fudge dipped *(Sunbelt Macaroo)*,
  1.4 oz. 23.0
coconut almond *(Barbara's)*, 2-oz. bar 23.0
oat bran-honey graham *(Nature Valley)*, 1 bar 16.0
oats'n honey *(Nature Valley)*, 1 bar 17.0
oats and honey, chewy *(Sunbelt)*, 1 bar 18.0
peanut butter:
  (Barbara's), 2-oz. bar 28.0
  (Barbara's Nature's Choice), .75-oz. bar 14.0
  (Kudos), 1 bar 18.0

Granola and cereal bars, peanut butter *(cont.)*
(Nature Valley), 1 bar 15.0
with raisins or fudge-dipped peanuts, chewy
(Sunbelt), 1 bar 24.0
trail mix *(Quaker Chewy)*, 1 bar 18.0
Grape:
fresh, American type (slipskin):
  10 medium 4.1
  peeled and seeded, ½ cup 7.9
fresh, European type (adherent skin):
  seeded, 1 lb 72.0
  seedless, 10 medium 8.9
  seedless or seeded, ½ cup 14.2
canned, Thompson seedless, in water, ½ cup 12.6
canned, Thompson seedless, in heavy syrup, ½ cup 25.2
Grape drink:
canned, bottled, chilled, or frozen*:
  (Crush), 11.5 fl. oz. 44.0
  (Hi-C), 6 fl. oz. 23.0
  (Kool-Aid Kool Bursts), 6.75 fl. oz. 30.0
  (Mott's), 10 fl. oz. 39.0
  (Tropicana), 6 fl. oz. 22.0
mix*:
  (Kool-Aid), 8 fl. oz. 25.0
  (Kool-Aid Presweetened), 8 fl. oz. 18.0
  wild *(Wyler's)*, 8 fl. oz. 21.0
Grape fruit roll, see "Fruit snack"
Grape juice:
canned or bottled:
  (R.W. Knudsen/R.W. Knudsen Concord), 8 fl. oz. 32.0
  (Tree Top), 6 fl. oz. 30.0
  blend *(Juicy Juice)*, 6 fl. oz. 22.0
  purple, red, or white *(Welch's)*, 6 fl. oz. 30.0
canned, sparkling, red *(Welch's)*, 6 fl. oz. 32.0
canned, sparkling, white *(Welch's)*, 6 fl. oz. 28.0
chilled or frozen* *(Minute Maid)*, 6 fl. oz. 24.0
frozen*:
  (Sunkist), 6 fl. oz. 17.1

(Welch's 100%), 6 fl. oz.	30.0
regular or white, sweetened *(Welch's)*, 6 fl. oz.	25.0
cocktail:	
(Welch's), 6 fl. oz.	26.0
(Welch's Orchard), 6 fl. oz.	27.0
frozen*, no sugar added *(Welch's)*, 6 fl. oz.	10.0

Grape juice drink:
canned or bottled:

(Kool-Aid Koolers), 8.45 fl. oz.	36.0
(Shasta Plus), 12 fl. oz.	44.0
(Tang Fruit Box), 8.45 fl. oz.	34.0
frozen* *(Bright & Early)*, 6 fl. oz.	24.0
frozen* *(Sunkist)*, 6 fl. oz.	17.0

Grape leaf, in jars, imported *(Krinos)*, 1 oz. ... 0
Grape punch, regular or Concord *(Minute Maid)*,
  6 fl. oz. ... 23.0
Grape-apple drink *(Mott's)*, 11.5 fl. oz. ... 44.0
Grape-apple juice *(Welch's)*, 6 fl. oz. ... 26.0
Grape-cranberry juice *(Welch's)*, 6 fl. oz. ... 28.0
Grape-peach juice, white grape *(Welch's)*, 6 fl. oz. ... 30.0
Grape-raspberry juice drink *(Boku)*, 8 fl. oz. ... 29.0
Grapefruit:
fresh, pink or red:

California or Arizona, ½ medium, 3¾" diameter	11.9
California or Arizona, sections with juice, ½ cup	11.1
Florida, ½ medium, 3¾" diameter	9.2
Florida, sections with juice, ½ cup	8.6
fresh, white:	
California, ½ medium, 3¾" diameter	10.7
California, sections with juice, ½ cup	10.5
Florida, ½ medium, 3¾" diameter	9.7
Florida, sections with juice, ½ cup	9.4
canned or chilled in water, ½ cup	11.2
canned or chilled in juice, ½ cup	11.4

Grapefruit juice:
fresh, 6 fl. oz. ... 17.0
canned, chilled, or bottled:
  unsweetened, 6 fl. oz. ... 16.6

Grapefruit juice, canned, chilled, or bottled *(cont.)*
(*Libby's*), 6 fl. oz. 17.0
(*Ocean Spray 100%*), 6 fl. oz. 18.0
(*R.W. Knudsen*), 8 fl. oz. 17.0
(*Minute Maid*), 6 fl. oz. 17.0
(*Mott's*), 11.5 oz. 37.0
(*Tree Top*), 6 fl. oz. 19.0
(*Welch's*), 6 fl. oz. 17.0
pink (*R.W. Knudsen*), 8 fl. oz. 18.0
chilled, regular or ruby red (*Tropicana*), 6 fl. oz. 14.0
frozen* (*Minute Maid*), 6 fl. oz. 18.0
cocktail, pink:
(*Minute Maid*), 6 fl. oz. 20.0
(*Ocean Spray*), 6 fl. oz. 20.0
(*Tropicana Twister*), 6 fl. oz. 19.0
(*Tropicana Twister* Light), 6 fl. oz. 6.0
(*Welch's*), 6 fl. oz. 22.0
Grapefruit juice drink:
(*Citrus Hill* Plus Calcium), 6 fl. oz. 19.0
(*Ocean Spray Ruby Red*), 6 fl. oz. 24.0
Gravy, see specific listings
Great northern beans:
dry, boiled, ½ cup 18.6
canned:
with liquid, ½ cup 27.6
(*Allens*), ½ cup 17.0
(*Eden*), ½ cup 20.0
(*Green Giant/Joan of Arc*), ½ cup 18.0
(*Hain*), 4 oz. 18.0
Green beans:
fresh, raw, ½ cup 3.9
fresh, boiled, drained, ½ cup 4.9
canned or packaged:
(*Green Giant Kitchen Sliced*), ½ cup 4.0
(*Stokely*), ½ cup 4.0
whole or cut (*Allens/Sunshine*), ½ cup 4.0
cut or French (*Green Giant/Green Giant* 50% Less
Salt), ½ cup 4.0

cut *(Green Giant Pantry Express)*, ½ cup 3.0
Almondine *(Green Giant)*, ½ cup 5.0
French *(Allens)*, ½ cup 4.0
Italian *(Allens/Sunshine)*, ½ cup 3.0
and potatoes *(Allen/Sunshine)*, ½ cup 5.0
shell outs *(Allens)*, ½ cup 6.0
freeze-dried* *(Mountain House)*, ½ cup 6.0
frozen:
   (Green Giant/Green Giant Harvest Fresh), ½ cup 4.0
   whole *(Seabrook)*, 3 oz. 5.0
   whole *(Southern)*, 3.5 oz. 6.8
   cut *(Seabrook)*, 3 oz. 6.0
   cut or French *(Frosty Acres)*, 3 oz. 6.0
   in butter sauce *(Green Giant* One Serving), 5.5 oz. 8.0
   in butter sauce, cut *(Green Giant)*, ½ cup 4.0
Green beans, combinations, frozen or packaged:
French, with toasted almonds *(Birds Eye)*, 3 oz. 8.0
mushroom, creamy *(Green Giant Garden Gourmet*
   Right for Lunch), 9.5 oz. 29.0
mushroom casserole *(Stouffer's)*, 4.75 oz. 13.0
potatoes and mushrooms, in sauce *(Green Giant*
   Pantry Express), ½ cup 8.0
Grenadine syrup *(Rose's)*, 1 tbsp. 8.0
Grits, see "Corn grits"
Ground cherry, trimmed, ½ cup 7.8
Grouper, without added ingredients 0
Guacamole, see "Avocado dip"
Guacamole seasoning:
(Lawry's Seasoning Blends), 1 pkg. 12.6
mix *(Old El Paso)*, ⅐ pkg. 2.0
Guanabana nectar *(Libby's)*, 6 fl. oz. 26.0
Guanabana punch *(R.W. Knudsen* Rain Forest),
   8 fl. oz. 29.0
Guava:
1 medium, 4 oz. 10.7
½ cup 9.8
strawberry, ½ cup 21.2
Guava fruit drink *(Ocean Spray Mauna La'I)*, 6 fl. oz. 24.0

Guava juice cocktail, frozen* *(Welch's Orchard
  Tropicals),* 6 fl. oz. 25.0
Guava nectar, canned:
(Kern's), 6 fl. oz. 28.0
(Libby's), 6 fl. oz. 26.0
(Libby's Ripe), 8 fl. oz. 35.0
Guava sauce, cooked, ½ cup 11.3
Guava-passion fruit drink *(Ocean Spray Mauna
  La'I),* 6 fl. oz. 25.0
Guinea hen, without added ingredients 0
Gumbo dinner mix *(Luzianne),* ⅕ pkg. 33.0

H

Food and Measure	Carbohydrate Grams

Häagen-Dazs Ice Cream Shop:

ice cream:

  cappuccino, ½ cup 22.0

  chocolate, Belgian, ½ cup 29.0

  chocolate Swiss almond, brandied cherry, or
    macadamia nut, ½ cup 24.0

  coffee or vanilla chip, ½ cup 26.0

  maple walnut, ½ cup 18.0

  pralines & cream, ½ cup 27.0

sorbet:

  lemon, ½ cup 35.0

  orange, ½ cup 36.0

  raspberry, ½ cup 27.0

yogurt, soft-serve:

  chocolate or strawberry, ½ cup 26.0

  coffee or vanilla, ½ cup 22.0

  raspberry, ½ cup 21.0

Haddock, fresh or smoked, without added
  ingredients 0

Haddock entree, frozen:

battered:

  (Gorton's Crispy), 2 pieces 16.0

  (Mrs. Paul's Crunchy Batter), 2 pieces 22.0

  (Van de Kamp's), 2 pieces 19.0

breaded:

  (Mrs. Paul's Light), 1 piece 15.0

  (Van de Kamp's), 2 pieces 19.0

  (Van de Kamp's Light), 1 piece 21.0

Hake, without added ingredients 0
Halibut, without added ingredients 0
Halibut entree, frozen, battered *(Van de Kamp's),*
    2 pieces 16.0
Halvah:
(Fantastic Foods), 1 bar 17.0
(Joyva), 1 oz. 12.0
Ham, fresh, without added ingredients 0
Ham, cured:
whole leg, unheated, 4 oz. 1
whole leg, roasted, 4 oz. or 1 cup chopped or diced 0
boneless:
    (11% fat), unheated, 4 oz. 3.5
    (11% fat), roasted, 4 oz. or 1 cup chopped or
      diced 0
    extra lean (5% fat), unheated, 4 oz. 1.1
    extra lean (5% fat), roasted, 4 oz. 1.7
    extra lean (5% fat), roasted, chopped or diced,
      1 cup 2.1
Ham, canned:
(Black Label/Cure 81 Half Ham), 1 oz. .... <2.0
(Hormel Curemaster/Light & Lean Half Ham), 2 oz. 1.0
(Oscar Mayer Jubilee), 3 oz. 0
"Ham," vegetarian, frozen *(Worthington Wham),*
    3 slices.. 3.0
Ham bologna *(Kahn's),* 1 slice 1.0
Ham entree, frozen or packaged:
and asparagus au gratin *(The Budget Gourmet* Light
    and Healthy), 8.7 oz. 26.0
and asparagus bake *(Stouffer's),* 9.5 oz. 32.0
scalloped potatoes *(Hormel Micro Cup),* 7.5 oz. 21.0
scalloped potatoes *(Swanson),* 9 oz. 25.0
Ham luncheon meat:
(Healthy Deli Deluxe), 1 oz. 1.0
(Healthy Deli Lessalt), 1 oz. 1.2
(Healthy Deli Light AM), 1 oz. 1.4
(Healthy Deli Old Tyme Taverne), 1 oz. 3
(Jones Dairy Farm Slices/Family Ham), 1 oz. .... tr.

(Kahn's Low Salt), 1 slice 1.0
(Oscar Mayer Jubilee), 3 oz. 0
baked:
  (Weight Watchers), 1 oz. 1.0
  (Oscar Mayer), 3 slices 1.0
  Virginia *(Healthy Deli)*, 1 oz. 1.6
Black Forest *(Healthy Deli)*, 1 oz. 7
boiled *(Oscar Mayer)*, 3 slices ...... <1.0
boiled *(Oscar Mayer Deli-Thin/Healthy Favorites)*,
  5 slices ...... <1.0
breakfast *(Oscar Mayer Healthy Favorites)*, 3 slices 2.0
Cajun *(Hillshire Farm* Deli Select), 1 oz. ...... <1.0
chopped:
  (Black Label), 1 oz. 1.0
  (Kahn's), 1 slice 1.0
  (Oscar Mayer), 1 oz. ...... <1.0
cooked:
  (Hormel Bread Ready/Hormel Deli), 1 oz. 1.0
  (Kahn's), 1 slice 1.0
  fresh *(Healthy Deli)*, 1 oz. 2
cooked or honey roasted *(Weight Watchers)*, 1 oz. 1.0
honey:
  (Healthy Deli Honey Valley), 1 oz. 1.7
  (Hillshire Farm Deli Select), 1 oz. ...... <1.0
  (Oscar Mayer), 3 slices 2.0
  (Oscar Mayer Deli-Thin/Healthy Favorites), 5 slices 2.0
minced, 1 oz. 5
slice *(Oscar Mayer* Jubilee), 3 oz. 0
smoked:
  (Hillshire Farm Deli Select), 1 oz. ...... <1.0
  (Oscar Mayer/Oscar Mayer Deli-Thin), 5 slices 0
  (Oscar Mayer Healthy Favorites), 5 slices ...... <1.0
steak *(Oscar Mayer* Jubilee), 2-oz. steak 0
Ham salad spread *(Libby's Spreadables)*, 1.9 oz. 6.0
Ham spread, deviled:
(Hormel), 1 oz. 1.0
(Underwood), 2⅛ oz. ...... <1.0
(Underwood Light), 2⅛ oz. 1.0

Ham and cheese breakfast bagel, frozen *(Weight Watchers)*, 3 oz... 28.0
Ham and cheese loaf:
(Kahn's), 1 slice.. 1.0
(Oscar Mayer), 1 slice 1.0
Ham and cheese pocket sandwich, frozen:
(Hot Pockets), 4.5 oz. 36.0
(Weight Watchers Ultimate 200), 4 oz. 24.0
Hamburger, see "Beef entree, frozen"
"Hamburger," vegetarian:
mix:
    (LaLoma Patty Mix), 1/4 cup............................... 4.0
    (Tofu Classics), 3.4 oz.*..................................... 14.0
    (Worthington Granburger), 6 tbsp. 7.0
    all varieties *(Nature's Burger)*, 3 oz.*................ 26.0
    chunk *(LaLoma Vita-Burger)*, 1/4 cup................. 6.0
    granules *(LaLoma Vita-Burger)*, 3 tbsp.............. 6.0
canned:
    (LaLoma Redi-Burger), 1/2" slice....................... 5.0
    (LaLoma Vege-Burger), 1/2 cup......................... 3.0
    (Worthington Vegetarian Burger), 1/2 cup 9.0
    (Worthington Vegetarian Burger No Salt), 1/2 cup 7.0
frozen, patties:
    (Ken & Robert's), 1 patty................................. 19.0
    (LaLoma Sizzle Burger), 1 patty....................... 10.0
    (Morningstar Farms Grillers), 1 patty................. 5.0
    (Morningstar Farms Prime), 1 patty 4.0
    (Worthington Fri-Pats), 1 patty......................... 5.0
    garden vegetable *(Morningstar Farms)*, 1 patty................ 9.0
    sandwich, with cheese *(Morningstar Farms)*,
    4.75 oz. 32.0
Hamburger entree mix*:
beef:
    noodle *(Hamburger Helper)*, 1 cup 29.0
    Romanoff *(Hamburger Helper)*, 1 cup................ 31.0
    teriyaki *(Hamburger Helper)*, 1 cup.................... 38.0
    cheddar'n bacon *(Hamburger Helper)*, 1 cup 30.0
    cheeseburger macaroni *(Hamburger Helper)*, 1 cup.......... 28.0

chili macaroni *(Hamburger Helper)*, 1 cup 32.0
hamburger hash *(Hamburger Helper)*, 1 cup 27.0
hamburger stew *(Hamburger Helper)*, 1 cup..................... 26.0
Italian, cheesy *(Hamburger Helper)*, 1 cup.......................... 31.0
Italian, zesty *(Hamburger Helper)*, 1 cup............................. 36.0
lasagne *(Hamburger Helper)*, 1 cup 33.0
meat loaf *(Hamburger Helper)*, 1 cup................................... 14.0
mushroom and wild rice *(Hamburger Helper)*, 1 cup......... 37.0
nacho cheese *(Hamburger Helper)*, 1 cup 35.0
pizza, dish *(Hamburger Helper)*, 1 cup................................. 37.0
Pizzabake (Hamburger Helper), 4.5 oz. 29.0
potato au gratin *(Hamburger Helper)*, 1 cup...................... 28.0
potato Stroganoff *(Hamburger Helper)*, 1 cup 27.0
rice Oriental *(Hamburger Helper)*, 1 cup 38.0
Sloppy Joe Bake (Hamburger Helper), 5 oz....................... 33.0
spaghetti *(Hamburger Helper)*, 1 cup................................... 32.0
Stroganoff or beef taco *(Hamburger Helper)*, 1 cup.......... 33.0
Tacobake (Hamburger Helper), 6 oz. 31.0
Hardee's, 1 serving:
Big Country Breakfast, bacon, ham, or sausage............... 51.0
Big Country Breakfast, country ham 52.0
Biscuit 'N' Gravy 45.0
blueberry muffin 56.0
breakfast bagel:
  plain 38.0
  with bacon, sausage, and/or egg 38.0
  with cheese and/or egg, bacon, sausage 39.0
breakfast biscuit:
  bacon, ham, or sausage 34.0
  bacon, ham, country ham, or sausage and egg
    and cheese 35.0
  Canadian Rise 'N' Shine 35.0
  chicken 42.0
  Cinnamon 'N' Raisin.. 37.0
  omelet, Ultimate 36.0
  Rise 'N' Shine... 34.0
  steak 46.0
  steak and egg.. 47.0

Hardee's, breakfast biscuit *(cont.)*
western omelet... 35.0
breakfast sandwich, *Frisco Ham* 46.0
breakfast sandwich, *Frisco Sausage* 43.0
Hash Rounds... 24.0
oat bran raisin muffin 59.0
pancakes, three, plain or with bacon or sausage............. 56.0
sandwiches and burgers:
Big Deluxe burger... 32.0
Big Roast Beef 29.0
Big Twin 34.0
cheeseburger.. 34.0
cheeseburger, bacon.. 31.0
chicken breast sandwich, grilled............................... 34.0
Chicken Fillet 44.0
combo sub 52.0
Fisherman's Fillet, bakery bun 50.0
Frisco Burger 43.0
Frisco Chicken 44.0
Frisco Club 46.0
ham sub 52.0
hamburger 33.0
hot dog 26.0
Hot Ham 'N' Cheese 32.0
Mushroom 'N' Swiss burger...................................... 33.0
New York Patty Melt.. 45.0
Real West bacon cheeseburger............................... 38.0
(Real West BBQ Beef 48.0
Reuben 48.0
roast beef, regular 29.0
roast beef sub 57.0
Turkey Club 32.0
turkey sub.. 53.0
chicken, fried:
breast, 4 oz.. 15.0
leg, 2 oz... 6.0
thigh, 3.8 oz... 13.0
wing, 1.9 oz. 9.0

Chicken Stix, 9 pieces... 20.0
Chicken Stix, 6 pieces... 13.0
side dishes:
  breadstick, 1.6 oz.. 24.0
  coleslaw, 4 oz... 13.0
  coleslaw, 12 oz... 38.0
  Crispy Curls, 3 oz... 36.0
  fries, *Big Fry* 66.0
  fries, large 48.0
  fries, regular 30.0
  gravy, 1.5 oz. 3.0
  gravy, 5 oz. 11.0
  mashed potato, 4 oz. 16.0
  mashed potato, 12 oz. 48.0
  potato salad, 5 oz. 18.0
Fixin's Cup 0
salads:
  chef... 5.0
  chicken, grilled 2.0
  garden... 3.0
  side 1.0
desserts and shakes:
  apple turnover 38.0
  Big Cookie 31.0
  Cool Twist cone, chocolate or vanilla, 4.2 oz................. 29.0
  Cool Twist sundae:
    caramel, 6 oz. 59.0
    hot fudge, 5.9 oz. 50.0
    strawberry, 5.9 oz. 48.0
  shake:
    Butterfinger 55.0
    chocolate.. 61.0
    strawberry 65.0
    vanilla 59.0
  strudel, strawberry cream cheese................................... 34.0
Hazelnut butter *(Roaster Fresh),* 1 oz............................. 5.0
Hazelnuts, see "Filberts"
Head cheese *(Oscar Mayer),* 1 slice 0

Heart, braised or simmered:
beef or pork, 4 oz. 5
chicken, broiler-fryer, 4 oz. 1
lamb, 4 oz. 2.2
turkey, 4 oz. 2.3
veal, 4 oz. 1
Herb garlic marinade, with lemon juice *(Lawry's),*
  2 tbsp. 3.8
Herb gravy mix* *(McCormick/Schilling),* ¼ cup 3.0
Herb seasoning and coating mix, Italian:
(McCormick/Schilling Bag'n Season), 1 pkg. 21.0
(Shake'n Bake), ¼ pkg. 14.0
Herbs, see specific listings
Herbs, mixed *(Lawry's Pinch of Herbs),* 1 tsp. 9
Herring, fresh, kippered, or smoked, without added
  ingredients 0
Herring, canned, see "Sardine"
Herring, pickled:
4 oz. 10.9
in jars:
  black pepper, cream sauce, or Cajun *(Elf),* 3 oz. 7.0
  cocktail sauce *(Elf),* 3 oz. 16.0
  dill sauce *(Elf),* 3 oz. 10.0
  horseradish sauce *(Elf),* 3 oz. 11.0
  lunch, sliced *(Elf),* 3 oz. 8.0
  rollmops, wine sauce *(Elf),* 3 oz. 13.0
  wine sauce *(Elf),* 3 oz. 12.0
Hibiscus cooler *(R.W. Knudsen),* 8 fl. oz. 24.0
Hibiscus-cranberry juice *(R.W. Knudsen),* 8 fl. oz. 28.0
Hickory nuts, dried, shelled, 1 oz. 5.2
Hollandaise sauce mix:
(French's), ⅕ pkg. 4.0
(Knorr), 1 serving 2.6
(McCormick/Schilling), ¼ pkg. 3.5
(McCormick/Schilling McCormick Collection), ¼ cup* 4.0
Homestyle gravy mix:
(French's), ¼ pkg. 3.0
(McCormick/Schilling), ¼ cup* 3.8

(Pillsbury), 1/4 cup*... 3.0
Hominy, canned, golden, white, or Mexican (Allens),
  1/2 cup 16.0
Hominy grits, see "Corn grits"
Honey (Sue Bee), 1 tbsp.. 16.0
Honey butter (Honey Butter), 1 tbsp.......................... 11.0
Honey loaf:
(Kahn's), 1 slice.. 1.0
(Oscar Mayer), 1 slice 1.0
Honey roll sausage, beef, 1 oz.................................. .6
Honeycomb, strained (Frieda's), 1 oz. 23.3
Honeydew:
1/10 of 7" diameter melon, 2" slice 11.8
pulp, cubed, 1/2 cup 7.8
Horseradish:
fresh:
  leafy tips, raw, chopped, 1/2 cup............................. .8
  leafy tips, boiled, drained, chopped, 1/2 cup 2.3
  pods, raw, sliced, 1/2 cup 4.3
  pods, boiled, drained, sliced, 1/2 cup..................... 4.8
prepared, regular or cream style (Kraft), 1 tbsp............ 1.0
prepared, red, white, or hot (Gold's), 1 tsp.............. <1.0
Horseradish sauce:
(Bennett's), 1 tbsp.. 3.0
(Heinz), 1 tbsp. 1.0
(Sauceworks), 1 tbsp. 2.0
Hot dog, see "Frankfurter"
Hot dog sauce, see "Chili sauce"
Hot sauce, see "Pepper sauce, hot" and specific
  listings
Hubbard squash:
raw (Frieda's), 1 oz. 3.3
baked, cubed, 1/2 cup 11.0
boiled, drained, mashed, 1/2 cup 7.6
Hummus mix (Fantastic Foods), 1/4 cup*................... 11.0
Hunter sauce mix* (McCormick/Schilling
  McCormick Collection), 1/4 cup 5.0

Hushpuppies:
frozen *(Stilwell)*, 3 pieces 19.0
frozen, jalapeño *(Stilwell)*, 3 pieces 4.0
mix, deluxe *(Golden Dipt)*, 1.25 oz. 26.0
mix, jalapeño or with onion *(Golden Dipt)*, 1.25 oz. 27.0
Hyacinth beans:
fresh, raw, trimmed, ½ cup 3.7
fresh, boiled, drained, ½ cup 4.1
dry, boiled, ½ cup 20.1

I

Food and Measure	Carbohydrate Grams

Ice, Italian (see also "Sorbet"):
all flavors (*Luigi's*), 6 fl. oz. 24.0
chocolate (*MamaTish's*), ½ cup... 36.0
lemon (*MamaTish's*), ½ cup 30.0
lemon-lime or orange-pineapple-banana
   (*MamaTish's*), ½ cup 26.0
raspberry (*MamaTish's*), ½ cup 34.0
strawberry (*MamaTish's*), ½ cup 28.0
Ice, bar (see also "Fruit bar, frozen"):
(*Blue Bell Rainbow Freeze*), 3.75 fl. oz. 23.0
(*Blue Bell* Twin Pop), 3 fl. oz... 18.0
Ice cream:
almond praline (*Dove* Bite Size), .75 oz. 8.0
almond praline (*Edy's Grand*), ½ cup 19.0
banana pudding (*Blue Bell* Supreme), ½ cup...................... 25.0
banana split (*Edy's Grand*), ½ cup...................................... 19.0
brownie, double fudge (*Edy's Grand*), ½ cup...................... 20.0
Brownie Overload, Triple (*Häagen-Dazs Exträas*),
   ½ cup 28.0
butter almond (*Breyers*), ½ cup 15.0
butter crunch (*Sealtest*), ½ cup 18.0
butter pecan:
   (*Blue Bell* Supreme), ½ cup... 17.0
   (*Breyers*), ½ cup... 15.0
   (*Chambord* French), ½ cup... 19.0
   (*Edy's Grand*), ½ cup 17.0
   (*Frusen Glädjé*), ½ cup 16.0
   (*Häagen-Dazs*), ½ cup.. 29.0

Ice cream, butter pecan *(cont.)*
  (Sealtest), ¹/₂ cup 16.0
Cappuccino Commotion (Häagen-Dazs Exträas),
  ¹/₂ cup 29.0
Caramel Cone Explosion (Häagen-Dazs Exträas),
  ¹/₂ cup 31.0
caramel nut sundae *(Häagen Dazs),* ¹/₂ cup 26.0
caramel pecan fudge *(Blue Bell* Supreme), ¹/₂ cup 21.0
caramel toasted almond *(Chambord* French), ¹/₂ cup........ 21.0
caramel toffee crunch *(Chambord* Lite), ¹/₂ cup 30.0
Carrot Cake Passion (Häagen-Dazs Exträas), ¹/₂ cup 26.0
cherry chocolate chip *(Edy's Grand),* ¹/₂ cup 18.0
cherry royale, chocolate coated *(Dove* Bite Size),
  .75 oz. 6.0
cherry vanilla *(Breyers),* ¹/₂ cup... 17.0
cherry vanilla, brandied *(Chambord* French), ¹/₂ cup 26.0
chocolate:
  (Breyers), ¹/₂ cup.. 20.0
  (Chambord French), ¹/₂ cup... 24.0
  (Edy's Grand), ¹/₂ cup 16.0
  (Frusen Glädjé), ¹/₂ cup... 17.0
  (Häagen-Dazs), ¹/₂ cup.. 24.0
  (Sealtest), ¹/₂ cup 18.0
  decadence *(Blue Bell* Supreme), ¹/₂ cup.......................... 20.0
  deep *(Häagen-Dazs),* ¹/₂ cup 30.0
  double *(Chambord* Lite), ¹/₂ cup....................................... 30.0
  Dutch *(Blue Bell* Supreme), ¹/₂ cup 17.0
  fudge mousse *(Edy's Grand),* ¹/₂ cup 16.0
  fudge sundae *(Edy's Grand),* ¹/₂ cup................................ 20.0
  milk *(Blue Bell* Supreme), ¹/₂ cup 21.0
  sundae *(Blue Bell* Supreme), ¹/₂ cup................................ 20.0
  swirl *(Borden),* ¹/₂ cup.. 18.0
  triple *(Blue Bell* Supreme), ¹/₂ cup................................... 21.0
  triple stripes *(Sealtest),* ¹/₂ cup 17.0
chocolate almond, Swiss *(Frusen Glädjé),* ¹/₂ cup 18.0
chocolate almond marshmallow *(Blue Bell* Supreme),
  ¹/₂ cup 22.0

chocolate chip:
   (Blue Bell Supreme), ½ cup.................................. 18.0
   (Edy's Grand Chocolate Chips!), ½ cup........................ 18.0
   (Sealtest), ½ cup 17.0
   mint *(Chambord* Lite), ½ cup................................... 29.0
   mint *(Edy's Grand* Chocolate Chips!), ½ cup.............. 18.0
   mint supreme *(Blue Bell)*, ½ cup 18.0
chocolate chocolate chip:
   (Chambord French), ½ cup................................... 26.0
   (Edy's Grand), ½ cup 17.0
   (Frusen Glädjé), ½ cup 21.0
   (Häagen-Dazs), ½ cup.. 28.0
chocolate chocolate mint *(Häagen-Dazs)*, ½ cup 26.0
chocolate fudge, deep *(Häagen-Dazs)*, ½ cup 28.0
chocolate marshmallow sundae *(Sealtest)*, ½ cup 21.0
chocolate mint *(Breyers)*, ½ cup 18.0
chocolate, deep, and peanut butter *(Häagen-Dazs)*,
   ½ cup 25.0
chocolate raspberry truffle *(Chambord* French),
   ½ cup 26.0
chocolate Swiss almond *(Chambord* Lite), ½ cup............. 30.0
coconut almond fudge *(Chambord* Lite), ½ cup 30.0
coffee:
   (Breyers), ½ *cup*.. 16.0
   (Chambord French), ½ cup................................... 21.0
   (Edy's Grand), ½ cup 15.0
   (Häagen-Dazs), ½ cup.. 23.0
   (Sealtest), ½ cup 16.0
coffee-toffee crunch *(Häagen-Dazs)*, ½ cup 27.0
cookie dough *(Edy's Grand)*, ½ cup 21.0
Cookie Dough Dynamo (Häagen-Dazs Exträas),
   ½ cup 31.0
cookies 'n cream:
   (Blue Bell Supreme), ½ cup.................................. 20.0
   (Breyers), ½ cup... 19.0
   (Edy's Grand), ½ cup 18.0
   (Häagen-Dazs), ½ cup.. 26.0
fruit special *(Blue Bell* Supreme), ½ cup 17.0

Ice cream *(cont.)*
fudge:
  brownie nut *(Blue Bell* Supreme), ½ cup 21.0
  marble *(Edy's Grand)*, ½ cup 18.0
  royale *(Sealtest)*, ½ cup 19.0
Heath candy crunch *(Edy's Grand)*, ½ cup 18.0
heavenly hash *(Sealtest)*, ½ cup 19.0
macadamia brittle *(Häagen-Dazs)*, ½ cup 25.0
malt ball'n fudge *(Edy's Grand)*, ½ cup 18.0
maple walnut *(Sealtest)*, ½ cup 17.0
mint supreme *(Dove* Bite Size), .75 oz. 8.0
mocha almond fudge *(Edy's Grand)*, ½ cup 17.0
mud pie *(Edy's Grand)*, ½ cup 18.0
Neapolitan *(Blue Bell* Supreme), ½ cup 17.0
peach *(Breyers)*, ½ cup 18.0
peaches & cream *(Chambord* French), ½ cup 24.0
peaches and vanilla *(Blue Bell* Homemade), ½ cup 24.0
Peanut Butter Burst (Häagen-Dazs Exträas), ½ cup 29.0
peanut butter cup *(Edy's Grand)*, ½ cup 16.0
peanut fudge sundae *(Sealtest)*, ½ cup 17.0
pecan pralines'n cream *(Blue Bell* Supreme), ½ cup 23.0
rocky road *(Edy's Grand)*, ½ cup 18.0
rum raisin *(Häagen-Dazs)*, ½ cup 21.0
strawberry:
  (Blue Bell Supreme), ½ cup 19.0
  (Borden), ½ cup 18.0
  (Breyers), ½ cup 16.0
  (Chambord French), ½ cup 22.0
  (Frusen Glädjé), ½ cup 20.0
  (Häagen-Dazs), ½ cup 23.0
  (Sealtest), ½ cup 18.0
  real *(Edy's Grand)*, ½ cup 16.0
tin roof *(Blue Bell* Supreme), ½ cup 21.0
vanilla:
  (Breyers), ½ cup 15.0
  (Chambord French), ½ cup 22.0
  (Edy's Grand), ½ cup 14.0
  (Frusen Glädjé), ½ cup 16.0

(Häagen-Dazs), ½ cup.. 23.0
(Sealtest), ½ cup 16.0
bean *(Chambord Lite),* ½ cup.................................... 26.0
bean *(Edy's Grand),* ½ cup....................................... 15.0
bean, natural, or homemade *(Blue Bell Supreme),*
  ½ cup.. 20.0
classic or French, chocolate coated *(Dove Bite*
  Size), .75 oz. 6.0
French *(Blue Bell Supreme),* ½ cup........................... 18.0
French *(Edy's Grand),* ½ cup..................................... 16.0
French *(Sealtest),* ½ cup 16.0
French, soft-serve, ½ cup.. 19.1
honey *(Häagen-Dazs),* ½ cup.................................... 22.0
vanilla and chocolate *(Breyers),* ½ cup 17.0
vanilla-chocolate-strawberry:
  (Breyers), ½ cup... 17.0
  (Edy's Grand), ½ cup 17.0
  (Sealtest), ½ cup 18.0
  (Sealtest Cubic Scoops), ½ cup 17.0
vanilla fudge:
  (Häagen-Dazs), ½ cup.. 26.0
  pecan *(Chambord Grand Indulgence),* ½ cup.............. 24.0
  twirl *(Breyers),* ½ cup 19.0
vanilla-orange *(Sealtest Cubic Scoops),* ½ cup............ 22.0
vanilla-peanut butter swirl *(Häagen-Dazs),* ½ cup 19.0
vanilla-red raspberry *(Sealtest Cubic Scoops),* ½ cup 22.0
vanilla Swiss almond:
  (Chambord French), ½ cup.. 24.0
  (Frusen Glädjé), ½ cup 18.0
  (Häagen-Dazs), ½ cup.. 24.0
"Ice cream," substitute or imitation:
almond praline *(Edy's Grand Light),* ½ cup 16.0
brownie chunk fudge swirl *(Simple Pleasures Light),*
  ½ cup 24.0
butter *Brickle (Edy's Grand Light),* ½ cup......................... 18.0
butter pecan *(Edy's Grand Light),* ½ cup......................... 16.0
butter pecan crunch *(Healthy Choice),* ½ cup.................. 26.0
café au lait *(Edy's Grand Light),* ½ cup 14.0

"Ice cream," substitute or imitation *(cont.)*

cappuccino *(Rice Dream)*, ½ cup...17.0
caramel *Brickle (Simple Pleasures Light)*, ½ cup 22.0
caramel cream, dreamy *(Edy's Grand Light)*, ½ cup.........15.0
carob, all varieties *(Rice Dream)*, ½ cup............................20.0
cherry, black *(Borden/Meadow Gold Fat Free)*,
  ½ cup 21.0
cherry, black *(Sealtest Free)*, ½ cup 25.0
chocolate:
  (Borden/Meadow Gold Fat Free), ½ cup.........................21.0
  (Edy's Sugar Free), ½ cup 13.0
  (Healthy Choice), ½ cup...24.0
  (Sealtest Free), ½ cup..23.0
  Dutch (Simple Pleasures Light), ½ cup 18.0
chocolate almond fudge *(Edy's Grand Light)*, ½ cup........15.0
chocolate caramel *(C'est Bon Chocolat)*, ½ cup...............30.0
chocolate caramel sundae *(Simple Pleasures Light)*,
  ½ cup 19.0
chocolate cherry/brandy *(C'est Bon Chocolat)*,
  ½ cup 53.0
chocolate chip:
  (Edy's Grand Light), ½ cup..15.0
  (Edy's Sugar Free), ½ cup 14.0
  (Healthy Choice), ½ cup...24.0
  cherry, Bordeaux *(Healthy Choice)*, ½ cup 24.0
  cookie dough *(Simple Pleasures Light)*, ½ cup..............20.0
  mint *(Healthy Choice)*, ½ cup 25.0
chocolate fudge mousse *(Edy's Grand Light)*, ½ cup 17.0
chocolate raspberry *(C'est Bon Chocolat)*, ½ cup 54.0
coffee toffee *(Healthy Choice)*, ½ cup................................25.0
cookies'n cream *(Edy's Grand Light)*, ½ cup.....................15.0
cookies'n cream *(Healthy Choice)*, ½ cup 24.0
cookies'n dream *(Rice Dream)*, ½ cup................................23.0
French silk *(Edy's Grand Light)*, ½ cup..............................18.0
fudge:
  (Edy's Grand Light), ½ cup..15.0
  brownie *(Healthy Choice)*, ½ cup 27.0
  chocolate or marble *(Edy's Fat Free)*, ½ cup.................22.0

cocoa marble *(Rice Dream)*, ½ cup.............................. 19.0
    marble, mint, or mocha *(Edy's Sugar Free)*, ½ cup 17.0
    mint *(Edy's Grand Light)*, ½ cup...................................... 16.0
    mocha almond *(Edy's Grand Light)*, ½ cup 15.0
    peanut butter *(Rice Dream)*, ½ cup................................ 19.0
fudge, double, swirl *(Healthy Choice)*, ½ cup.................... 24.0
fudgescotch swirl *(Edy's Grand Light)*, ½ cup................... 16.0
lemon *(Rice Dream)*, ½ cup... 17.0
malt ball'n fudge *(Edy's Grand Light)*, ½ cup............... 15.0
Neapolitan *(Healthy Choice)*, ½ cup................................ 22.0
Neapolitan *(Rice Dream)*, ½ cup 21.0
peach *(Sealtest Free)*, ½ cup 23.0
peach or strawberry *(Borden/Meadow Gold* Fat
    Free), ½ cup 21.0
peanut butter cookie dough'n fudge *(Healthy*
    Choice), ½ cup... 24.0
praline and caramel *(Healthy Choice)*, ½ cup.................... 26.0
rocky road:
    (Edy's Grand Light), ½ cup.. 17.0
    (Healthy Choice), ½ cup.. 32.0
    (Simple Pleasures Light), ½ cup................................. 20.0
S'mores *(Edy's Grand Light)*, ½ cup.................................. 17.0
strawberry:
    (Edy's Fat Free), ½ cup... 20.0
    (Edy's Sugar Free), ½ cup 13.0
    (Sealtest Free), ½ cup 23.0
    swirl *(Earle Swensen's* Gourmet Sugar Free),
        ½ cup.. 17.0
strawberry or wildberry *(Rice Dream)*, ½ cup..................... 17.0
tin roof sundae *(Earle Swensen's* Gourmet Sugar
    Free), ½ cup 18.0
toffee crunch *(Simple Pleasures* Light), ½ cup.................. 21.0
vanilla:
    (Blue Bell Diet), ½ cup 12.0
    (Blue Bell Free), ½ cup 16.0
    (Borden/Meadow Gold Fat Free), ½ cup........................ 20.0
    (Edy's Fat Free), ½ cup... 20.0
    (Edy's Grand Light), ½ cup.. 15.0

"Ice cream," substitute or imitation, vanilla *(cont.)*
   (Edy's Sugar Free), 1/2 cup 13.0
   (Healthy Choice), 1/2 cup... 21.0
   (Rice Dream), 1/2 cup 17.0
   (Sealtest Free), 1/2 cup 24.0
   (Simple Pleasures Light), 1/2 cup 17.0
vanilla'n caramel *(Edy's* Sugar Free), 1/2 cup 16.0
vanilla fudge:
   (Rice Dream), 1/2 cup 21.0
   royale *(Sealtest Free),* 1/2 cup 24.0
   swirl *(Simple Pleasures* Light), 1/2 cup 21.0
vanilla-chocolate-strawberry *(Sealtest Free),* 1/2 cup.......... 23.0
vanilla-strawberry royale *(Sealtest Free),* 1/2 cup................ 25.0
vanilla Swiss almond *(Earle Swensen's* Gourmet
   Sugar Free), 1/2 cup 15.0
vanilla Swiss almond *(Rice Dream),* 1/2 cup 20.0
Ice cream bar:
(Heath), 1 bar 16.0
(Kool-Aid Pops), 1 bar 9.0
(Snickers), 2 fl.-oz. bar... 20.0
(Snickers), 1 fl.-oz. bar... 10.0
almond *(Dove),* 1 bar 32.0
almond *(Mars),* 1 bar.. 19.0
chocolate, chocolate coated:
   (Klondike), 1 bar 23.0
   (3 Musketeers), 1 bar... 16.0
   (3 Musketeers Snack), 1 bar 6.0
chocolate, dark chocolate coated *(Dove),* 1 bar................. 34.0
chocolate, dark chocolate coated *(Häagen-Dazs),*
   1 bar 38.0
chocolate, milk chocolate coated:
   (Dove), 1 bar 35.0
   (Milky Way), 1 bar 21.0
   (Milky Way Snack), 1 bar... 8.0
coconut, milk or dark chocolate coated *(Bounty),*
   .84-fl.-oz. bar.. 7.0
coconut, cherry, dark chocolate coated *(Bounty),*
   .84-fl.-oz. bar.. 8.0

crunch:
  caramel almond *(Häagen-Dazs)*, 1 bar............................ 17.0
  chocolate-peanut butter or vanilla crisp *(Häagen-
    Dazs)*, 1 bar.. 16.0
  coffee almond *(Häagen-Dazs)*, 1 bar 28.0
crunchy cookies *(Dove)*, 1 bar.. 34.0
fudge *(Häagen-Dazs)*, 1 bar.. 19.0
fudge, double *(Blue Bell)*, 1 bar.. 24.0
peanut *(Dove)*, 1 bar 32.0
peanut butter-chocolate crisp *(Häagen-Dazs)*, 1 bar......... 29.0
vanilla, caramel brittle *(Häagen-Dazs)*, 1 bar...................... 32.0
vanilla, chocolate coated:
  (Blue Bell), 1 bar.. 27.0
  (Klondike), 1 bar 23.0
  (3 Musketeers), 1 bar.. 16.0
  (3 Musketeers Snack), 1 bar 6.0
  with almonds *(Häagen-Dazs)*, 1 bar............................... 26.0
  with popcorn *(Klondike Krispy)*, 1 bar 26.0
vanilla, dark chocolate coated:
  (Dove), 1 bar.. 33.0
  (Häagen-Dazs), 1 bar.. 38.0
  (Klondike), 1 bar 23.0
  (Milky Way), 1 bar 22.0
  (Milky Way Snack), 1 bar.. 8.0
vanilla, milk chocolate coated *(Dove)*, 1 bar 33.0
vanilla, milk chocolate coated *(Häagen-Dazs)*, 1 bar......... 25.0
"Ice cream" bar, substitute or imitation:
(Blue Bell Bullet), 1 bar.. 11.0
chocolate:
  (Rice Dream), 1 bar 33.0
  fudge *(Blue Bell)*, 1 bar 20.0
  fudge *(Blue Bell Sugar Free)*, 1 bar 5.0
  fudge, double *(Light n' Lively)*, 1 bar............................. 11.0
  fudge swirl *(Sealtest Free)*, 1 bar.................................. 19.0
  malt, chocolate crisp coated *(Blue Bell Grizzly
    Bar)*, 1 bar... 20.0
  mousse *(Light n' Lively)*, 1 bar....................................... 12.0
orange vanilla *(Blue Bell Dream Bar)*, 1 bar........................ 16.0

"Ice cream" bar, substitute or imitation *(cont.)*
orange vanilla *(Light n' Lively)*, 1 bar.................................. 10.0
strawberry *(Light n' Lively)*, 1 bar 12.0
strawberry *(Rice Dream)*, 1 bar... 31.0
vanilla *(Rice Dream)*, 1 bar... 33.0
vanilla, chocolate coated:
  (Blue Bell Mooo Bar), 1 bar 17.0
  (Klondike Lite), 1 bar 13.0
  (Light n' Lively), 1 bar.. 14.0
vanilla fudge swirl *(Sealtest Free)*, 1 bar 18.0
vanilla strawberry swirl *(Sealtest Free)*, 1 bar 17.0
Ice cream cone or cup:
plain or rainbow *(Comet)*, 1 piece 4.0
sugar *(Comet)*, 1 piece 11.0
waffle *(Comet)*, 1 piece... 15.0
filled, chocolate, vanilla, or strawberry *(Blue Bell)*,
  3 fl. oz.. 12.0
filled, vanilla *(Blue Bell* Homemade), 3 fl. oz...................... 19.0
Ice cream, mix*:
chocolate *(Salada)*, 1 cup 31.0
strawberry or vanilla *(Salada)*, 1 cup 32.0
Ice cream sandwich:
(Blue Bell), 1 piece.. 27.0
(Klondike Lite), 1 piece 17.0
chocolate chip *(Klondike)*, 1 piece 35.0
vanilla *(Klondike)*, 1 piece 33.0
"Ice cream" sandwich, imitation, all varieties *(Rice
  Dream* Pie), 1 piece.. 47.0
Ice cream and sorbet, see "Sorbet"
Ice milk:
almond praline *(Edy's* Low Fat), 1/2 cup 22.0
almond praline delight *(Swensen's)*, 1/2 cup...................... 20.0
caramel nut *(Light n' Lively)*, 1/2 cup.................................. 18.0
caramel turtle fudge *(Swensen's)*, 1/2 cup 18.0
chocolate *(Borden)*, 1/2 cup.. 18.0
chocolate *(Breyers Light)*, 1/2 cup...................................... 18.0
chocolate chip *(Light n' Lively)*, 1/2 cup 18.0

chocolate chip *(Weight Watchers Grand Collection)*,
½ cup 19.0
chocolate fudge twirl *(Breyers Light)*, ½ cup 21.0
coffee *(Light n' Lively)*, ½ cup 16.0
cookies n' cream:
    (Edy's Low Fat), ½ cup 20.0
    (Light n' Lively), ½ cup 18.0
    (Swensen's), ½ cup 20.0
heavenly hash *(Breyers Light)*, ½ cup 21.0
heavenly hash *(Light n' Lively)*, ½ cup 20.0
mocha almond fudge *(Edy's* Low Fat), ½ cup 20.0
peaches 'n cream *(Blue Bell* Light), ½ cup 21.0
pecan pralines'n creme *(Weight Watchers Grand
    Collection)*, ½ cup 20.0
praline almond *(Breyers Light)*, ½ cup 19.0
rocky road *(Edy's* Low Fat), ½ cup 20.0
strawberry *(Borden)*, ½ cup 17.0
strawberry *(Breyers Light)*, ½ cup 18.0
toffee fudge parfait *(Breyers Light)*, ½ cup 22.0
vanilla:
    (Blue Bell Light), ½ cup 17.0
    (Borden), ½ cup 17.0
    (Breyers Light), ½ cup 18.0
    (Edy's Low Fat), ½ cup 18.0
    (Light n' Lively), ½ cup 16.0
    soft serve, ½ cup 19.2
vanilla chocolate almond *(Light n' Lively)*, ½ cup 17.0
vanilla-chocolate-strawberry *(Breyers Light)*, ½ cup 18.0
vanilla-chocolate-strawberry *(Light n' Lively)*, ½ cup 17.0
vanilla fudge twirl *(Light n' Lively)*, ½ cup 18.0
vanilla-red raspberry parfait *(Breyers Light)*, ½ cup 23.0
vanilla-red raspberry swirl *(Light n' Lively)*, ½ cup 19.0
Icing, cake, see "Frosting"
Italian sausage, see "Sausage"
Italian seasoning:
(McCormick/Schilling Spice Blends), 1 tsp. 6
(Tone's), 1 tsp. 7

J

Food and Measure	Carbohydrate Grams

Jack-in-the-Box, 1 serving:
breakfast dishes:
  Breakfast Jack 30.0
  crescent, sausage 28.0
  crescent, supreme 27.0
  hash browns 14.0
  pancake platter 87.0
  pancake syrup, 1.5 oz. 30.0
  scrambled egg platter 50.0
  scrambled egg pocket 31.0
  sourdough sandwich 31.0
burgers and sandwiches:
  bacon bacon cheeseburger 41.0
  cheeseburger, regular, double, or ultimate 33.0
  chicken, spicy crispy 55.0
  chicken fajita pita 29.0
  chicken fillet, grilled 36.0
  chicken supreme 47.0
  chicken and mushroom 40.0
  fish supreme 44.0
  gyro, beef 55.0
  hamburger 28.0
  Jumbo Jack 42.0
  Jumbo Jack, with cheese 46.0
  sirloin steak 49.0
  sourdough burger, grilled 34.0
  steak, country fried 42.0

Mexican food:
    chimichangas, mini, 4 pieces.. 57.0
    chimichangas, mini, 6 pieces.. 85.0
    guacamole, .9 oz.. 2.0
    salsa, 1 oz. 2.0
    taco 15.0
    taco, super.. 22.0
salads:
    chef 10.0
    side .... <1.0
    taco... 28.0
finger foods:
    chicken strips, 4 pieces 18.0
    chicken strips, 6 pieces 28.0
    chicken wings, 6 pieces.. 78.0
    chicken wings, 9 pieces.. 117.0
    egg rolls, 3 pieces... 54.0
    egg rolls, 5 pieces... 92.0
    ravioli, toasted, 7 pieces 57.0
    ravioli, toasted, 10 pieces.. 81.0
side dishes:
    fries, regular... 45.0
    fries, small 28.0
    fries, jumbo.. 51.0
    fries, seasoned, curly 39.0
    onion rings.. 38.0
    sesame breadsticks... 12.0
    tortilla chips, 1 oz... 18.0
sauces:
    BBQ or sweet and sour, 1 oz. 11.0
    hot, .5 oz. 1.0
    Italian, 1.5 oz. 6.0
dressings:
    bleu cheese, 2.5 oz... 14.0
    buttermilk, house, 2.5 oz. 8.0
    Italian, low calorie, 2.5 oz. 2.0
    Thousand Island, 2.5 oz.. 12.0

Jack-in-the-Box (cont.)
desserts:
   apple turnover 48.0
   cheesecake 29.0
   double fudge cake 49.0
shake, chocolate or strawberry 55.0
shake, vanilla 57.0
Jackfruit, trimmed, 1 oz. 6.8
Jalapeño, see "Pepper, jalapeño"
Jalapeño dip:
(Kraft), 2 tbsp. 3.0
cheddar *(Breakstone's* Gourmet), 2 tbsp. 2.0
cheese *(Kraft* Premium), 2 tbsp. 3.0
nacho *(Price's)*, 1 oz. 2.0
Jalapeño loaf:
(Kahn's), 1 slice 2.0
(Oscar Mayer), 1 oz. 2.4
Jam and preserves (see also "Fruit spreads" and
  "Jelly"):
all varieties:
   (Knott's Berry Farm), 1 tsp. 4.0
   (Kraft), 1 tsp. 4.0
   (Polaner), 2 tsp. 9.0
   (Smucker's), 1 tsp. 4.0
   except organic *(R. W. Knudsen)*, 2 tsp. 8.0
   organic *(R. W. Knudsen)*, 2 tsp. 7.0
apricot *(Chambord)*, 1 tbsp. 11.0
blueberry or peach *(Chambord)*, 1 tbsp. 13.0
cherry, black *(Chambord)*, 1 tbsp. 11.0
currant, black *(Chambord)*, 1 tbsp. 12.0
four fruit *(Chambord)*, 1 tbsp. 11.0
grape *(Welch's)*, 2 tsp. 9.0
orange:
   (Chambord), 1 tbsp. 11.6
   marmalade *(R. W. Knudsen)*, 2 tsp. 8.0
   marmalade *(Smucker's)*, 1 tsp. 4.0
plum *(Chambord* Fancy), 1 tbsp. 12.0

raspberry, black or red, or strawberry *(Chambord)*,
  1 tbsp. 12.0
strawberry *(Kraft* Reduced Calorie), 1 tsp. 2.0
strawberry *(Smucker's* Imitation), 1 tsp. 1.0
Jamaican jerk:
dipping sauce *(Helen's Tropical Exotics)*, 2 tbsp. 10.0
seasoning and marinade *(Helen's Tropical Exotics)*,
  1 tbsp. dry 7.0
Jambalaya dinner mix *(Luzianne)*, ¼ pkg. 43.0
Java plum:
3 medium, .4 oz. 1.4
seeded, ½ cup 10.5
Jelly:
all flavors:
  (Knott's Berry Farm), 1 tsp. 4.0
  (Kraft), 1 tsp. 4.0
  (Polaner), 2 tsp. 9.0
  (Smucker's), 1 tsp. 4.0
  (Welch's), 2 tsp. 9.0
grape:
  (Kraft Reduced Calorie), 1 tsp. 2.0
  (Smucker's Imitation), 1 tsp. 1.0
  (Welch's), 2 tsp. 9.0
Jelly and peanut butter *(Smucker's Goober Grape/*
  Strawberry), 2 tbsp. 18.0
Jerusalem artichoke:
sliced, ½ cup 13.1
stored *(Frieda's Sunchoke)*, 1 oz. 16.7
Jicama, see "Yam bean tuber"
Jujube:
raw, seeded, 1 oz. 5.7
dried, 1 oz. 20.1
Jute, potherb:
raw, ½ cup 8
boiled, drained, ½ cup 3.1

K

Food and Measure	Carbohydrate Grams

Kale:
fresh, raw, chopped, ½ cup 3.4
fresh, boiled, drained, chopped, ½ cup 3.7
canned (Allens/Sunshine), ½ cup 3.0
frozen, chopped:
  (Frosty Acres), 3.3 oz. 5.0
  (Seabrook), 3.3 oz. 5.0
  (Southern), 3.5 oz. 4.8
Kale, Scotch:
raw, chopped, ½ cup 2.8
boiled, drained, chopped, ½ cup 3.7
Kamut:
flakes (Arrowhead Mills), 1 oz. 22.0
grain, rolled, or flour (Arrowhead Mills), 2 oz. 41.0
Kasha, see "Buckwheat groats"
Kauai punch (Santa Cruz Natural), 8 fl. oz. 28.0
Kelp, see "Seaweed"
KFC, 1 serving:
Original Recipe:
  breast, center 8.0
  breast, side 9.0
  drumstick 3.0
  thigh 8.0
  wing, whole 5.0
Extra Tasty Crispy:
  breast, center 14.0
  breast, side 19.0
  drumstick 6.0

thigh.. 7.0
wing, whole... 8.0
Hot & Spicy:
   breast, center 13.0
   breast, side... 16.0
   drumstick... 6.0
   thigh.. 10.0
   wing, whole... 5.0
Hot Wings, 6 pieces 18.0
Kentucky Nuggets, 6 pieces... 15.0
Kentucky Nuggets sauce:
   barbeque, 1 oz. 7.0
   honey, .5 oz... 12.0
Chicken Littles sandwich 14.0
Colonel's chicken sandwich 39.0
side dishes:
   biscuit 26.0
   coleslaw.. 13.0
   corn on the cob... 21.0
   fries, crispy 33.0
   mashed potatoes with gravy... 15.0
Kidney beans:
dry *(Arrowhead Mills),* 2 oz.. 35.0
dry, boiled, 1/2 cup 20.1
canned, red:
   with liquid, 1/2 cup 20.0
   (Hunt's), 4 oz. 20.0
   (Progresso), 4 oz. 21.0
   (Stokely), 1/2 cup 20.0
   dark *(Allens/East Texas Fair),* 1/2 cup............................ 20.0
   dark *(Hain),* 4 oz. 16.0
   dark or light *(Green Giant/Joan of Arc),* 1/2 cup 20.0
   light *(Allens),* 1/2 cup 20.0
canned, white *(Progresso* Cannellini), 4 oz. 19.0
Kidney beans, sprouted:
raw, 1/2 cup.. 3.8
boiled, drained, 4 oz.. 5.4

Kidneys, braised:

beef or lamb, 4 oz. 1.1

pork or veal, 4 oz. 0

Kielbasa (see also "Polish sausage"):

(Hillshire Farm Bun Size/Polska Flavorseal/Polska

    Links), 2 oz. 2.0

(Hillshire Farm Polska Flavorseal Lite), 2 oz. 1.0

(Kahn's Bun Size Polska), 1 link 2.0

beef *(Hillshire Farm* Polska Flavorseal), 2 oz. 1.0

Kiwi nectar *(R. W. Knudsen),* 8 fl. oz. 14.0

Kiwifruit:

1 large, 3.7 oz. 13.5

1 medium, 3.1 oz. 11.3

fuzzless *(Frieda's),* 1 oz. 2.1

Knockwurst:

(Hillshire Farm), 2 oz. 1.0

beef *(Hebrew National),* 1 link .... <1.0

Kohlrabi:

raw, sliced, ½ cup 4.3

boiled, drained, sliced, ½ cup 5.5

Kumquat:

1 medium, .7 oz. 3.1

seeded, 1 oz. 4.7

seeded *(Frieda's),* 1 oz. 4.8

L

Food and Measure	Carbohydrate Grams

Lamb, without added ingredients 0
Lamb quarters, boiled, drained, chopped, ½ cup 4.5
Lard 0
Lasagna entree, canned or packaged:
(Hormel Micro Cup), 7.5 oz. 25.0
Italian *(Hormel Top Shelf)*, 10 oz. 30.0
with meat sauce:
   (Dinty Moore American Classics), 10 oz. 33.0
   (Healthy Choice), 7.5 oz. 29.0
   (Libby's Diner), 7.75 oz. 29.0
Lasagna entree, freeze-dried* *(Mountain House)*,
  1 cup 23.0
Lasagna entree, frozen:
(Celentano), 10 oz. 51.0
(Celentano Great Choice), 10 oz. 42.0
(Dining Lite), 9 oz. 36.0
(Freezer Queen), 10 oz. 41.0
(On-Cor), 8 oz. 34.0
(Stouffer's), 10 oz. 40.0
(Tyson Gourmet Selection), 11.5 oz. 47.0
(Weight Watchers), 10.25 oz. 29.0
cheese:
   (Dining Lite), 9 oz. 36.0
   Italian *(Weight Watchers)*, 11 oz. 29.0
   three *(The Budget Gourmet)*, 10 oz. 36.0
Florentine *(Weight Watchers Smart Ones)*, 11 oz. 34.0
garden *(Weight Watchers)*, 11 oz. 30.0

Lasagna entree, frozen *(cont.)*
with meat sauce:
   (Banquet Family), 7 oz. 30.0
   (The Budget Gourmet Light and Healthy), 9.4 oz. 30.0
   (Dining Lite), 9 oz. 36.0
   (Freezer Queen Family), 7 oz. 28.0
   (Healthy Choice), 10 oz. 37.0
   (Lean Cuisine), 10.25 oz. 36.0
   (Swanson), 10 oz. 44.0
primavera *(Celentano* Great Choice), 10 oz. 33.0
sausage, Italian *(The Budget Gourmet)*, 10 oz. 34.0
tuna, with spinach noodles and vegetables *(Lean
  Cuisine)*, 9.75 oz. 29.0
vegetable:
   (The Budget Gourmet Light and Healthy), 10.5 oz. 36.0
   (On-Cor), 8 oz. 34.0
   (Stouffer's), 10.5 oz. 35.0
zucchini *(Healthy Choice* Quick Meal), 11.5 oz. 41.0
zucchini *(Lean Cuisine)*, 11 oz. 34.0
Lasagna sheets, frozen, precooked *(Aunt Vi's)*, 4 oz. 36.0
Leeks:
fresh:
   raw, 9.9-oz. leek 17.6
   raw, trimmed, chopped, ½ cup 7.4
   boiled, drained, chopped, ½ cup 4.0
freeze-dried, 1 tbsp. 2
Lemon:
1 medium, 2⅛"-diameter, 3.9 oz. with peel 11.6
1 wedge, ¼ medium 2.9
peeled, 2⅛"-diameter 5.4
peel, 1 tbsp. 1.0
Lemon dill seasoning *(McCormick/Schilling* Bag'n
  Season), 1 pkg. 15.0
Lemon herb seasoning *(McCormick/Schilling* Spice
  Blends), 1 tsp. 7
Lemon juice:
fresh, 1 tbsp. 1.3

bottled or chilled *(ReaLemon)*, 1 tbsp. 2.0
frozen *(Minute Maid)*, 1 fl. oz. 2.0
frozen *(Sunkist)*, 1 fl. oz. 2.0
Lemon pepper:
(Lawry's Spice Blends), 1 tsp. 1.2
(McCormick/Schilling Parsley Patch), 1 tsp. 2.0
(McCormick/Schilling Spice Blends), 1 tsp. 8
Lemon pepper marinade *(Lawry's)*, 1 oz. 2.1
Lemon-lime drink mix* *(Kool-Aid)*, 8 fl. oz. 25.0
Lemonade:
canned or bottled:
  (Crush), 11.5 fl. oz. 35.0
  (R. W. Knudsen Natural), 8 fl. oz. 26.0
  (Kool-Aid Koolers), 8.45 fl. oz. 32.0
  (Santa Cruz Natural), 8 fl. oz. 21.0
  (Shasta), 12 fl. oz. 42.0
  (Shasta Plus), 12 fl. oz. 43.0
  (Sunkist), 8 fl. oz. 36.0
  (Welch's), 6 fl. oz. 24.0
  (Wylers), 6 fl. oz. 16.0
chilled *(Tropicana)*, 6 fl. oz. 22.0
chilled, regular, country style or pink *(Minute Maid)*,
  6 fl. oz. 21.0
frozen* *(Sunkist)*, 8 fl. oz. 24.2
mix*:
  (Kool-Aid), 8 fl. oz. 25.0
  (Kool-Aid Presweetened), 8 fl. oz. 17.0
  regular or pink *(Wyler's* Crystals), 8 fl. oz. 20.0
Lemonade fruit blends:
cherry:
  (Boku), 8 fl. oz. 29.0
  (R. W. Knudsen), 8 fl. oz. 31.0
  dark sweet *(Santa Cruz Natural)*, 8 fl. oz. 20.0
cranberry:
  (R. W. Knudsen), 8 fl. oz. 29.0
  (Minute Maid), 6 fl. oz. 23.0

Lemonade fruit blends, cranberry *(cont.)*
(Santa Cruz Natural), 8 fl. oz. 24.0
Concord grape-wild blackberry *(Santa Cruz Natural),*
8 fl. oz. 22.0
raspberry *(R. W. Knudsen),* 8 fl. oz. 28.0
raspberry *(Minute Maid),* 6 fl. oz. 23.0
raspberry or strawberry *(Santa Cruz Natural),* 8 fl. oz. 20.0
strawberry *(R. W. Knudsen),* 8 fl. oz. 21.0
Lentil, dry:
green *(Arrowhead Mills),* 2 oz. 35.0
red *(Arrowhead Mills),* 2 oz. 34.0
boiled, 1/2 cup 19.9
Lentil, sprouted, raw, 1/2 cup 8.4
Lentil dishes:
canned, hearty, with vegetables *(Health Valley Fast
Menu Fat Free),* 5 oz. 12.0
mix*:
and couscous *(Fantastic Only a Pinch),* 10 oz. 47.0
curried, with rice *(Fantastic),* 10 oz. 44.0
pilaf, with couscous *(Fantastic Leapin' Lentils),*
10 oz. 42.0
Lentil rice loaf, frozen *(Natural Touch),* 2 1/2" slice 18.0
Lettuce:
bibb, Boston, or butterhead, 1 head, 5" diameter 3.8
bibb, Boston, or butterhead, 2 inner leaves 4
cos or romaine, 1 inner leaf 2
cos or romaine, shredded, 1/2 cup 7
iceberg, 1 head, 6" diameter 11.3
iceberg, 1 leaf, .7 oz. 4
limestone *(Frieda's),* 1 oz. 7
looseleaf, shredded, 1/2 cup 1.0
Lima beans:
fresh, raw, trimmed, 1/2 cup 15.7
fresh, boiled, drained, 1/2 cup 20.1
canned:
(Green Giant/Joan of Arc Butter Beans), 1/2 cup 12.0
(Stokely), 1/2 cup 16.0
green *(Allens/Butterfield/Sunshine),* 1/2 cup 15.0

green and white *(Allens)*, ½ cup 15.0
large *(Allens Butterbeans)*, ½ cup 18.0
frozen:
baby *(Green Giant Harvest Fresh)*, ½ cup 18.0
baby *(Seabrook)*, 3.3 oz. 24.0
baby, butter *(Seabrook)*, 3.3 oz. 26.0
Fordhook *(Seabrook)*, 3.3 oz. 19.0
speckled *(Seabrook)*, 3.3 oz. 23.0
tiny *(Seabrook)*, 3.3 oz. 21.0
in butter sauce *(Green Giant)*, ½ cup 17.0
Lima beans, mature:
baby, boiled, ½ cup 21.2
large, boiled, ½ cup 19.6
canned, with liquid, ½ cup 17.9
Lime:
1 medium, 2″-diameter 7.1
peeled, seeded, 1 oz. 3.0
Lime cooler, tropical *(R. W. Knudsen)*, 8 fl. oz. 32.0
Lime juice:
fresh, 1 tbsp. 1.4
bottled *(ReaLime)*, 1 tbsp. 1.0
sweetened *(Rose's)*, 1 tbsp. 6.0
Limeade:
(Minute Maid), 6 fl. oz. 19.0
Key lime *(Boku)*, 8 fl. oz. 28.0
Ling, without added ingredients.................................... 0
Ling cod, without added ingredients............................... 0
Linguine, see "Pasta"
Linguine entree, frozen:
with clam sauce *(Lean Cuisine)*, 9⅝ oz. 36.0
with scallops and clams *(The Budget Gourmet Light
and Healthy)*, 9.5 oz. 34.0
with shrimp *(Healthy Choice)*, 9.5 oz. 40.0
with shrimp and clams *(The Budget Gourmet)*, 10 oz. 35.0
Liquor[1], all proofs, 1 fl. oz. .... tr.

---

[1] *Includes all pure distilled liquors: bourbon, brandy, gin, rum, Scotch, tequila, vodka, whiskey, etc.*

Little Caesars, 1 serving:
Baby Pan!Pan! 53.0
Crazy Bread, 1 piece 18.0
Crazy Sauce 11.0
Pizza!Pizza!, cheese, 1 slice:
  round, small 14.0
  round, medium 16.0
  round, large 18.0
  square, small, medium, or large 22.0
Pizza!Pizza!, cheese and pepperoni, 1 slice:
  round, small 14.0
  round, medium 16.0
  round, large 18.0
  square, small, medium, or large 22.0
Slice!Slice! 71.0
salads:
  antipasto, small 8.0
  Greek, small 6.0
  tossed, small 7.0
sandwiches:
  ham and cheese or Italian 47.0
  tuna 51.0
  turkey 49.0
  veggie 48.0
Liver:
beef, pan-fried, 4 oz. 8.9
chicken, simmered, 4 oz. 1.0
chicken, simmered, chopped, 1 cup 1.2
duck, raw, 1 oz. 1.0
goose, raw, 1 oz. 1.8
lamb or pork, pan-fried or braised, 4 oz. 4.3
turkey, simmered, 4 oz. 3.9
turkey, simmered, chopped, 1 cup 4.8
veal (calves), braised, 4 oz. 3.1
Liver cheese *(Oscar Mayer),* 1 slice .... <1.0
Liver loaf *(Kahn's),* 1 slice 3.0
Liver pâté, see "Pâté"

Liver sausage (see also "Braunschweiger"):
(Jones Dairy Farm/Jones Dairy Farm Chub/Lowfat),
  1 oz. ....tr.
Lobster, northern, meat only:
raw, 4 oz. 6
boiled or steamed, 4 oz. 1.5
boiled or steamed, 1 cup, 5.1 oz. 1.9
"Lobster," imitation *(Louis Kemp* Lobster Delights),
  2 oz. 5.0
Lobster, spiny, see "Spiny lobster"
Lobster Newburg, frozen *(Stouffer's),* 6.5 oz. 9.0
Lobster sauce, rock, canned *(Progresso),* ½ cup 11.0
Loganberries:
fresh, 1 cup 21.5
frozen, ½ cup 9.6
Long John Silver's:
à la carte:
  chicken, light herb, 3.5 oz. ....<1.0
  Chicken Planks, 1 piece 11.0
  fish, batter dipped, 1 piece 12.0
  fish, lemon crumb, baked, 5 oz. 4.0
  shrimp, batter dipped, 1 piece 2.0
  Chicken Planks, with fries, 2 pieces 50.0
sandwiches, 1 serving:
  chicken, batter dipped, without sauce 39.0
  fish, batter dipped, without sauce 40.0
soup and side dishes:
  coleslaw, fork drained, 3.4 oz. 20.0
  Corn Cobette, with prep, 1 piece 18.0
  fries, 3 oz. 28.0
  green beans, 3.5 oz. 3.0
  hushpuppy, 1 piece 10.0
  rice, 4 oz. 30.0
  roll, 1 piece 23.0
  seafood chowder, with cod, 7 oz. 10.0
  seafood gumbo, with cod, 7 oz. 4.0
finger food:
  Chicken Planks, 2 pieces 22.0

Long John Silver's, finger food *(cont.)*
fish, batter dipped, 1 piece 12.0
salads, without dressing or crackers, 1 serving:
  ocean chef 13.0
  seafood 12.0
  small 3.0
condiments and dressings:
  catsup, .32 oz. 2.0
  honey mustard sauce, .42 oz. 5.0
  Italian dressing, creamy, 1 oz. .... <1.0
  malt vinegar, .28 oz. 0
  ranch dressing, 1 oz. .... <1.0
  sea salad dressing, 1 oz. 2.0
  seafood sauce, .42 oz. 3.0
  sweet'n sour sauce, .42 oz. 5.0
  tartar sauce, .42 oz. 2.0
desserts, 1 serving:
  apple pie 45.0
  brownie, walnut 54.0
  cherry pie 55.0
  cookie, chocolate chip 35.0
  cookie, oatmeal raisin 15.0
  lemon pie 60.0
Longan, shelled:
fresh, seeded, 1 oz. 4.3
dried, 1 oz. 21.0
Loquat:
1 medium, .6 oz. 1.2
peeled, seeded, 1 oz. 3.4
Lotus root:
raw, trimmed, 1 oz. 4.9
boiled, drained, 4 oz. 18.2
Lotus seed:
raw, 1 oz. 4.9
dried, 1 oz. 18.3
fried, 1 cup 20.6
Lox, without added ingredients 0

Lunch combinations:
bologna and American cheese *(Lunchables)*, 1 pkg.......... 18.0
chicken and:
  Monterey jack cheese *(Lunchables)*, 1 pkg. 17.0
  Monterey jack cheese and fudge *(Lunchables)*,
    1 pkg. 31.0
  roast beef or turkey, deluxe *(Lunchables)*, 1 pkg........... 21.0
ham and:
  cheddar cheese *(Lunchables)*, 1 pkg............................. 18.0
  honey, American cheese and pudding
    (Lunchables), 1 pkg. 34.0
  honey, chicken, deluxe *(Lunchables)*, 1 pkg. 24.0
  roast beef, deluxe *(Lunchables)*, 1 pkg......................... 21.0
  Swiss cheese *(Lunchables)*, 1 pkg................................. 17.0
  Swiss cheese and cookies *(Lunchables)*, 1 pkg............. 27.0
salami and mozzarella cheese *(Lunchables)*, 1 pkg.......... 17.0
turkey and:
  cheddar cheese *(Lunchables)*, 1 pkg............................. 17.0
  ham, deluxe *(Lunchables)*, 1 pkg................................... 21.0
  smoked, Monterey jack cheese *(Lunchables)*,
    1 pkg. 19.0
spreadable:
  ham, garden vegetable *(Lunchables)*, 1 pkg. 33.0
  honey ham, herb and chive *(Lunchables)*, 1 pkg. 33.0
  turkey, green onion *(Lunchables)*, 1 pkg. 34.0
  smoked turkey, ranch and herb *(Lunchables)*,
    1 pkg. 31.0
Luncheon meat (see also specific listings):
spiced loaf *(Oscar Mayer)*, 1 slice 2.0
spiced loaf *(Kahn's)*, 1 slice.. 1.0
canned *(Spam/Deviled Spam)*, 1 oz. ....<2.0
canned *(Spam Less Salt/Lite)*, 2 oz. 1.0
Luncheon "meat," vegetarian, canned:
(LaLoma Nuteena), ½" slice 6.0
(Worthington Numete), ½" slice 7.0
(Worthington Protose), ½" slice.. 9.0
Lupin, boiled, ½ cup... 8.2

Lychee, shelled:
raw, seeded, 1 oz. 4.7
raw, peeled *(Frieda's)*, 1 oz. 4.6
dried, 1 oz. 20.0

M

Food and Measure	Carbohydrate Grams

Macadamia nuts, shelled:
raw *(Frieda's),* 1 oz. 4.5
dried, 1 oz. 3.9
dried, 1 cup 18.4
oil-roasted, 1 oz. 3.7
roasted, salted *(Master Choice),* 1 oz. 4.0
Macaroni (see also "Pasta"):
uncooked, 2 oz. 42.6
uncooked, elbow, 1 cup 78.4
cooked:
  4 oz. 32.1
  elbow, 1 cup 39.7
  small shells, 1 cup 32.6
  spirals, 1 cup 38.0
  vegetable (tricolor), 4 oz. 30.2
  whole-wheat, 4 oz. 30.1
Macaroni and cheese, see "Macaroni dinner" and
  "Macaroni entree"
Macaroni dinner, and cheese, frozen *(Swanson),*
  12.25 oz. 49.0
Macaroni entree, canned or packaged:
and beef, in sauce *(Libby's Diner),* 7.75 oz. 34.0
and cheese:
  (Franco-American), 7.35 oz. 24.0
  (Hormel Micro Cup), 7.5 oz. 28.0
  (Libby's Diner), 7.5 oz. 27.0
small, with tomato sauce *(Mother's Choice),* 7.5 oz. 29.0

Macaroni entree, frozen:
and beef:
(Healthy Choice Quick Meal), 8.5 oz. 32.0
(Weight Watchers), 9 oz. 31.0
with cheese (Swanson), 9 oz. 26.0
with tomatoes (Stouffer's), 11.5 oz. 38.0
in tomato sauce (Lean Cuisine), 10 oz. 35.0
and cheese:
(Banquet Casserole), 6.5 oz. 30.0
(Banquet Family), 7 oz. 28.0
(The Budget Gourmet Side Dish), 5.75 oz. 22.0
(Freezer Queen), 11.5 oz. 59.0
(Freezer Queen Family), 4.5 oz. 19.0
(Green Giant One Serving), 5.7 oz. 27.0
(Healthy Choice Quick Meal), 9 oz. 45.0
(Lean Cuisine), 9 oz. 37.0
(Morton Casserole), 6.5 oz. 30.0
(On-Cor), 8 oz. 27.0
(Stouffer's), 6 oz. 23.0
(Swanson), 7 oz. 24.0
(Swanson Entrees), 9 oz. 25.0
(Weight Watchers), 9 oz. 43.0
cheddar/Parmesan (The Budget Gourmet),
   10.5 oz. 49.0
nacho (Healthy Choice Quick Meal), 9 oz. 44.0
Macaroni entree mix*:
and cheese:
(Fantastic Foods), 1/2 cup 20.0
(Kraft Deluxe Dinner), 3/4 cup 36.0
(Kraft Dinner/Family Size Dinner), 3/4 cup 34.0
Parmesan, with whole milk (Fantastic Foods),
   1/2 cup 21.0
Parmesan, with skim milk (Fantastic Foods),
   1/2 cup 20.0
rotini, with broccoli (Velveeta), 1/2 cup 24.0
shells (Velveeta Dinner), 3/4 cup 25.0
shells, with bacon or Mexican (Velveeta Bits of
   Bacon/Touch of Mexico), 1/2 cup 27.0

spiral *(Kraft* Dinner), ¾ cup...36.0
salad, creamy *(Suddenly Salad),* ½ cup.............................21.0
Mace, ground, 1 tsp.. .9
Mackerel, fresh or canned, meat only...............................0
Mahi mahi, raw or cooked without added
   ingredients 0
Mai tai mixer:
bottled *(Holland House),* 4.5 fl. oz....................................36.0
instant *(Holland House),* .56 oz. 16.0
Malt cooler:
berry or peach *(Bartles & Jaymes),* 6 fl. oz.......................16.2
berry or tropical, light *(Bartles & Jaymes),* 6 fl. oz............15.6
cherry, black *(Bartles & Jaymes),* 6 fl. oz.........................15.0
cherry, black, light *(Bartles & Jaymes),* 6 fl. oz.................14.4
strawberry *(Bartles & Jaymes),* 6 fl. oz.............................15.6
tropical *(Bartles & Jaymes),* 6 fl. oz..................................18.0
Malted milk powder:
(Carnation Original), 3 heaping tsp...................................16.0
natural, 3 heaping tsp...15.9
chocolate, 3 heaping tsp...18.4
chocolate *(Carnation),* 3 heaping tsp.................................18.0
Mammy apple, peeled, seeded, 1 oz...............................3.5
Mango:
1 medium, 10.6 oz...35.2
peeled *(Frieda's),* 1 oz...4.8
peeled, sliced, ½ cup 14.0
Mango flavored drink mix* *(Tang),* 6 fl. oz. 20.0
Mango nectar:
(Kern's), 6 fl. oz...28.0
(Libby's), 6 fl. oz...26.0
Mango-peach juice *(R. W. Knudsen),* 8 fl. oz. 29.0
Manhattan mixer, bottled *(Holland House),* 1 fl. oz. 7.0
Manicotti, frozen *(Celentano),* 7 oz. 31.0
Manicotti entree, frozen:
(Celentano Great Choice), 10 oz. 41.0
cheese *(Healthy Choice),* 9.25 oz. 34.0
cheese *(Weight Watchers),* 9.25 oz. 31.0
cheese *(The Budget Gourmet),* 10 oz. 36.0

Manicotti entree *(cont.)*
Florentine *(Celentano* Great Choice), 10 oz. 29.0
with sauce *(Celentano),* 10 oz. 41.0
vegetable, marinara *(On-Cor),* 8 oz. 26.0
Maple sugar, see "Sugar, maple"
Maple syrup:
(Cary's/Maple Orchards/MacDonald's), 1 tbsp. 13.0
imitation *(Cary's* Sugar Free), 1 tbsp. 2.0
Margarine, all varieties and blends 0
Margarita mixer:
bottled *(Holland House),* 3 fl. oz. 18.0
bottled, strawberry *(Holland House),* 3.5 fl. oz. 24.0
frozen, with liquor* *(Bacardi),* 7 fl. oz. 24.0
instant *(Holland House),* .56 oz. dry 14.0
instant, strawberry *(Holland House),* .56 oz. dry 16.0
Marinade, see specific listings
Marjoram, dried, 1 tsp. 4
Marmalade, see "Jam and preserves"
Marrow squash, raw, trimmed, 1 oz. 1.0
Marshmallow topping:
(Smucker's), 2 tbsp. 29.0
creme *(Kraft),* 1 oz. 23.0
plain or raspberry *(Marshmallow Fluff),* 1 heaping
   tsp. 15.0
Matzo, see "Crackers"
Matzo meal, see "Cracker crumbs and meal"
Mayonnaise:
(Bennett's Real), 1 tbsp. 1.0
(Blue Plate), 1 tbsp. 0
(Cains All Natural), 1 tbsp. 0
(Hain/Hain Real No Salt), 1 tbsp. 0
(Hain Light Low Sodium), 1 tbsp. 2.0
(Hellmann's/Best Foods), 1 tbsp. 0
(Hellmann's/Best Foods Light), 1 tbsp. 1.0
(Kraft), 1 tbsp. 0
(Kraft Light), 1 tbsp. 1.0
(Master Choice), 1 tbsp. 0
(Rokeach), 1 tbsp. 0

(Smartbeat Fat Free), 1 tbsp... 3.0
canola *(Hain)*, 1 tbsp... <1.0
canola *(Hain* Reduced Calorie), 1 tbsp. 2.0
canola, corn, or soy *(Smartbeat* Light), 1 tbsp. 1.0
cholesterol free *(Hellmann's)*, 1 tbsp. 1.0
eggless or safflower *(Hain/Hain* No Salt), 1 tbsp..................... 0
soy *(Featherweight Soyamaise)*, 1 tbsp............................... 0
tofu *(Nasoya Nayonaise)*, 1 tbsp...................................... 1.0
McDonald's, 1 serving:
breakfast biscuit:
   with bacon, egg, and cheese... 33.0
   with biscuit spread or sausage....................................... 32.0
   with sausage and egg... 33.0
breakfast dishes:
   burrito 21.0
   eggs, scrambled.. 1.0
   hash browns... 15.0
   hotcakes, with syrup and margarine.............................. 74.0
   sausage 0
breakfast muffin:
   Egg McMuffin 28.0
   English, with spread 26.0
   Sausage McMuffin, with or without egg...................... 27.0
danish:
   apple.. 51.0
   cinnamon raisin 58.0
   iced cheese 42.0
   raspberry.. 62.0
muffin, fat-free, apple bran 40.0
sandwiches:
   Big Mac 42.0
   cheeseburger... 30.0
   chicken fajita.. 20.0
   Filet-O-Fish 38.0
   hamburger 30.0
   McChicken.. 39.0
   McLean Deluxe, with or without cheese...................... 35.0
   McRib 44.0

McDonald's, sandwiches *(cont.)*
Quarter Pounder, with or without cheese......................... 34.0
Chicken McNuggets:
4 piece.. 11.0
6 piece.. 17.0
9 piece.. 25.0
McNuggets sauces:
barbeque, 1.12 oz. 12.0
honey, ½ oz. 12.0
hot mustard, 1.05 oz. 8.0
sweet and sour, 1.12 oz. 14.0
french fries:
small.. 26.0
medium.. 36.0
large 46.0
salads:
chef.. 8.0
chicken, chunky.. 7.0
garden.. 6.0
side 4.0
salad dressing:
blue cheese, ½ oz. or ⅕ packet 1.0
ranch, ½ oz. or ¼ packet 1.0
red French, reduced calorie, ½ oz. or ¼ packet 5.0
Thousand Island, ½ oz. or ⅕ packet 4.0
vinaigrette, lite, ½ oz. or ¼ packet 2.0
pies and cookies:
baked apple pie... 35.0
cookies, Chocolaty Chip 42.0
cookies, *McDonaldland* 47.0
shakes, lowfat, 10.4 oz.:
chocolate 66.0
strawberry 67.0
vanilla.. 60.0
yogurt, frozen, lowfat:
cone, vanilla.. 22.0
sundae, hot caramel... 59.0
sundae, hot fudge 50.0

sundae, strawberry.. 49.0
Meat, see specific listings
Meat, potted, canned:
(Hormel), 1 oz..<2.0
(Libby's), 1.83 oz. 0
"Meat" loaf, vegetarian, mix:
(LaLoma Savory Dinner Loaf), 1/4 cup 4.0
(Natural Touch), 4 oz. 7.0
Meat loaf dinner, frozen:
(Armour Classics), 11.25 oz...................................... 32.0
(Banquet Extra Helping), 16.25 oz.............................. 60.0
(Freezer Queen), 9.5 oz.. 23.0
(Swanson 4 Compartment), 10 oz. 38.0
(Swanson Hungry Man), 16.5 oz. 60.0
Meat loaf entree, frozen:
(Banquet Healthy Balance), 11 oz. 36.0
(Banquet Meals), 9.5 oz... 32.0
(On-Cor), 8 oz. 15.0
gravy, whipped potato *(Stouffer's* Homestyle),
   9 7/8 oz.. 20.0
with macaroni and cheese *(Lean Cuisine),* 9 3/8 oz. 26.0
with tomato sauce *(Banquet Entree Express),* 7 oz........... 16.0
Meat loaf seasoning mix:
(French's), 1/7 pkg. 3.0
(French's Roasting Bag),* 1/6 pkg.................................... 3.0
(Lawry's Seasoning Blends),* 1 pkg. 64.5
(McCormick/Schilling Bag'n Season),* 1 pkg...................... 26.0
Meat marinade mix *(French's),* 1/16 pkg. 1.0
Meat tenderizer, unseasoned *(Tone's),* 1 tsp. 1.2
"Meatball," vegetarian:
canned *(LaLoma Tender Rounds),* 6 pieces....................... 7.0
canned *(Worthington Non-Meat Balls),* 3 pieces 5.0
frozen *(LaLoma Savory Meatballs),* 7 pieces 7.0
Meatball dinner, Swedish, frozen *(Armour Classics),*
   11.25 oz.. 23.0
Meatball entree, Swedish, frozen:
(On-Cor), 8 oz. 7.0
in cream sauce *(Swanson),* 8.5 oz. 26.0

Meatball entree *(cont.)*
in gravy with pasta *(Lean Cuisine)*, 9¹/₈ oz. 31.0
in gravy with parsley noodles *(Stouffer's)*, 9.25 oz. 42.0
with noodles *(The Budget Gourmet)*, 10 oz. 37.0
sauce and *(Dining Lite)*, 9 oz. 34.0
Meatball seasoning mix, Swedish *(McCormick/*
 Schilling), ¹/₄ pkg. 11.0
Meatball stew, canned, *(Dinty Moore)*, 8 oz. 14.0
Melon balls, cantaloupe and honeydew, frozen,
 ¹/₂ cup 6.9
Menudo seasoning mix *(Gebhardt)*, 1 tsp. 1.0
Mesquite marinade *(Lawry's)*, 2 tbsp. 3.0
Mesquite seasoning *(Tone's)*, 1 tsp. 3.2
Mexican beans, canned:
(Allens/Brown Beauty), ¹/₂ cup 24.0
(Old El Paso Mexe-Beans), ¹/₂ cup 31.0
Mexican bean dip *(Hain)*, 4 tbsp. 9.0
Mexican dinner, frozen (see also specific listings):
(Patio Fiesta), 12 oz. 54.0
(Swanson Hungry Man), 20 oz. 88.0
style:
  (Banquet Extra Helping), 19 oz. 102.0
  (Patio), 13.25 oz. 64.0
  combination *(Swanson* 4 Compartment), 13.25 oz. 61.0
Mexican entree, frozen (see also specific listings):
combination *(Banquet Meals)*, 11 oz. 54.0
style *(Banquet Meals)*, 11 oz. 53.0
Mexican seasoning:
(Tone's), 1 tsp. 1.3
rice *(Lawry's Seasoning Blends)*, 1 pkg. 17.0
Milk:
buttermilk, cultured, 1 cup 11.7
whole, 3.3% fat, 1 cup 11.4
lowfat:
  2% or 1% fat, 1 cup 11.7
  2%, protein fortified, 1 cup 13.5
  1%, protein fortified, 1 cup 13.6
skim, 1 cup 11.9

Milk, canned:
condensed, sweet:
  1 tbsp. 10.4
  (Borden), ⅓ cup 54.0
  (Carnation), ⅓ cup.. 56.0
  (Eagle/Meadow Gold), 3 tbsp. 32.0
  filled dairy blend *(Magnolia)*, 3 tbsp................ 33.0
evaporated:
  (Carnation/Carnation Lowfat), ½ cup.............. 12.0
  (Pet/Dairymate), ½ cup 12.0
  imitation, filled *(Diehl)*, ½ cup 12.0
  skim *(Carnation Lite)*, ½ cup........................... 14.0
  skim *(Pet/Dairymate Light)*, ½ cup 14.0
Milk, chocolate, see "Chocolate milk"
Milk, dry:
buttermilk, sweet cream, 1 cup........................... 58.8
buttermilk, sweet cream, 1 tbsp. 3.2
whole, 1 oz.. 10.9
whole, 1 cup 49.2
nonfat:
  regular, 1 cup 62.4
  instant, 3.2-oz. packet 35.5
  instant *(Carnation)*, 5 level tbsp. 12.0
Milk, goat's, 1 cup... 10.9
"Milk," imitation:
fluid[1], 1 cup.. 15.0
soy, see "Soy milk"
Milk, sheep's, 1 cup.. 13.1
Milk beverage, see "Milk shake" and specific
  flavors
Milkfish, without added ingredients 0
Milk shake, frozen, chocolate *(Micro-Magic)*,
  1 shake.. 46.0
Milk shake mix:
chocolate fudge *(Weight Watchers)*, 1 packet 11.0
orange sherbet *(Weight Watchers)*, 1 packet..................... 12.0

---
[1] *Containing a blend of hydrogenated vegetable oils.*

Millet:
uncooked, 1 oz. 20.7
cooked, 4 oz. 26.8
hulled, uncooked *(Arrowhead Mills)*, 1 oz. 21.0
Millet flour *(Arrowhead Mills)*, 2 oz. 41.0
Mincemeat, see "Pie filling"
Miso:
1 oz. 7.9
½ cup 38.6
Molasses:
bead *(La Choy)*, ½ tsp. 2.0
dark or light *(Brer Rabbit)*, 1 tbsp. 14.0
gold or green *(Grandma's)*, 1 tbsp. 17.0
Monkfish, without added ingredients 0
Monosodium glutamate *(Tone's)*, 1 tsp. 0
Mortadella, beef and pork, 1 oz. 9
Mostaccioli entree, frozen:
with meat sauce *(Banquet Family)*, 7 oz. 28.0
with meatballs *(On-Cor)*, 8 oz. 30.0
Mothbeans, boiled, 4 oz. 23.8
Mother's loaf, pork, 1 oz. 2.1
Mousse, frozen:
chocolate *(Weight Watchers Sweet Celebrations)*,
   1 serving 26.0
chocolate caramel, triple *(Weight Watchers Sweet*
   Celebrations), 1 serving 31.0
praline pecan *(Weight Watchers Sweet Celebrations)*,
   1 serving 25.0
Mousse mix, chocolate:
dark or white *(Knorr)*, 1 serving dry 8.2
milk *(Knorr)*, 1 serving dry 9.9
Muffin:
(Arnold Bran'nola), 1 piece 30.0
(Arnold Extra Crisp), 1 piece 26.0
apple:
   (Awrey's), 1.5-oz. piece 17.0
   spice *(Health Valley)*, 1 piece 30.0
   streusel *(Awrey's)*, 1 piece 50.0

streusel *(Hostess* 97% Fat Free), 1 piece...................... 23.0
banana:
  (Health Valley), 1 piece.................................... 29.0
  nut *(Awrey's* Grande), 1 piece 55.0
  walnut, mini *(Hostess)*, 5 pieces 27.0
blueberry:
  (Awrey's), 1.5-oz. piece... 18.0
  (Awrey's Grande), 1 piece.. 52.0
  (Hostess 97% Fat Free), 1 piece 21.0
  apple *(Health Valley* Twin Pack), 1 piece 32.0
  mini *(Hostess)*, 5 pieces 29.0
carrot *(Health Valley* Twin Pack), 1 piece 30.0
cinnamon apple, mini *(Hostess)*, 5 pieces............... 17.0
cranberry *(Awrey's)*, 1 piece 20.0
corn *(Awrey's)*, 1.5-oz. piece.................................... 20.0
English:
  (Pepperidge Farm), 1 piece.................................... 27.0
  (Roman Meal), 1 piece 24.6
  (Tastykake), 1 piece 26.0
  (Thomas'), 1 piece 25.0
  (Wonder Rounds), 1 piece 24.0
  bran nut *(Thomas')*, 1 piece 23.0
  cinnamon raisin *(Oatmeal Goodness)*, 1 piece.............. 26.0
  cinnamon raisin *(Pepperidge Farm)*, 1 piece.................. 29.0
  cinnamon raisin *(Tastykake)*, 1 piece............................... 31.0
  cinnamon-raisin bran *(Pepperidge Farm*
    Wholesome Choice), 1 piece.................................. 28.0
  honey & oatmeal *(Oatmeal Goodness)*, 1 piece 24.0
  honey wheat *(Thomas')*, 1 piece................................. 21.0
  oat bran *(Thomas'* 12 Pack), 1 piece............................. 26.0
  onion *(Thomas')*, 1 piece... 27.0
  raisin *(Thomas')*, 1 piece 30.0
  raisin *(Wonder* Rounds), 1 piece.................................. 26.0
  rye *(Thomas')*, 1 piece... 24.0
  sandwich size *(Thomas')*, 1 piece................................... 42.0
  sourdough *(Tastykake)*, 1 piece.................................... 25.0
  sourdough *(Thomas')*, 1 piece 26.0
  sourdough *(Wonder* Rounds), 1 piece............................. 24.0

Muffin, English *(cont.)*
  white, country *(Pepperidge Farm* Wholesome
    Choice), 1 piece.. 26.0
  oat bran:
    (Hostess), 1 piece.. 21.0
    almond date or raisin *(Health Valley* Fancy Fruit),
      1 piece 31.0
    banana nut *(Hostess),* 1 piece 20.0
    blueberry *(Health Valley* Fancy Fruit), 1 piece 32.0
  raisin:
    (Arnold), 1 piece 33.0
    bran *(Awrey's),* 1.5-oz. piece 18.0
    bran *(Awrey's* Grande), 1 piece 50.0
  raspberry *(Health Valley* Twin Pack), 1 piece 30.0
  sourdough *(Arnold),* 1 piece 25.0
Muffin, frozen or refrigerated:
  apple oatmeal *(Pepperidge Farm* Wholesome
    Choice), 1 piece 28.0
  apple spice *(Healthy Choice),* 1 piece................................. 40.0
  banana nut *(Healthy Choice),* 1 piece 32.0
  banana nut *(Weight Watchers),* 1 piece 32.0
  blueberry:
    (Healthy Choice), 1 piece 39.0
    (Pepperidge Farm Wholesome Choice), 1 piece 27.0
    (Weight Watchers), 1 piece 32.0
  bran, harvest honey *(Weight Watchers),* 1 piece 32.0
  corn *(Pepperidge Farm* Wholesome Choice), 1 piece 28.0
  English *(Roman Meal),* 1 piece 28.7
  English, honey nut oat bran *(Roman Meal),* 1 piece.......... 31.5
  raisin bran *(Pepperidge Farm* Wholesome Choice),
    1 piece 30.0
Muffin mix*:
  apple cinnamon *(Betty Crocker),* 1 piece 18.0
  apple cinnamon *(Robin Hood/Gold Medal* Pouch),
    1 piece 24.0
  banana *(Robin Hood/Gold Medal* Pouch), 1 piece 22.0
  banana nut *(Betty Crocker),* 1 piece.................................... 18.0

blueberry:
   (Betty Crocker Twice the Blueberries), 1 piece 18.0
   (Duncan Hines), 1 piece 21.0
   (Duncan Hines Bakery Style), 1 piece 32.0
   (Pillsbury Lovin' Lites), 1 piece... 21.0
   (Robin Hood/Gold Medal Pouch), 1 piece..................... 25.0
   wild *(Betty Crocker),* 1 piece.. 19.0
   wild *(Betty Crocker* Light), 1 piece.................................... 20.0
caramel *(Robin Hood/Gold Medal* Pouch), 1 piece 24.0
cinnamon streusel *(Betty Crocker),* 1 piece 27.0
cinnamon swirl *(Duncan Hines* Bakery Style), 1 piece 32.0
corn:
   (Dromedary), 1 piece 20.0
   (Robin Hood/Gold Medal Pouch), 1 piece..................... 27.0
   blue *(Arrowhead Mills),* 1 piece... 15.0
honey bran *(Robin Hood/Gold Medal* Pouch), 1 piece...... 25.0
oat bran:
   (Arrowhead Mills Wheat Free), 1 piece............................ 11.0
   (Betty Crocker), 1 piece 26.0
   apple spice *(Arrowhead Mills),* 1 piece............................ 15.0
wheat bran *(Arrowhead Mills),* 1 piece................................ 43.0
Mulberries:
10 berries, ½ oz... 1.5
½ cup... 6.9
Mullet, without added ingredients 0
Mung beans, dry:
(Arrowhead Mills), 2 oz. 7.0
boiled, ½ cup.. 19.3
Mung beans, sprouted, fresh:
raw, 1 oz. 1.7
boiled, drained, ½ cup 2.6
Mungo beans, boiled, ½ cup.. 16.5
Mushroom:
fresh, raw, pieces, ½ cup.. 1.6
fresh, boiled, drained, pieces, ½ cup 4.0
canned:
   all cuts, plain or with garlic *(B in B),* ¼ cup..................... 2.0
   all cuts *(Green Giant),* ¼ cup.. 2.0

Mushroom, canned *(cont.)*
in butter sauce *(Green Giant)*, ½ cup 4.0
straw *(Green Giant)*, ¼ cup 2.0
frozen:
whole *(Birds Eye* Deluxe), 2.6 oz. 4.0
battered *(Qwik Krisp)*, 7 pieces 13.0
breaded *(Ore-Ida)*, 2.67 oz. 12.0
breaded *(Stilwell)*, 5 pieces 13.0
Mushroom, enoki:
1 large, 4⅛" long 4
trimmed, 1 oz. 2.2
Mushroom, Japanese honey, trimmed *(Frieda's)*,
1 oz. 1.2
Mushroom, oyster, fresh or dried *(Frieda's)*, 1 oz. 1.3
Mushroom, shiitake:
fresh, raw *(Frieda's)*, 1 oz. 3.2
fresh, cooked, 4 medium or ½ cup pieces 10.4
dried, 4 medium, ½ oz. 11.3
Mushroom, Yamabiko honshimeji *(Frieda's)*, 1 oz. 1.2
Mushroom gravy:
canned:
(Franco-American), 2 oz. 3.0
(Heinz HomeStyle), 2 oz. 3.0
with wine *(Pepperidge Farm)*, ¼ cup 4.0
mix:
(French's), ¼ pkg. 3.0
(LaLoma Gravy Quik), 2 tbsp.* 2.0
(McCormick/Schilling), ¼ cup* 3.0
Mushroom and herb dip *(Breakstone's* Gourmet),
2 tbsp. 2.0
Mussels, blue, meat only:
raw, 4 oz. 4.2
raw, 1 cup 5.5
boiled or steamed, 4 oz. 8.4
Mustard, prepared:
(Kraft Pure), 1 tbsp. 1.0
blend *(Hellmann's* Dijonnaise), 1 tsp. 1.0
brown *(Heinz* Spicy), 1 tbsp. 1.0

creamy mild or spicy brown *(Gulden's)*, ¼ oz. 0
Dijon *(French's)*, 1 tsp... 0
Dijon *(Grey Poupon)*, 1 tbsp. 0
with horseradish *(French's)*, 1 tbsp. 1.0
with horseradish *(Kraft)*, 1 tbsp. 1.0
hot *(Gulden's* Diablo), ¼ oz. 0
mild, yellow *(Heinz)*, 1 tbsp.. 1.0
with onion *(French's)*, 1 tsp. 2.0
spicy *(French's* Bold'n Spicy), 1 tsp. 0
stone ground *(Hain/Hain* No Salt), 1 tbsp. 1.0
yellow or Medford *(French's)*, 1 tbsp. 1.0
Mustard greens:
fresh, raw, chopped, 1 oz., ½ cup.............................. 1.4
fresh, boiled, drained, chopped, ½ cup...................... 1.5
canned *(Allens/Sunshine)*, ½ cup 2.0
frozen, chopped *(Frosty Acres)*, 3.3 oz. 3.0
frozen, chopped *(Seabrook)*, 3.3 oz. 3.0
Mustard powder *(Spice Islands)*, 1 tsp. 3
Mustard seeds, yellow, 1 tsp.................................... 1.2
Mustard spinach:
raw, chopped, ½ cup.. 2.9
boiled, drained, chopped, ½ cup................................ 2.5
Mustard tallow.. 0

N

Food and Measure	Carbohydrate Grams

Nacho dip, see "Cheese dip"
Nachos, mix, regular or jalapeño:
(Tio Sancho Microwave Snacks):
    chips, 4 oz. 74.4
    cheese sauce, 3.5 oz. 2.3
Natto, ½ cup 12.6
Navy beans:
dry, boiled, ½ cup 24.0
canned, with liquid, ½ cup 26.8
canned *(Allens),* ½ cup 24.0
Navy beans, sprouted:
raw, ½ cup 6.8
boiled, drained, 4 oz. 17.0
Nectarine:
1 medium, 2½" diameter 16.0
sliced, ½ cup 8.1
New England Brand sausage *(Oscar Mayer),*
    2 slices .... <1.0
New Zealand spinach:
raw, chopped, 1 oz. or ½ cup 7
boiled, drained, chopped, ½ cup 2.0
Newberg sauce, canned, with sherry *(Snow's),*
    ⅓ cup 10.0
Newberg sauce mix *(Knorr),* 1 serving 2.9
Noodle, egg:
uncooked, 2 oz.:
    (Creamette), 2 oz. 40.0
    (Herb's Organic), 2 oz. 40.0

(Prince), 2 oz... 40.0
cooked, 1 cup 39.7
cooked, spinach, 1 cup 38.8
precooked, frozen *(Aunt Vi's)*, 4 oz. 13.0
Noodle, Chinese:
(Azumaya), 1 oz... 16.6
cellophane or long rice, dry, 2 oz. 48.8
chow mein, ½ cup... 13.0
chow mein, narrow or wide *(La Choy)*, ½ cup................... 16.0
fried *(Frieda's Crispy)*, 1 oz... 18.0
rice *(La Choy)*, ½ cup 21.0
Noodle, Japanese:
(Azumaya), 1 oz... 16.6
soba, dry, 2 oz... 42.5
soba, cooked, 1 cup 24.4
somen, dry, 2 oz.. 42.2
somen, cooked, 1 cup 48.5
udon, dry, 2 oz.. 32.3
udon, cooked, 4 oz... 23.0
Noodle and chicken dinner, frozen *(Swanson)*,
  10.5 oz... 31.0
Noodle and chicken dishes:
canned *(Dinty Moore American Classics)*, 10 oz. 24.0
canned *(Hormel Micro Cup)*, 7.5 oz. 19.0
freeze-dried* *(Mountain House)*, 1 cup............................. 28.0
Noodle dishes, mix*:
Alfredo, Alfredo broccoli, or carbonara Alfredo
  (Lipton Noodles and Sauce), ½ cup............................... 22.0
beef *(Lipton* Noodles and Sauce), ½ cup 22.0
broccoli au gratin *(Noodle Roni)*, ½ cup 23.0
butter or butter and herb *(Lipton* Noodles and
  Sauce), ½ cup 22.0
cheddar, white, shells *(Noodle Roni)*, ½ cup..................... 23.0
cheddar bacon *(Lipton* Noodles and Sauce), ½ cup 22.0
cheese:
  (Lipton Noodles and Sauce), ½ cup.............................. 24.0
  with egg noodles *(Kraft* Dinner), ¾ cup 37.0
  fettuccine *(Noodle Roni)*, ½ cup..................................... 22.0

Noodle dishes, mix *(cont.)*
chicken:
   (Lipton Noodles and Sauce), ½ cup.............................. 22.0
   broccoli *(Lipton* Noodles and Sauce), ½ cup................ 24.0
   creamy *(Lipton* Noodles and Sauce), ½ cup................. 23.0
   with egg noodles *(Kraft* Dinner), ¾ cup 32.0
garlic, creamy *(Noodle Roni)*, ½ cup.................................. 24.0
Parmesan *(Noodle Roni Parmesano)*, ½ cup..................... 24.0
Parmesan or with herbs, angel hair *(Noodle Roni)*,
  ½ cup 26.0
Parmesan or Romanoff *(Lipton* Noodles and Sauce),
  ½ cup 22.0
sour cream and chive *(Lipton* Noodles and Sauce),
  ½ cup 23.0
Stroganoff *(Lipton* Noodles and Sauce), ½ cup 20.0
Noodle entree, frozen:
and beef, with gravy *(Banquet* Family), 7 oz. 20.0
Romanoff *(Stouffer's)*, 6 oz.. 22.0
Nut topping (see also specific listings):
(Fisher Fancy), 1 oz.. 7.0
oil-roasted, with peanuts *(Fisher)*, 1 oz. 7.0
Nutmeg, ground, 1 tsp.. 1.1
Nuts, see specific listings
Nuts, mixed:
(Flavor House Deluxe), 1 oz.. 5.0
dry-roasted:
   with peanuts, 1 oz.. 7.2
   (Fisher), 1 oz. 7.0
   (Flavor House), 1 oz. 8.0
oil-roasted:
   with peanuts, 1 oz.. 6.1
   (Fisher/Fisher Lightly Salted), 1 oz............................... 6.0
   (Flavor House), 1 oz. 4.0
cashews and almonds, oil-roasted *(Fisher)*, 1 oz. 6.0
peanuts and cashews, honey-roasted *(Fisher)*, 1 oz. 6.0

O

Food and Measure   Carbohydrate Grams

Oat bran:
raw, 1 oz. 18.8
cooked, 1 cup 25.1
Oat flour *(Arrowhead Mills)*, 2 oz. 43.0
Oat groats *(Arrowhead Mills)*, 2 oz. 38.0
Oats (see also "Cereal"):
whole-grain, 1 oz. 18.8
flakes *(Arrowhead Mills)*, 2 oz. 39.0
rolled or oatmeal, dry, 1 oz. 19.0
rolled or oatmeal, cooked, 1 cup 25.2
steel cut *(Arrowhead Mills)*, 2 oz. 37.0
Ocean perch, without added ingredients 0
Ocean perch entree, frozen:
battered *(Gorton's Crispy)*, 2 pieces 19.0
breaded *(Van de Kamp's Light)*, 1 piece 21.0
Octopus, meat only:
raw, 4 oz. 2.5
boiled or steamed, 4 oz. 5.0
Oheloberries, ½ cup 4.8
Oil, all varieties 0
Okara, see "Tofu"
Okra:
fresh:
  raw, sliced, ½ cup 3.8
  boiled, drained, 8 pods, 3″ × ⅝″ 6.1
  boiled drained, sliced, ½ cup 5.8
canned, cut *(Allens)*, ½ cup 2.0

Okra *(cont.)*
canned, with tomatoes *(Allens)*, ½ cup............................... 3.0
frozen:
  boiled, drained, sliced, ½ cup 7.5
  whole *(Seabrook)*, 3.3 oz............................... 7.0
  whole *(Stilwell)*, 9 pieces............................... 6.0
  whole, baby *(Frosty Acres)*, 3.3 oz. 7.0
  cut *(Seabrook)*, 3.3 oz. 6.0
  cut *(Stilwell)*, ¾ cup or 3 oz............................... 4.0
  breaded *(Ore-Ida)*, 3 oz............................... 17.0
  breaded *(Stilwell* Light), 21 pieces or 3 oz. 14.0
Old-fashioned mixer, bottled *(Holland House)*,
  1 fl. oz............................... 8.0
Old-fashioned loaf *(Oscar Mayer)*, 1 slice 2.0
Olive, pickled:
Alfonso *(Krinos)*, ½ oz. 1.0
Calamata or Nafplion *(Krinos)*, ½ oz. 2.0
green, with pits:
  10 small 4
  10 large............................... .5
  10 giant............................... .9
green, pitted, 1 oz............................... .4
green, Greek, cracked *(Krinos)*, ½ oz. 1.0
ripe, all varieties, except Spanish *(Vlasic)*, ½ oz............................... 1.0
ripe, oil-cured *(Progresso)*, 5 medium 3.0
ripe, imported *(Krinos)*, ½ oz............................... 3.0
ripe, salt-cured, Greek style:
  10 medium............................... 1.7
  10 extra large............................... 2.3
  pitted, 1 oz. 2.5
  imported *(Krinos)*, ½ oz............................... 1.0
ripe, Spanish, all varieties *(Vlasic)*, ½ oz............................... 1.0
royal *(Krinos)*, ½ oz............................... 1.0
Olive loaf *(Oscar Mayer)*, 1 slice............................... 3.0
Olive oil............................... 0
Olive salad *(Progresso)*, ½ cup 5.0
Omelet, see "Egg breakfast"

Onion, mature:
fresh or stored:
  raw, 1 oz... 2.4
  raw, chopped, ½ cup.. 6.9
  raw, chopped, 1 tbsp... .9
  boiled, drained, chopped, ½ cup 10.7
in jars:
  cocktail, regular or spiced *(Vlasic),* 1 oz. 1.0
  sweet *(Heinz),* 1 oz. 9.0
  wild, marinated *(Krinos* Volvi), 1 oz.................. 2.0
frozen:
  whole, small *(Seabrook),* 3.3 oz. 8.0
  chopped, boiled, drained, 1 tbsp. 1.0
  chopped *(Ore-Ida),* 2 oz..................................... 4.0
  chopped *(Seabrook),* 1 oz.................................. 2.0
  with cream sauce *(Birds Eye),* 5 oz. 12.0
  rings, see "Onion rings"
Onion, dried:
flakes, 1 tbsp. 4.2
minced *(Lawry's* Spice Blends), 1 tsp..................... 1.6
Onion, green (scallion), raw, trimmed, with tops:
chopped, ½ cup 3.7
chopped, 1 tbsp. 4
Onion, Welsh, trimmed, 1 oz............................... 1.8
Onion dip:
creamy *(Kraft* Premium), 2 tbsp............................ 2.0
French:
  (Breakstone's/Sealtest), 2 tbsp. 2.0
  (Frito-Lay's), 2 tbsp. 3.0
  (Kraft Premium), 2 tbsp. 2.0
French or green onion *(Kraft),* 2 tbsp...................... 3.0
toasted *(Breakstone's* Gourmet), 2 tbsp. 2.0
Onion chive dip mix *(Knorr),* 1 serving.................. .7
Onion flavor snack, rings *(Tom's),* ¾ oz. 12.0
Onion gravy:
canned *(Heinz),* 2 oz. 4.0
mix:
  (French's), ¼ pkg...4.0

Onion gravy, mix *(cont.)*
(*LaLoma Gravy Quik*), 2 tbsp.* 2.0
(*McCormick/Schilling*), ¼ cup* 3.6
Onion powder *(Spice Islands)*, 1 tsp. 1.7
Onion ring batter mix *(Golden Dipt)*, 1 oz. 22.0
Onion rings, frozen:
(*Ore-Ida Onion Ringers*), 2 oz. 17.0
(*Qwik-Krisp* Natural Cut), 4 pieces 22.0
(*Stilwell* Crispy Crunchy), 6 pieces 30.0
battered:
  (*Farm Rich*), 4 oz. 32.0
  (*Mrs. Paul's* Crispy), 2 oz. 15.0
  beer (*Stilwell*), 4 pieces 21.0
Onion salt *(Tone's)*, 1 tsp. 4
Orange:
California:
  navel, 1 medium, 2⅞"-diameter 16.3
  navel, sections without membrane, ½ cup 9.6
  Valencia, 1 medium, 2⅝" diameter 14.4
  Valencia, sections without membrane, ½ cup 10.7
Florida, 1 medium, 2¹¹⁄₁₆"-diameter 17.4
Florida, sections without membrane, ½ cup 10.7
peel, 1 tbsp. 1.5
Orange, canned, Mandarin, see "Tangerine"
Orange drink:
canned *(Hi-C)*, 6 fl. oz. 23.0
canned *(Kool-Aid Kool Bursts)*, 6.75 oz. 34.0
mix*:
  (Kool-Aid), 8 fl. oz. 25.0
  (Kool-Aid Presweetened), 8 fl. oz. 18.0
  (Tang), 6 fl. oz. 19.0
  (Tang Sugar Free), 6 fl. oz. 1.0
Orange float *(R.W. Knudsen)*, 8 fl. oz. 27.0
Orange fruit juice blend *(Mott's)*, 11.5 fl. oz. 46.0
Orange juice:
fresh, 6 fl. oz. 19.3
canned or bottled:
  (Libby's), 6 fl. oz. 20.0

(Minute Maid), 6 fl. oz. 20.0
(Ocean Spray 100%), 6 fl. oz. 19.0
(R.W. Knudsen), 8 fl. oz. 22.0
(Tree Top), 6 fl. oz. 22.0
blend *(Minute Maid)*, 6 fl. oz. 22.0
blend *(Welch's)*, 6 fl. oz. 22.0
chilled:
  6 fl. oz. 18.8
  (Tropicana), 6 fl. oz. 16.0
  (Tropicana Pure Premium), 6 fl. oz. 19.0
  all varieties, except Premium Choice *(Minute
    Maid)*, 6 fl. oz. 20.0
  regular or country style *(Minute Maid* Premium
    Choice)*, 6 fl. oz. 21.0
frozen*:
  6 fl. oz. 20.1
  (TreeSweet), 6 fl. oz. 20.0
  all varieties *(Minute Maid)*, 6 fl. oz. 20.0
cocktail *(Ocean Spray)*, 6 fl. oz. 25.0
Orange juice drink:
(Kool-Aid Koolers), 8.45 fl. oz. 30.0
(Shasta Plus), 12 fl. oz. 46.0
(Tang Fruit Box), 8.45 fl. oz. 32.0
tropical *(Tang Fruit Box)*, 8.45 fl. oz. 37.0
chilled *(Bright & Early)*, 6 fl. oz. 21.0
chilled *(Tropicana)*, 6 fl. oz. 22.0
frozen* *(Bright & Early)*, 6 fl. oz. 21.0
Orange sauce, Mandarin *(La Choy)*, 1 tbsp. 6.1
Orange-banana juice:
(Chiquita), 6 fl. oz. 22.0
(Smucker's Naturally 100%), 8 fl. oz. 30.0
Orange-banana juice drink *(Boku)*, 6 fl. oz. 22.0
Orange-banana nectar *(Kern's)*, 6 fl. oz. 25.0
Orange-cranberry juice *(Master Choice Tropical
  Shakers)*, 6 fl. oz. 25.0
Orange-cranberry juice drink:
(Ocean Spray Refreshers), 6 fl. oz. 26.0
(Tropicana), 6 fl. oz. 23.0

Orange-cranberry juice drink *(cont.)*
(Tropicana Twister Light), 6 fl. oz. 4.0
Orange-grapefruit juice, canned, 6 fl. oz. 19.1
Orange-kiwi-passion fruit juice *(Tropicana),* 6 fl. oz. 17.0
Orange-mango juice:
(R.W. Knudsen), 8 fl. oz. 24.0
drink *(Tropicana Twisters),* 6 fl. oz. 21.0
Orange-passion fruit juice drink *(Tropicana*
Twister), 6 fl. oz. 19.0
Orange-peach juice *(Master Choice Tropical*
Shakers), 6 fl. oz. 25.0
Orange-peach juice drink:
(Boku), 6 fl. oz. 22.0
(Tropicana Twister), 6 fl. oz. 21.0
Orange-peach-mango juice *(Tropicana),* 6 fl. oz. 19.0
Orange-pineapple juice *(Tropicana),* 6 fl. oz. 19.0
Orange-raspberry juice *(Master Choice Tropical*
Shakers), 6 fl. oz. 25.0
Orange-raspberry juice drink:
(Tropicana Twister), 6 fl. oz. 20.0
(Tropicana Twister Light), 6 fl. oz. 6.0
Orange-strawberry-banana juice:
(Master Choice Tropical Shakers), 6 fl. oz. 25.0
(Tropicana), 6 fl. oz. 18.0
Orange-strawberry-banana juice drink:
(Tropicana Twister), 6 fl. oz. 20.0
(Tropicana Twister Light), 6 fl. oz. 6.0
Orange-strawberry-guava juice drink *(Tropicana*
Twister), 6 fl. oz. 20.0
Oregano, dried *(Spice Islands),* 1 tsp. 1.0
Oriental 5-spice *(Tone's),* 1 tsp. 1.9
Oriental seasoning and coating mix *(McCormick/*
Schilling Bag'n Season), 1 pkg. 31.0
Oyster plant, see "Salsify"
Oyster stew, see "Soup"
Oysters, meat only:
Eastern, wild:
    raw, 1 lb. 17.7

    raw, 6 medium, 3 oz. 3.3
    baked, broiled, or microwaved, 4 oz. 5.4
    steamed or poached, 4 oz. 8.9
Eastern, farmed, raw, 4 oz. 6.3
Eastern, farmed, baked, broiled, or microwaved,
    4 oz. 8.3
Pacific:
    raw, 4 oz. 5.6
    raw, boiled, or steamed, 1 medium 2.5
    boiled or steamed, 4 oz. 11.2
Oysters, canned, Eastern:
(Bumble Bee), 1 cup 15.4
wild, with liquid, 4 oz. 4.4
wild, with liquid, 1 cup 9.7

P

Food and Measure	Carbohydrate Grams

P&B loaf *(Kahn's)*, 1 slice.. 1.0
Pancake, frozen:
(Aunt Jemima Original), 3 pieces............................. 38.0
(Hungry Jack Microwave Original), 3 pieces 49.0
blueberry *(Hungry Jack Microwave)*, 3 pieces 47.0
buttermilk *(Hungry Jack Microwave)*, 3 pieces 51.0
buttermilk or plain *(Downyflake)*, 3 pieces 45.0
oat bran *(Hungry Jack Microwave)*, 3 pieces.................... 45.0
wheat, harvest *(Hungry Jack Microwave)*, 3 pieces........... 46.0
Pancake batter, frozen *(Aunt Jemima Original/*
Buttermilk), 3 cakes*, 4″ each.............................. 36.0
Pancake breakfast, frozen:
with bacon *(Swanson Great Starts)*, 4.5 oz........................ 43.0
blueberry, with sausage, on a stick *(Jimmy Dean*
Flapsticks), 1 piece... 15.0
mini *(Swanson Breakfast Blast)*, 4.25 oz. 51.0
with sausages *(Swanson Great Starts)*, 6 oz. 53.0
with sausage, on a stick *(Jimmy Dean Flapsticks)*,
1 piece.. 13.0
silver dollar, with sausages *(Swanson* Budget),
3.75 oz.. 36.0
and vegetarian links *(Morningstar Farms)*, 4 oz. 31.0
Pancake and waffle mix:
(Bisquick Shake'n Pour Original), 3 cakes*, 4″ each 49.0
(Hungry Jack Extra Lights), 3 cakes*, 4″ each................... 28.0
(Hungry Jack Extra Lights Complete), 3 cakes*,
4″ each 38.0

apple cinnamon *(Bisquick Shake'n Pour)*, 3 cakes*,
  4″ each 47.0
blueberry *(Bisquick Shake'n Pour)*, 3 cakes*, 4″ each 52.0
blueberry, wild *(Hungry Jack)*, 3 cakes*, 4″ each 41.0
buttermilk:
  (Betty Crocker), 3 cakes*, 4″ each................................... 39.0
  (Bisquick Shake'n Pour), 3 cakes*, 4″ each 49.0
  (Hungry Jack), 3 cakes*, 4″ each.................................. 28.0
  (Hungry Jack Complete), 3 cakes*, 4″ each.................. 38.0
  (Robin Hood/Gold Medal Pouch), ⅛ mix 16.0
kamut *(Arrowhead Mills)*, ¼ cup 26.0
whole grain *(Arrowhead Mills)*, ½ cup............................. 58.0
wild rice *(Arrowhead Mills)*, 2.5 oz. dry 53.0
Pancake syrup (see also "Maple syrup"):
table blends:
  1 tbsp. 15.1
  with butter, 1 tbsp. 14.8
  with 2% maple, 1 tbsp. 13.9
  (Country Kitchen), 2 tbsp.. 27.0
  (Country Kitchen Lite), 2 tbsp.................................... 13.0
  (Hungry Jack), 2 tbsp... 26.0
  (Hungry Jack Lite), 2 tbsp... 14.0
  (Log Cabin), 2 tbsp.. 26.0
  (Log Cabin Lite), 2 tbsp.. 13.0
  (Vermont Maid), 1 tbsp.. 13.0
  butter flavor *(Country Kitchen)*, 2 tbsp......................... 27.0
Pancreas, without added ingredients.................................. 0
Papaya:
1-lb. papaya, 3½″ × 5⅛″... 29.8
peeled, cubed, ½ cup 6.9
peeled *(Frieda's)*, 1 oz. 2.8
Papaya concentrate:
(R.W. Knudsen), 1.5 fl. oz... 22.0
cream *(R.W. Knudsen)*, 2 fl. oz...................................... 6.0
Papaya nectar:
canned, 6 fl. oz. 27.2
(Kern's), 6 fl. oz... 27.0
(R.W. Knudsen), 8 fl. oz. 26.0

Papaya nectar *(cont.)*
(Libby's), 6 fl. oz. 28.0
Papaya-lime juice *(R.W. Knudsen)*, 8 fl. oz. 29.0
Paprika, 1 tsp. 1.2
Parsley:
fresh, 10 sprigs 6
fresh, chopped, ½ cup 1.9
dried, 1 tsp. 2
freeze-dried, 1 tbsp. 2
Parsley root, 1 oz. 7
Parsley seasoning, all purpose *(McCormick/*
Schilling Parsley Patch), ½ tsp. 5
Parsnip:
raw, sliced, ½ cup 12.1
boiled, drained, 1 medium, 9″ × 2¼″ diameter 31.3
boiled, drained, sliced, ½ cup 15.2
Passion fruit, purple:
1 medium 4.2
trimmed, 1 oz. 6.6
trimmed *(Frieda's)*, 1 oz. 6.0
Passion fruit juice:
fresh, purple, 6 fl. oz. 25.2
fresh, yellow, 6 fl. oz. 26.8
cocktail, frozen* *(Welch's Orchard Tropicals)*, 6 fl. oz. 25.0
Passion fruit-orange nectar *(Libby's Ripe)*, 8 fl. oz. 36.0
Passion fruit-raspberry juice *(R.W. Knudsen)*,
8 fl. oz. 32.0
Pasta, dry (see also "Macaroni" and specific
listings):
uncooked:
plain, 2 oz. 42.6
all varieties *(Master Choice)*, 2 oz. 42.0
(Ronzoni), 2 oz. 41.0
kamut ribbons *(Eden)*, 2 oz. 31.0
pepper, bell, and basil fettuccine *(Herb's* Organic),
2 oz. 40.0
sesame rice spirals or spinach ribbons *(Eden)*,
2 oz. 40.0

vegetable spirals *(Eden)*, 2 oz..44.0
cooked, spaghetti:
    plain, 1 cup..39.7
    corn, 1 cup...39.1
    spinach, 1 cup...36.6
    whole wheat, 1 cup...37.2
Pasta, refrigerated:
uncooked:
    with egg, 2 oz..31.0
    fettuccine or linguine *(Contadina)*, 3 oz. 45.0
    spaghetti style *(Contadina)*, 3 oz. 48.0
    spinach, with egg, 2 oz...31.6
cooked, with egg, 4 oz..28.3
cooked, spinach, with egg, 4 oz. 28.4
Pasta, frozen (see also specific listings) yolkless,
    precooked *(Aunt Vi's)*, 4 oz...29.0
Pasta dinner (see also specific listings), frozen, with
    turkey and vegetables *(Swanson)*, 11.25 oz....................36.0
Pasta dishes, canned or packaged (see also
    specific listings):
broccoli marinara *(Del Monte Pasta Classics)*, ¾ cup 13.0
Italian style *(Del Monte Pasta Classics)*, ¾ cup.................11.0
with meatballs, in tomato sauce *(Franco-American
    CircusO's)*, 7⅜ oz..26.0
spirals, and chicken *(Libby's Diner)*, 7.75 oz. 16.0
in tomato and cheese sauce *(Franco-American
    CircusO's)*, 7.5 oz...31.0
Pasta dishes, frozen (see also "Pasta entree" and
    specific listings):
Alfredo, with broccoli *(The Budget Gourmet* Side
    Dish)*, 5.5 oz..22.0
creamy cheddar *(Green Giant Pasta Accents)*, ½ cup 14.0
Dijon *(Green Giant Garden Gourmet Right for
    Lunch)*, 9.5 oz..21.0
garden herb seasoning *(Green Giant Pasta Accents)*,
    ½ cup 12.0
garlic seasoning *(Green Giant Pasta Accents)*, ½ cup 14.0

Pasta dishes, frozen *(cont.)*

Florentine *(Green Giant Garden Gourmet Right for Lunch)*, 9.5 oz. 27.0

Parmesan, with sweet peas *(Green Giant One Serving)*, 5.5 oz. 21.0

primavera *(Green Giant Pasta Accents)*, ½ cup 15.0

Pasta dishes, mix* (see also "Salad mix" and specific listings):

Alfredo *(McCormick/Schilling Pasta Prima)*, ½ cup 27.0

cheese:

    cheddar, tangy *(Hain Pasta & Sauce)*, ½ cup 19.0

    cheddar broccoli, Parmesan, or three cheese with vegetables *(Kraft Pasta & Cheese)*, ½ cup 19.0

    cheddar broccoli *(Lipton Pasta and Sauce)*, ½ cup 25.0

    Parmesan, creamy *(Hain Pasta & Sauce)*, ½ cup 20.0

chicken with herbs *(Kraft Pasta & Cheese)*, ½ cup 21.0

dill, creamy, multibran *(Hain Pasta & Sauce)*, ½ cup 22.0

garlic, creamy *(Lipton Pasta & Sauce)*, ½ cup 28.0

garlic, creamy *(McCormick/Schilling Pasta Prima)*, ½ cup 44.0

herb and garlic *(McCormick/Schilling Pasta Prima)*, ½ cup 45.0

herb tomato *(Lipton Pasta & Sauce)*, ½ cup 26.0

Italian, herb *(Hain Pasta & Sauce)*, ½ cup 18.0

Italian, multibran *(Hain Pasta & Sauce)*, ½ cup 17.0

marinara *(McCormick/Schilling Pasta Prima)*, ½ cup. 55.0

pesto *(McCormick/Schilling Pasta Prima)*, ½ cup 29.0

primavera *(Hain Pasta & Sauce)*, ½ cup 19.0

primavera *(McCormick/Schilling Pasta Prima)*, ¾ cup 32.0

salsa, multibran *(Hain Pasta & Sauce)*, ½ cup 18.0

seafood, creamy *(McCormick/Schilling Pasta Prima)*, ½ cup 9.0

sour cream with chives *(Kraft Pasta & Cheese)*, ½ cup 22.0

Swiss, creamy *(Hain Pasta & Sauce)*, ½ cup 20.0

tomato basil *(McCormick/Schilling Pasta Prima)*, ¾ cup 21.0

Pasta entree, frozen (see also "Pasta dishes, frozen" and specific listings):
baked, and cheese *(Celentano)*, 10 oz.................................... 63.0
with chicken cacciatore *(Healthy Choice Extra Portion)*, 12.5 oz. 47.0
with chicken teriyaki *(Healthy Choice Extra Portion)*, 12.6 oz. 58.0
Italiano *(Healthy Choice Extra Portion)*, 12 oz.................... 59.0
Italiano *(Weight Watchers Ultimate 200)*, 8 oz. 19.0
Portafino *(Weight Watchers Smart Ones)*, 9.5 oz. 30.0
Romanoff supreme *(Weight Watchers)*, 9 oz....................... 29.0
with shrimp and vegetables *(Healthy Choice Extra Portion)*, 12.5 oz. 44.0
trio *(Tyson Gourmet Selection)*, 11 oz. 53.0
vegetable, Italiano *(Healthy Choice Quick Meal)*, 10 oz.. 46.0
Pasta salad, see "Pasta dishes" and "Salad mix"
Pasta sauce (see also "Tomato sauce" and specific listings):
(Eden), 4 oz. 14.0
(Hunt's Chunky/Traditional), 4 oz....................................... 12.0
(Hunt's Homestyle), 4 oz. 10.0
(Pastorelli Italian Chef), 4 oz. 13.0
(Prego), 4 oz.. 20.0
(Prego Low Sodium), 4 oz. 11.0
(Progresso), 4 oz.. 13.0
(Ragú Old World), 4 oz. 9.0
(Ragú Thick & Hearty), 4 oz... 15.0
with beef and pork *(Classico D'Abruzzi)*, 4 oz. 7.0
cheese:
    four *(Classico Di Parma)*, 4 oz. 7.0
    four *(Master Choice Quattro Formaggi)*, 4 oz................... 8.0
    three *(Prego)*, 4 oz.. 17.0
garden combination *(Prego Extra Chunky)*, 4 oz. 14.0
garden harvest or chunky mushroom *(Ragú Today's Recipe)*, 4 oz. 8.0
garden medley or garlic and basil *(Ragú Fino Italian)*, 4 oz.. 12.0

Pasta sauce *(cont.)*
marinara:
  ½ cup 12.7
  (Hain), 4 oz. 9.0
  (Master Choice), 4 oz. 10.0
  (Prego), 4 oz. 10.0
  (Progresso), 4 oz. 9.0
  (Ragú Old World), 4 oz. 7.0
  (Rokeach), 3 oz. 9.0
meat or meat flavor:
  (Hunt's), 4 oz. 12.0
  (Hunt's Homestyle), 4 oz. 9.0
  (Master Choice Bolognese), 4 oz. 14.0
  (Prego), 4 oz. 20.0
  (Progresso), 4 oz. 13.0
  (Ragú Old World), 4 oz. 7.0
meatless *(Master Choice* Pomodoro), 4 oz. 12.0
mushroom:
  (Hain), 4 oz. 8.0
  (Hunt's), 4 oz. 12.0
  (Hunt's Homestyle), 4 oz. 10.0
  (Prego), 4 oz. 20.0
  (Progresso), 4 oz. 13.0
  (Ragú Thick & Hearty), 4 oz. 15.0
  super *(Ragú* Chunky Garden Style), 4 oz. 15.0
mushroom and green pepper *(Prego* Extra Chunky),
  4 oz. 14.0
mushroom and onion *(Prego* Extra Chunky), 4 oz. 13.0
mushroom and pepper *(Master Choice* Giardino),
  4 oz. 12.0
mushroom with extra spice *(Prego* Extra Chunky),
  4 oz. 17.0
mushroom and tomato *(Prego* Extra Chunky), 4 oz. 16.0
with olives and mushrooms *(Classico* Di Sicilia), 4 oz. 7.0
onion and garlic *(Prego)*, 4 oz. 15.0
Parmesan *(Ragú Fino* Italian), 4 oz. 12.0
with pepper, spicy red *(Classico* Di Roma
  Arrabbiata), 4 oz. 6.0

with peppers, sweet, and onions (Classico Di
   Salerno), 4 oz. 7.0
sausage and green pepper (Prego Extra Chunky),
   4 oz. 19.0
tomato:
   and basil (Classico Di Napoli), 4 oz. 6.0
   and basil (Prego), 4 oz. 18.0
   garlic and onions (Ragú Chunky Garden Style),
      4 oz. 15.0
   and herbs (Ragú Fino Italian), 4 oz. 13.0
   and herbs (Ragú Today's Recipe), 4 oz. 8.0
   onion, garlic (Prego Extra Chunky), 4 oz. 14.0
with zinfandel (Sutter Home), 4 oz. 11.0
Pasta sauce, frozen or refrigerated:
meatless (Bodin's), 3.4 oz. 10.0
tomato, chunky (Contadina Light), 5 oz. 9.0
Pasta sauce mix:
(Lawry's Rich & Thick), 1 pkg. 28.1
(McCormick/Schilling), ¼ pkg. 6.0
(Spatini), 1 cup* 10.0
with mushrooms (Lawry's), 1 pkg. 26.0
Pastrami:
(Healthy Deli), 1 oz. 8
(Hillshire Farm Deli Select), 1 oz. .... <1.0
turkey, see "Turkey pastrami"
Pastry dough
(see also "Pie crust"):
sheet, puff pastry (Pepperidge Farm), ¼ piece 22.0
shell:
   patty (Pepperidge Farm), 1 piece 16.0
   puff pastry, mini (Pepperidge Farm), 1 piece 4.0
   tart (Stilwell), 1 piece 9.0
Pâté, canned:
1 oz. 4
1 tbsp. 2
chicken liver, 1 oz. 1.9
chicken liver, 1 tbsp. 9
goose liver, smoked, 1 oz. 1.3

Pâté *(cont.)*
goose liver, smoked, 1 tbsp... .6
liver *(Sells)*, 2¼ oz.. 3.0
Pea pod, Chinese, see "Peas, edible-podded"
Peach:
fresh, 1 medium, 2½"-diameter, 4 per lb.......................... 9.7
fresh, pulp, sliced, ½ cup... 9.4
canned, halves or slices, except as noted:
   (Hunt's), 4 oz... 23.0
   (Stokely), ½ cup 18.0
   cling, in water, ½ cup 7.5
   cling, in water *(Libby's)*, ½ cup................... 8.0
   cling, in juice, ½ cup.................................... 14.3
   cling, in juice, diced *(Del Monte Fruit Naturals)*,
    ½ cup.. 16.0
   cling, in extra light syrup, diced *(Del Monte Lite)*,
    ½ cup.. 16.0
   cling, in light syrup, ½ cup 18.3
   cling, in heavy syrup *(Libby's)*, ½ cup........... 25.0
   cling, in heavy syrup, diced *(Del Monte)*, ½ cup 24.0
   cling or freestone, in heavy syrup, ½ cup........... 25.5
   freestone, in extra heavy syrup, ½ cup............. 34.1
   spiced, heavy syrup, whole, ½ cup.................. 24.3
dried:
   (Del Monte), 2 oz....................................... 35.0
   sulfured, halves, ½ cup.................................. 49.1
   sulfured, 10 halves, 4.6 oz............................. 79.7
freeze-dried *(Mountain House Fruit Crisps)*, ¼ cup........... 15.0
frozen, sliced, sweetened, ½ cup 30.0
Peach butter *(Smucker's)*, 1 tsp............................ 4.0
Peach daiquiri mixer, frozen*, with rum *(Bacardi)*,
  7 fl. oz.. 33.0
Peach drink, canned *(Hi-C)*, 6 fl. oz..................... 24.0
Peach juice:
(Smucker's Naturally 100%), 8 fl. oz........................... 30.0
orchard blend *(Dole Pure & Light)*, 6 fl. oz.................. 24.0
Peach nectar:
canned, 6 fl. oz. 26.0

(Kern's), 6 fl. oz.	26.0
(R.W. Knudsen), 8 fl. oz.	32.0
(Libby's), 6 fl. oz.	24.0
(Libby's Ripe), 8 fl. oz.	32.0

Peanut:

(Beer Nuts), 1 oz.	7.0
unroasted, 1 oz.	4.5
boiled, salted, 1 oz.	6.0

dry-roasted:

1 oz.	6.0
½ cup	15.7
(Fisher/Fisher Lightly Salted), 1 oz.	6.0
(Flavor House), 1 oz.	4.0

honey-roasted:

(Eagle Honey Roast), 1 oz.	7.0
(Fisher), 1 oz.	5.0
dry-roasted *(Fisher)*, 1 oz.	4.0
dry- or oil-roasted *(Flavor House)*, 1 oz.	8.0

oil-roasted:

1 oz.	5.3
½ cup	13.6
(Fisher/Fisher Lightly Salted), 1 oz.	6.0
butter toffee *(Flavor House)*, 1 oz.	20.0
flavored, hot *(Tom's)*, 1 oz.	5.0
party, oil-roasted *(Flavor House)*, 1 oz.	4.0
red skin *(Tom's)*, 1⅛-oz. pkg.	5.0

Spanish:

(Flavor House), 1 oz.	3.0
raw or roasted *(Fisher)*, 1 oz.	5.0
dry-roasted *(Planters)*, 1 oz.	6.0
toasted *(Tom's)*, 1⅛-oz. pkg.	6.0

Peanut butter:

chunky, 2 tbsp.	6.9

chunky or creamy:

(Arrowhead Mills), 2 tbsp.	6.0
(Jif/Jif Extra Chunky), 2 tbsp.	6.0
(Peter Pan Chunky/Peter Pan Creamy Salt Free), 2 tbsp.	5.0

Peanut butter, chunky or creamy *(cont.)*
   (Roaster Fresh), 2 tbsp... 5.0
   (Simply Jif/Simply Jif Extra Chunky), 2 tbsp. 5.0
   (Skippy Creamy/Super Chunk), 2 tbsp. 4.0
   (Smucker's Chunky Natural/Creamy Natural/No
      Salt Added), 2 tbsp.. 6.0
creamy:
   2 tbsp. 6.6
   (Peter Pan Creamy), 2 tbsp.. 6.0
   honey sweetened *(Smucker's)*, 2 tbsp............................ 7.0
jelly and, see "Jelly and peanut butter"
Peanut butter flavor baking chips *(Reese's)*, ¼ cup...... 19.0
Peanut butter-caramel topping *(Smucker's)*,
   2 tbsp. 29.0
Peanut flour:
defatted, 1 cup... 20.8
lowfat, 1 cup 18.8
Pear:
fresh, unpeeled, Bartlett, 1 medium, 2½ per lb................. 25.1
fresh, unpeeled, sliced, ½ cup.. 12.5
canned, halves or slices, except as noted:
   (Hunt's), 4 oz. 22.0
   (Stokely), ½ cup 23.0
   in water, ½ cup 9.5
   in water *(Libby's)*, ½ cup 10.0
   in juice, ½ cup 16.0
   in extra light syrup, diced *(Del Monte* Lite), ½ cup 15.0
   in light syrup, ½ cup 19.0
   in heavy syrup, ½ cup 24.4
   in heavy syrup, diced *(Del Monte)*, ½ cup 24.0
   in heavy syrup *(Libby's)*, ½ cup.................................... 23.0
dried, sulfured, 2 oz.. 39.5
dried, sulfured, halves, ½ cup... 62.7
freeze-dried *(Mountain House Fruit Crisps)*, ¼ cup........... 14.0
Pear, Asian, whole, 1 medium, 2¼″ × 2½″ diameter · 13.0
Pear juice, *(R.W. Knudsen)*, 8 fl. oz. 28.0
Pear nectar:
canned, 6 fl. oz. 29.6

(Kern's), 6 fl. oz. 28.0
(Libby's), 6 fl. oz. 28.0
Peas, see specific listings
Peas, cream, canned *(Allens/East Texas Fair)*, ½ cup 14.0
Peas, crowder:
canned *(Allens/East Texas Fair)*, ½ cup 15.0
frozen *(Seabrook)*, 3 oz. 23.0
Peas, edible-podded:
fresh:
   raw, ½ cup 5.4
   boiled, drained, ½ cup 5.6
   sugar snap *(Frieda's)*, 1 oz. 3.4
frozen:
   boiled, drained, ½ cup 7.2
   (Green Giant Sugar Snap), ½ cup 8.0
   Chinese *(Chun King)*, 1.5 oz. 3.0
   Chinese *(Seabrook)*, 2 oz. 4.0
   snow *(La Choy)*, 3 oz. 6.0
mix*, Oriental snow, with rice *(Fantastic)*, 10 oz. 30.0
Peas, field, canned:
(Allens), ½ cup 18.0
with snaps *(Allens)*, ½ cup 13.0
Peas, green or sweet:
fresh:
   raw, in pod, 1 lb. 24.9
   raw, shelled, ½ cup 10.4
   boiled, drained, ½ cup 12.5
canned:
   dry early June *(Crest Top)*, ½ cup 15.0
   sweet *(Green Giant 50% Less Salt)*, ½ cup 11.0
   sweet *(Stokely)*, ½ cup 10.0
   sweet, with pearl onions *(Green Giant)*, ½ cup 11.0
   very young, small, early or sweet *(Green Giant)*,
   ½ cup 12.0
   very young, tender, sweet *(Green Giant)*, ½ cup 11.0
freeze-dried* *(Mountain House)*, ½ cup 12.0
frozen:
   (Frosty Acres), 3.3 oz. 13.0

Peas, green or sweet, frozen *(cont.)*
   (Seabrook), 3.3 oz. 13.0
   Le Sueur baby, early *(Green Giant Harvest Fresh),*
     1/2 cup 12.0
   Le Sueur baby, early *(Green Giant Select),* 1/2 cup 13.0
   sweet *(Green Giant),* 1/2 cup 11.0
   sweet *(Green Giant Harvest Fresh),* 1/2 cup 12.0
   tiny *(Frosty Acres),* 3.3 oz. 11.0
frozen in butter sauce:
   Le Sueur baby, early *(Green Giant),* 1/2 cup 14.0
   Le Sueur baby, early *(Green Giant* One Serving*),*
     4.5 oz. 17.0
   sweet *(Green Giant),* 1/2 cup 14.0
   tender, sweet *(Bird's Eye),* 1/2 cup 12.0
Peas, green, combinations, frozen or packaged:
and carrots, see "Peas and carrots"
Le Sueur style *(Green Giant Valley Combinations),*
   1/2 cup 12.0
and mushrooms *(Del Monte Vegetable Classics),*
   1/2 cup 9.0
and mushrooms, *Le Sueur* early peas *(Green Giant*
   Select*),* 1/2 cup 11.0
and water chestnuts, Oriental *(The Budget Gourmet*
   Side Dish*),* 1 serving 14.0
Peas, lady, canned, with or without snaps *(Allens/*
   Sunshine), 1/2 cup 14.0
Peas, pepper, canned *(Allens/East Texas Fair),*
   1/2 cup 15.0
Peas, purple hull:
canned *(Allens/East Texas Fair),* 1/2 cup 18.0
frozen *(Frosty Acres),* 3.3 oz. 23.0
Peas, snow, see "Peas, edible-podded"
Peas, sprouted, mature seeds:
raw, 1/2 cup 17.0
boiled, drained, 4 oz. 24.8
Peas, sugar snap, see "Peas, edible-podded"
Peas, white acre, canned *(Allens/East Texas Fair),*
   1/2 cup 14.0

Peas and carrots:
canned (Stokely), ½ cup.. 9.0
frozen (Frosty Acres), 3.3 oz................................... 11.0
frozen (Seabrook), 3.3 oz....................................... 11.0
Pecan, shelled:
raw, ground or chopped (Fisher), 1 oz............................... 5.0
dried:
  1 oz.. 5.2
  halves, 1 cup 19.7
  chopped, 1 cup 21.7
dry-roasted, 1 oz.. 6.3
oil-roasted, 1 oz... 4.6
Pecan flour, 1 oz. 14.4
Pecan topping, in syrup (Smucker's), 2 tbsp. 28.0
Pectin, unsweetened, dry, 1.75-oz. pkg...................... 45.2
Penne entree, frozen, with Italian sausage (The
  Budget Gourmet), 10 oz... 54.0
Pepper, ground:
black, 1 tsp. 1.4
chili (Spice Islands), 1 tsp.. 1.2
red or cayenne, 1 tsp. 1.0
white, 1 tsp. 1.7
seasoned (see also specific listings):
  (Lawry's Spice Blends), 1 tsp. 1.8
  (McCormick/Schilling All Pepper), 1 tsp. 1.0
  pizza (Lawry's Spice Blends), 1 tsp............................. 3.2
Pepper, banana, 1 oz.:
hot or mild, chunks or rings (Vlasic), 1 oz. 1.0
sweet, rings (Vlasic), 1 oz. 2.0
Pepper, bell, see "Pepper, sweet":
Pepper, cherry:
(Progresso/Progresso Pickled), ½ cup............................. 3.0
(Vlasic), 1 oz. 2.0
Pepper, chili:
raw, green and red, without seeds, 1 medium,
  1.6 oz.. 4.3
raw, green and red, without seeds, chopped, ½ cup 7.1

Pepper, chili *(cont.)*
canned or in jars:
  with liquid, chopped, ½ cup 4.2
  green, whole *(Old El Paso)*, 1 chili 1.0
  green, chopped *(Old El Paso)*, 2 tbsp. 2.0
  hot, Mexican, or mild *(Vlasic)*, 1 oz. 2.0
Pepper, jalapeño:
all styles *(Ortega)*, 1 oz. 3.0
marinated *(La Victoria)*, 1½ pieces 2.0
nacho *(La Victoria)*, 14 pieces 1.0
Pepper, pepperoncini:
(Progresso Tuscan), ½ cup 7.0
salad *(Vlasic)*, 1 oz. 1.0
Pepper, piccalilli *(Progresso)*, ½ cup 4.0
Pepper, stuffed, entree, frozen:
(On-Cor), 8 oz. 15.0
(Stouffer's Single Serving), 10 oz. 28.0
green, with beef, tomato sauce *(Stouffer's)*, 7.75 oz. 22.0
sweet red *(Celentano)*, 13 oz. 28.0
Pepper, sweet:
fresh, green and red:
  raw, 1 medium, 3¾" × 3" diameter 4.8
  raw, chopped, ½ cup 3.2
  boiled, drained, 1 medium 4.9
  boiled, drained, chopped, ½ cup 4.6
fresh, yellow, raw, 1 large, 5" × 3" diameter 11.8
fresh, yellow, raw, 10 strips, 1.8 oz. 3.3
canned or in jars (see also "Pimiento"):
  roasted *(Progresso)*, ½ cup 5.0
  fried *(Progresso)*, ½ jar 4.0
  salad *(B&G)*, 1 oz. 3.0
freeze-dried, 1 tbsp. 3
frozen, chopped, 1 oz. 1.3
frozen, chopped, green or red *(Seabrook)*, 1 oz. 1.0
Pepper rings, hot *(Vlasic)*, 1 oz. 1.0
Pepper sauce, hot:
(Gebhardt), ½ tsp. .... <1.0
(Pickapeppa), 1 tbsp. 4.0

(Tabasco), 2 fl. oz. 7
cayenne *(Maull's)*, 1 tsp. 1.0
Pepper sauce mix *(Knorr)*, 1 serving dry 3.4
Peppercorn sauce mix*, green *(McCormick/
    Schilling McCormick Collection)*, ¼ cup 4.0
Peppered loaf:
(Kahn's), 1 slice 1.0
(Oscar Mayer), 1 oz. 1.3
Pepperoni:
(Hormel/Rosa Grande), 1 oz. ....<2.0
(Oscar Mayer), 15 slices 0
sliced *(Hormel Deli)*, 1 oz. ....<2.0
sliced *(Pillow Pack)*, 1 oz. 1.0
Perch, without added ingredients 0
Perch, frozen, battered *(Van de Kamp's)*, 2 pieces 18.0
Persimmon:
Japanese, fresh, 1 medium, 2½″ × 3½″ 31.2
Japanese, dried, 1 oz. 20.8
California, dried *(Frieda's)*, 1 oz. 1
fuyu, fresh *(Frieda's)*, 1 oz. 5.6
hachiya, fresh, trimmed *(Frieda's)*, 1 oz. 10.1
native, fresh, 1 medium, 1.1 oz. 8.4
Pesto dip mix* *(Knorr)*, 1 tbsp. 1.0
Pheasant, without added ingredients 0
Phyllo, see "Fillo pastry"
Picante beans, canned *(Allens/East Texas Fair)*,
    ½ cup 15.0
Picante sauce (see also "Salsa"):
(Frito-Lay's), 1 oz. 3.0
(Gebhardt), 1 tbsp. 1.0
(Old El Paso Thick'n Chunky), 2 tbsp. 1.0
(Tabasco), 1 oz. 2.9
hot, medium, or mild *(Chi-Chi's)*, 1 oz. 2.0
hot or medium *(Rosarita Chunky)*, 3 tbsp. 4.0
mild *(Rosarita Chunky)*, 3 tbsp. 5.0
Pickle:
bread and butter:
    (Mrs. Fanning's), 2 slices, ⅔ oz. 3.0

Pickle, bread and butter *(cont.)*
   slices *(Claussen),* 1 oz. 4.0
   chips or chunks *(Vlasic/Vlasic* Old Fashioned),
     1 oz. 6.0
   stix *(Vlasic),* 1 oz. 5.0
   sweet *(Vlasic* Sweet Butter Chips Half Salt), 1 oz. 7.0
   zesty chips *(Vlasic),* 1 oz. 11.0
dill:
   all varieties *(New Morning* Kosher/*New Morning*
     Kosher No Salt), 1.1 oz. 1.0
   all varieties *(Vlasic* Original/Deli/Kosher), 1 oz. 1.0
   whole, 3¾" long, 2.3 oz. 2.7
sour, 1 oz. 6
sweet, all varieties *(Vlasic),* 1 oz. 10.0
Pickle loaf:
(Kahn's/Kahn's Family Pack), 1 slice 2.0
beef *(Kahn's* Family Pack), 1 slice 1.0
Pickle and pimiento loaf *(Oscar Mayer),* 1 slice 4.0
Pickle relish, see "Relish"
Pickling spice *(Tone's),* 1 tsp. 1.2
Pie, frozen:
apple:
   (Banquet Family Size), ⅙ pie 37.0
   (Mrs. Smith's 8"), ⅙ pie 40.0
   (Mrs. Smith's 9"), ⅛ pie 50.0
   (Mrs. Smith's 10"), ⅒ pie 43.0
   (Sara Lee Homestyle), 3.7 oz. 37.0
apple, Dutch:
   (Mrs. Smith's 8"), ⅙ pie 48.0
   (Mrs. Smith's 10"), ⅒ pie 50.0
   (Sara Lee Homestyle), 3.7 oz. 41.0
   crumb *(Mrs. Smith's* 9"), ⅑ pie 48.0
apple-cranberry *(Mrs. Smith's* 8"), ⅙ pie 43.0
banana cream *(Banquet),* ⅙ pie 21.0
banana cream *(Pet-Ritz),* ⅙ pie 22.0
berry *(Mrs. Smith's* 8"), ⅙ pie 44.0
blackberry *(Mrs. Smith's* 8"), ⅙ pie 43.0
blackberry or blueberry *(Banquet* Family Size), ⅙ pie 40.0

blueberry *(Mrs. Smith's 8")*, 1/6 pie 39.0
blueberry cheese yogurt *(Mrs. Smith's 7")*, 1/4 pie 48.0
Boston cream, see "Cake, frozen"
cherry:
   (Banquet Family Size), 1/6 pie 36.0
   (Mrs. Smith's 8"), 1/6 pie 41.0
   (Mrs. Smith's 9"), 1/8 pie 48.0
   (Mrs. Smith's 10"), 1/10 pie 44.0
chocolate cream *(Banquet)*, 1/6 pie 24.0
chocolate cream *(Pet-Ritz)*, 1/6 pie 27.0
coconut cream *(Banquet)*, 1/6 pie 22.0
coconut cream *(Pet-Ritz)*, 1/6 pie.. 27.0
coconut custard *(Mrs. Smith's 8")*, 1/6 pie 30.0
coconut custard *(Mrs. Smith's 10")*, 1/10 pie 30.0
French silk cream *(Mrs. Smith's 8")*, 1/5 pie 55.0
lemon cream *(Banquet)*, 1/6 pie 23.0
lemon cream *(Pet-Ritz)*, 1/6 pie 26.0
lemon meringue *(Mrs. Smith's 8")*, 1/5 pie 54.0
mince *(Mrs. Smith's 8")*, 1/6 pie 48.0
mince *(Mrs. Smith's 10")*, 1/10 pie 51.0
mincemeat *(Banquet* Family Size), 1/6 pie 38.0
Neapolitan cream *(Pet-Ritz)*, 1/6 pie 17.0
peach:
   (Banquet Family Size), 1/6 pie 35.0
   (Mrs. Smith's 8"), 1/6 pie 37.0
   (Mrs. Smith's 9"), 1/8 pie 46.0
peach cheese yogurt *(Mrs. Smith's 7")*, 1/4 pie 46.0
pecan *(Mrs. Smith's 8")*, 1/5 pie... 73.0
pecan *(Mrs. Smith's 10")*, 1/8 pie... 68.0
pumpkin:
   (Banquet Family Size), 1/6 pie 29.0
   (Mrs. Smith's 8"), 1/6 pie 36.0
   (Mrs. Smith's), 1/10 pie 38.0
   hearty *(Mrs. Smith's 8")*, 1/6 pie 37.0
raspberry, red *(Mrs. Smith's 8")*, 1/6 pie 43.0
strawberry *(Mrs. Smith's 8")*, 1/5 pie................................... 44.0
strawberry banana yogurt *(Mrs. Smith's 7")*, 1/4 pie 48.0
strawberry cream *(Banquet)*, 1/6 pie 22.0

Pie, frozen *(cont.)*
strawberry cream *(Pet-Ritz)*, 1/6 pie.................................... 20.0
strawberry-rhubarb *(Mrs. Smith's 8")*, 1/6 pie...................... 44.0
Pie, snack:
apple:
   (Drake's), 1 piece... 29.0
   (Hostess), 1 piece.. 60.0
   (Tastykake), 1 piece... 46.0
   French *(Hostess)*, 1 piece................................... 60.0
   French *(Tastykake)*, 1 piece............................... 63.0
banana creme *(Tastykake)*, 1 piece 54.0
blackberry or blueberry *(Hostess)*, 1 piece 59.0
blueberry *(Drake's)*, 1 piece... 30.0
blueberry *(Tastykake)*, 1 piece.. 55.0
cherry:
   (Drake's), 1 piece... 30.0
   (Hostess), 1 piece.. 65.0
   (Tastykake), 1 piece... 49.0
coconut creme *(Tastykake)*, 1 piece 46.0
lemon:
   (Drake's), 1 piece... 27.0
   (Hostess), 1 piece.. 60.0
   (Tastykake), 1 piece... 48.0
lemon lime *(Tastykake)*, 1 piece 49.0
marshmallow, banana *(Little Debbie)*, 1 piece.................. 28.0
marshmallow, chocolate *(Little Debbie)*, 1 piece.............. 27.0
oatmeal creme *(Little Debbie)*, 1 piece........................... 24.0
peach *(Hostess)*, 1 piece 60.0
peach *(Tastykake)*, 1 piece... 47.0
pineapple cheese *(Tastykake)*, 1 piece 54.0
pumpkin *(Tastykake)*, 1 piece.. 46.0
raisin creme *(Little Debbie)*, 1 piece............................... 23.0
strawberry *(Hostess)*, 1 piece 56.0
strawberry *(Tastykake)*, 1 piece...................................... 57.0
(Tastykake Tasty Klair), 1 piece...................................... 51.0
Pie, snack, frozen:
chocolate mocha *(Weight Watchers Sweet*
   Celebrations), 1 piece.. 29.0

Mississippi mud *(Weight Watchers Sweet
    Celebrations)*, 1 piece.. 28.0
Pie crust, shell (see also "Pastry dough"), frozen or
    refrigerated:
(Oronoque), 1/6 shell 9.0
(Pet-Ritz), 1/6 shell... 9.0
(Pet-Ritz, 95/8"), 1/6 shell 15.0
(Pillsbury All Ready), 1/8 of 2-crust pie 24.0
(Stilwell), 1/8 shell 9.0
cookie crumb *(Nilla/Oreo)*, 3/4 oz. 14.0
deep dish *(Pet-Ritz/Oronoque)*, 1/6 shell 11.0
deep dish *(Stilwell)*, 1/8 shell 10.0
graham cracker:
    (Honeymaid), 3/4 oz. 15.0
    (Pet Ritz), 1/6 shell 8.0
    (Stilwell), 1/6 shell... 17.0
vegetable shortening *(Pet-Ritz)*, 1/6 shell................... 11.0
vegetable shortening, deep dish *(Pet-Ritz)*, 1/6 shell 12.0
Pie crust mix:
(Betty Crocker), 1/16 pkg. 10.0
(Pillsbury), 1/8 mix* 20.0
Pie filling, canned (see also "Pudding, mix"):
apple *(Comstock)*, 1/3 cup 22.0
blueberry *(Comstock)*, 1/3 cup 25.0
cherry *(Comstock)*, 1/3 cup 23.0
mincemeat:
    (Borden None Such), 1/3 cup 48.0
    with brandy and rum *(Borden None Such)*, 1/3 cup........ 49.0
    condensed *(Borden None Such)*, 1/4 pkg. 50.0
pumpkin, mix *(Libby's)*, 1 cup 64.0
Pierogi, frozen:
potato cheese *(Golden)*, 3 pieces 38.0
potato onion *(Golden)*, 3 pieces 36.0
Pigeon peas:
fresh, raw, 1/2 cup.. 18.4
fresh, boiled, drained, 1/2 cup 15.0
mature, boiled, 1/2 cup 19.5
Pig's feet, without added ingredients............................ 0

Pig's feet, pickled:
1 oz. .... <.1
(Penrose), 6 oz. 2.0
Pig's knuckles, pickled, *(Penrose)*, 6 oz. 1.0
Pike, without added ingredients 0
Pili nuts, dried:
shelled, 1 oz. 1.1
shelled, 1 cup 4.8
Pimiento, all varieties, drained *(Dromedary)*, 1 oz. 2.0
Pimiento spread *(Price's/Price's Light)*, 1 oz. 2.0
Piña colada mixer:
bottled *(Holland House)*, 4.5 fl. oz. 36.0
frozen*, with rum *(Bacardi)*, 7 fl. oz. 37.0
instant *(Holland House)*, .56 oz. dry 12.0
Pine nuts, dried:
pignolias:
  1 oz. 4.0
  1 tbsp. 1.4
  (Progresso), 1 tbsp. 1.0
pinyons, 1 oz. 5.5
pinyons, 10 kernels 2
Pineapple:
fresh, diced, 1/2 cup 9.6
fresh, baby, trimmed *(Frieda's Sugarloaf)*, 1 oz. 3.9
canned:
  in juice, 4 oz. 17.8
  in juice *(Dole)*, 1/2 cup 18.0
  in heavy syrup, 4 oz. 22.9
  in heavy syrup *(Dole)*, 1/2 cup 23.0
  in heavy syrup, chunks, tidbits, or crushed, 1/2 cup 25.8
  with mandarin orange *(Dole)*, 1/2 cup 19.0
frozen, sweetened, chunks, 1/2 cup 27.1
Pineapple float *(R.W. Knudsen)*, 8 fl. oz. 31.0
Pineapple juice:
canned or bottled:
  6 fl. oz. 25.9
  (R.W. Knudsen), 8 fl. oz. 25.0
  (Mott's), 11.5 fl. oz. 51.0

(Tree Top), 6 fl. oz. 24.0
chilled or frozen* *(Dole)*, 6 fl. oz. 22.0
chilled or frozen* *(Minute Maid)*, 6 fl. oz. 23.0
frozen*, 6 fl. oz. 23.9
Pineapple juice drink, frozen* *(Bright & Early)*,
  6 fl. oz. 23.0
Pineapple nectar *(Libby's)*, 6 fl. oz. 27.0
Pineapple topping:
(Kraft), 1 tbsp. 13.0
(Smucker's), 2 tbsp. 32.0
Pineapple-banana juice cocktail, frozen* *(Welch's*
  Orchard Tropicals), 6 fl. oz. 24.0
Pineapple-coconut juice *(R.W. Knudsen)*, 8 fl. oz. 24.0
Pineapple-grapefruit juice *(Dole)*, 6 fl. oz. 22.0
Pineapple-grapefruit juice drink:
(Tropicana), 6 fl. oz. 24.0
regular or pink *(Del Monte)*, 6 fl. oz. 24.0
Pineapple-orange drink:
(Crush), 11.5 fl. oz. 39.0
(Mott's), 10 fl. oz. 39.0
Pineapple-orange juice:
(Dole), 6 fl. oz. 22.0
chilled or frozen* *(Minute Maid)*, 6 fl. oz. 23.0
Pineapple-orange-banana juice:
chilled *(Dole)*, 6 fl. oz. 23.0
frozen* *(Dole)*, 6 fl. oz. 21.0
Pineapple-orange-guava juice:
chilled *(Dole)*, 6 fl. oz. 21.0
frozen* *(Dole)*, 6 fl. oz. 22.0
Pineapple-passion-fruit-banana juice *(Dole)*,
  6 fl. oz. 21.0
Pink beans, boiled, ½ cup 23.5
Pinto bean mix*, and rice *(Fantastic)*, 10 oz. 44.0
Pinto beans:
dry *(Arrowhead Mills)*, 2 oz. 36.0
dry, boiled, ½ cup 21.8
canned:
  with liquid, ½ cup 17.5

Pinto beans, canned *(cont.)*
(Eden), 1/2 cup...20.0
(Eden No Salt Added), 1/2 cup..........................17.0
(Gebhardt), 4 oz...19.0
(Green Giant/Joan of Arc), 1/2 cup 20.0
(Hain), 4 oz...15.0
(Old El Paso), 1/2 cup......................................19.0
(Progresso), 1/2 cup...21.0
dry, 1/2 cup..17.5
dry *(Allens/East Texas Fair)*, 1/2 cup...............18.0
frozen *(Seabrook)*, 3.2 oz..................................29.0
Pinto beans, sprouted, boiled, drained, 4 oz......4.6
Pistachio nuts:
dried, in shell, 1 lb...56.3
dried, shelled, 1 oz. 7.1
dry-roasted:
   in shell, salted, 1 lb..64.9
   shelled, 1 oz. 7.8
   shelled, 1 cup...35.2
natural or red tint *(Fisher)*, 1 oz. 7.0
Pitanga:
1 medium, .3 oz. 5
1/2 cup..6.5
Pizza, frozen:
Canadian bacon *(Totino's Party)*, 1/2 pie............42.0
Canadian bacon *(Jeno's Crisp'N Tasty)*, 1/2 pie....28.0
cheese:
   (Ellio's Healthy Slices), 1 slice.......................25.0
   (Ellio's 9 Slice), 1/9 pie................................24.0
   (Ellio's Round 16"), 1/6 pie 24.0
   (Ellio's 3 Slice), 1/3 pie................................24.0
   (Jeno's Crisp'N Tasty), 1/2 pie.......................28.0
   (Pillsbury Oven Lovin'), 1/2 pie 24.0
   (Totino's Microwave), 1 pie 30.0
   (Totino's Pan Pizza), 1/6 pie..........................35.0
   (Totino's Party), 1/2 pie 40.0
   (Totino's Party Family Size), 1/3 pie...............43.0
   (Weight Watchers), 6.03-oz. pkg......................36.0

double *(Ellio's* 6 Slice), 1/6 pie 22.0
extra *(Ellio's* 3 Slice), 1/3 pie 26.0
cheese, four *(Master Choice)*, 1/4 pie 30.0
cheese, three:
   (Pappalo's 9"), 1/2 pie................................ 47.0
   (Pappalo's 12"), 1/4 pie............................... 41.0
   (Pappalo's Pan), 1/5 pie 39.0
Chicken Suprema (Ellio's Healthy Slices), 1 slice 24.0
combination:
   (Jeno's Crisp'N Tasty), 1/2 pie...................... 27.0
   (MicroMagic Deep Dish), 1 pie...................... 60.0
   (Pillsbury Oven Lovin'), 1/2 pie 26.0
   (Totino's Microwave), 1 pie 34.0
   (Totino's Party), 1/2 pie 43.0
   (Totino's Party Family Size), 1/3 pie................. 47.0
   (Weight Watchers Deluxe), 7.32 oz. 36.0
garden style *(Ellio's Healthy Slices)*, 1 slice 25.0
hamburger *(Jeno's Crisp'N Tasty)*, 1/2 pie 28.0
hamburger *(Totino's Party)*, 1/2 pie 37.0
Mexican style *(Master Choice)*, 1/4 pie.................... 28.0
pepperoni:
   (Banquet), 1 pie 45.0
   (Ellio's 3 Slice), 1/3 pie 24.0
   (Jeno's Crisp'N Tasty), 1/2 pie...................... 28.0
   (MicroMagic Deep Dish), 1 pie...................... 65.0
   (Pappalo's 9"), 1/2 pie................................ 47.0
   (Pappalo's 12"), 1/4 pie 40.0
   (Pappalo's Pan), 1/5 pie 40.0
   (Pillsbury Oven Lovin'), 1/2 pie 25.0
   (Tombstone Light), 1/2 pie 22.0
   (Totino's Microwave), 1 pie 29.0
   (Totino's Pan Pizza), 1/6 pie......................... 35.0
   (Totino's Party), 1/2 pie 41.0
   (Totino's Party Family Size), 1/3 pie................. 44.0
   (Weight Watchers), 6.08 oz. 36.0
sausage:
   (Banquet), 1 pie 48.0
   (Jeno's Crisp'N Tasty), 1/2 pie...................... 27.0

Pizza, sausage *(cont.)*
  (MicroMagic Deep Dish), 1 pie...62.0
  (Pappalo's 9"), ½ pie..47.0
  (Pappalo's 12"), ¼ pie..39.0
  (Pappalo's Pan), ⅕ pie..39.0
  (Pillsbury Oven Lovin'), ½ pie 26.0
  (Totino's Microwave), 1 pie 31.0
  (Totino's Pan Pizza), ⅙ pie..35.0
  (Totino's Party), ½ pie...44.0
  (Totino's Party Family Size), ⅓ pie.....................................48.0
sausage and pepperoni:
  (Banquet), 1 pie 43.0
  (Master Choice), ¼ pie...28.0
  (Pappalo's 9"), ½ pie..45.0
  (Pappalo's 12"), ¼ pie..40.0
  (Pappalo's Pan), ⅕ pie..40.0
  (Totino's Pan Pizza), ⅙ pie..35.0
supreme:
  (Pappalo's 9"), ½ pie..46.0
  (Pappalo's 12"), ¼ pie..38.0
  (Pappalo's Pan), ⅕ pie..37.0
  (Pillsbury Oven Lovin'), ½ pie 27.0
  (Tombstone Light), ½ pie..23.0
  (Tombstone Light, 12"), ⅕ pie 30.0
spinach *(Master Choice* Gourmet), ¼ pie 29.0
vegetable:
  (Tombstone Light), ½ pie..22.0
  (Tombstone Light, 12"), ⅕ pie 31.0
  mixed *(Ellio's Healthy Slices),* 1 slice..............................24.0
Pizza, croissant crust, frozen:
cheese *(Pepperidge Farm),* 1 pie 41.0
deluxe or pepperoni *(Pepperidge Farm),* 1 pie 43.0
Pizza, French bread, frozen:
Canadian bacon *(Stouffer's),* ½ pkg. 40.0
cheese:
  (Healthy Choice), 5.6 oz. 46.0
  (Lean Cuisine), 5⅛ oz..38.0
  (Pillsbury Oven Lovin'), 1 piece...40.0

(Stouffer's), ¹/₂ pkg. 40.0
double *(Stouffer's)*, ¹/₂ pkg. 43.0
double *(Stouffer's Lunch Express)*, 1 piece.................. 48.0
three *(Lean Cuisine)*, 5.5 oz. 38.0
combination *(Pillsbury Oven Lovin')*, 1 piece 41.0
deluxe:
    (Healthy Choice), 6.35 oz. 41.0
    (Lean Cuisine), 6¹/₈ oz... 40.0
    (Stouffer's), ¹/₂ pkg... 40.0
    (Stouffer's Lunch Express), 1 piece 41.0
hamburger *(Stouffer's)*, ¹/₂ pkg.................................... 39.0
pepperoni:
    (Healthy Choice), 6 oz. 38.0
    (Lean Cuisine), 5.25 oz.. 41.0
    (Pillsbury Oven Lovin'), 1 piece............................ 40.0
    (Stouffer's), ¹/₂ pkg... 39.0
pepperoni and mushroom *(Stouffer's)*, ¹/₂ pkg. 40.0
sausage:
    (Lean Cuisine), 6 oz.. 42.0
    (Pillsbury Oven Lovin'), 1 piece............................ 41.0
    (Stouffer's), ¹/₂ pkg... 40.0
    Italian turkey *(Healthy Choice)*, 6.35 oz. 48.0
sausage and pepperoni or vegetable deluxe
    (Stouffer's), ¹/₂ pkg... 41.0
Pizza chips, cheese *(Keebler Pizzarias)*, 1 oz. 18.0
Pizza crust (see also "Bread shell"):
(Pillsbury All Ready), ¹/₈ crust 16.0
mix *(Robin Hood Pouch)*, ¹/₆ mix.................................. 22.0
Pizza Hut:
hand-tossed, 1 slice (¹/₈ pie):
    beef.. 19.8
    cheese 27.5
    Meat Lover's... 28.0
    pepperoni.. 27.7
    Pepperoni Lover's or pork 27.9
    sausage, Italian... 27.5
    supreme or super supreme..................................... 28.3
    Veggie Lover's 28.2

Pizza Hut (cont.)
pan pizza, 1 slice (⅛ pie)

beef	26.6
cheese	26.2
Meat Lover's or pork	26.7
pepperoni	26.4
Pepperoni Lover's	26.6
sausage, Italian	26.2
supreme or super supreme	27.0
Veggie Lover's	26.9

Thin'n Crispy, 1 slice (⅛ pie):

beef or pork	19.8
cheese	19.4
Meat Lover's	20.0
pepperoni	19.6
Pepperoni Lover's	19.9
sausage, Italian	19.4
supreme	20.2
super supreme	20.3
Veggie Lover's	20.1

Pizza mix:
Mexican *(Tio Sancho):*

sauce, 2 oz.	.2
tortilla, 1 piece	24.0

Pizza pocket, frozen:

combo *(Hot Pockets),* 4.5 oz.	38.0
deluxe *(Lean Pockets),* 4.5 oz.	34.0
deluxe *(Weight Watchers Ultimate 200),* 4 oz.	25.0
pepperoni *(Hot Pockets),* 4.5 oz.	39.0
pepperoni, sausage, or sausage and pepperoni *(Jeno's),* 4.5 oz.	35.0
sausage *(Hot Pockets),* 4.5 oz.	36.0
supreme *(Jeno's),* 4.5 oz.	36.0

Pizza roll, frozen:

cheese *(Jeno's Pizza Rolls),* 3 oz.	30.0
combination *(Jeno's Pizza Rolls),* 3 oz.	26.0
hamburger *(Jeno's Pizza Rolls),* 3 oz.	28.0
pepperoni or sausage *(Jeno's Pizza Rolls),* 3 oz.	26.0

Pizza sauce:
(Contadina Pizza Squeeze/Contadina Quick & Easy),
  1/4 cup 5.0
(Master Choice), 3 tbsp. 4.0
(Pastorelli Continental Chef/Italian Chef), 2 oz. or
  1/4 cup 5.0
(Ragú), 3 tbsp.. 3.0
with cheese, garlic and basil, or traditional *(Ragú
  Pizza Quick),* 3 tbsp.. 3.0
with Italian cheese or pepperoni *(Contadina),* 1/4 cup.......... 5.0
pepperoni *(Master Choice),* 3 tbsp............................. 4.0
tomato, chunky *(Ragú Pizza Quick),* 3 tbsp. 5.0
Plantain:
raw:
  1 medium, 9.7 oz. 57.1
  sliced, 1/2 cup... 23.6
  (Frieda's), 1 oz. 8.8
cooked, sliced, 1/2 cup 24.0
Plum:
fresh, pitted, sliced, 1/2 cup.................................... 10.7
fresh, Japanese or hybrid, 1 medium, 2 1/8" diameter.......... 8.6
canned:
  in juice, 1/2 cup 19.1
  in juice, 3 plums and 2 tbsp. liquid 14.4
  in light syrup, 1/2 cup... 20.5
  in light syrup, 3 plums and 2 3/4 tbsp. liquid 21.7
  in heavy syrup, 1/2 cup 30.0
  in heavy syrup, 3 plums and 2 3/4 tbsp. liquid................ 30.9
  (Stokely), 1/2 cup 30.0
Plum sauce, tangy *(La Choy),* 1 oz. 10.8
Poi, 1/2 cup 32.7
Poke greens, canned *(Allens),* 1/2 cup 2.0
Pokeberry shoots:
raw, 1/2 cup... 3.0
boiled, drained, 1/2 cup 2.5
Polenta mix *(Fantastic),* 4 oz. 19.0
Polish sausage (see also "Kielbasa") *(Hillshire
  Farm),* 2 oz. 2.0

Pollock, without added ingredients 0
Pomegranate:
1 medium, 9.7 oz. 26.4
trimmed *(Frieda's)*, 1 oz. 4.6
Pomegranate juice *(R.W. Knudsen)*, 8 fl. oz. 21.0
Pompano, without added ingredients 0
Popcorn, popped:
(Chesters), ½ oz. 9.0
(Jiffy Pop Pan Popcorn), 4 cups 16.0
(Kettle Poppins), ½ oz. 9.0
(Orville Redenbacher's Gourmet Original/Hot Air/
  White), 3 cups 10.0
(Tom's Natural), ¾ oz. 13.0
air popped, white *(Jolly Time)*, 3 cups 15.0
air popped, yellow *(Jolly Time)*, 3 cups 14.0
brewer's yeast *(Kettle Poppins)*, ½ oz. 8.0
butter flavor *(Jiffy Pop* Pan Popcorn), 4 cups 16.0
butter flavor *(Smartfood* Light), ½ oz. 9.0
butter toffee, with peanuts *(Cracker Jack)*, 1 oz. 20.0
caramel:
  (Barbara's Nature's Choice Original), 1 oz. 25.0
  (Flavor House Crunch), 1.1 oz. 26.0
  (Tom's), 1.6 oz. 40.0
  with peanuts *(Barbara's Nature's Choice)*, 1 oz. 23.0
  with peanuts *(Cracker Jack)*, 1 oz. 22.0
cheddar, white:
  (Flavor House), 1.1 oz. 13.0
  (Kettle Poppins), ½ oz. 9.0
  (Smartfood), ½ oz. 7.0
  (Tom's), 1¼ oz. 12.0
cheese flavor:
  (Tom's), 1.5-oz. pkg. 14.0
  cheddar *(Chee•tos)*, ½ oz. 6.0
  cheddar *(Chesters)*, ½ oz. 7.0
honey caramel *(Keebler* Pop Deluxe), 1 oz. 22.0
Popcorn, microwave, popped:
(Chesters Natural), 3 cups 13.0
(Jolly Time Natural), 3 cups 15.0

(Jolly Time Natural Light), 3 cups 13.0
(Orville Redenbacher's Gourmet Natural/Gourmet
  Salt Free), 3 cups 11.0
(Orville Redenbacher's Light Natural), 3 cups 8.0
(Pop•Secret), 3 cups 11.0
(Pop•Secret Light), 3 cups 12.0
(Pop Weaver's Natural/Butter), 4 cups 20.0
plain or butter flavor *(Jiffy Pop)*, 4 cups 17.0
plain or butter flavor *(Jiffy Pop* Pan), 4 cups 16.0
butter flavor:
  (Chesters), 3 cups 13.0
  (Jolly Time), 3 cups 13.0
  (Jolly Time Light), 3 cups 12.0
  (Orville Redenbacher's Gourmet/Gourmet Salt
    Free), 3 cups 11.0
  (Orville Redenbacher's Lite), 3 cups 8.0
  (Pop•Secret/Pop•Secret Salt Free), 3 cups 11.0
  (Pop•Secret Light), 3 cups 12.0
butter toffee *(Orville Redenbacher's* Gourmet),
  2½ cups 26.0
caramel *(Orville Redenbacher's* Gourmet), 2½ cups 29.0
cheddar *(Jolly Time)*, 3 cups 17.0
cheddar *(Orville Redenbacher's* Gourmet), 3 cups 14.0
cheese *(Chesters)*, 3 cups 11.0
sour cream 'n onion *(Orville Redenbacher's*
  Gourmet), 3 cups 12.0
Popcorn cake, plain or butter flavor *(Quaker)*,
  1 piece 7.0
Popcorn seasoning:
(Tone's), 1 tsp. 0
(McCormick/Schilling Parsley Patch), 1 tsp. 3.0
Poppyseeds, 1 tsp. 7
Porgy, without added ingredients 0
Pork (see also "Ham"), fresh, without added
  ingredients 0
Pork, cured (see also "Ham, cured"):
arm (picnic), roasted, 4 oz. 0
blade roll, lean with fat, roasted, 4 oz. 4

Pork, cured *(cont.)*
smoked, shoulder, butt, boneless *(Oscar Mayer Sweet Morsel)*, 3 oz. 2.0
Pork dinner, loin of, frozen *(Swanson)*, 10.75 oz. 26.0
Pork entree, canned:
chow mein *(La Choy* Bi-Pack), ¾ cup 7.0
sweet and sour *(La Choy)*, ¾ cup 48.0
Pork entree, freeze-dried*, sweet and sour, with
rice *(Mountain House)*, 1 cup 44.0
Pork entree, frozen, sweet and sour *(Chun King)*,
13 oz. 78.0
Pork entree sauce, see "Entree sauce"
Pork fat 0
Pork gravy:
canned *(Franco-American)*, 2 oz. 3.0
canned *(Heinz* Home Style), 2 oz. 3.0
mix *(French's)*, ¼ pkg. 3.0
mix *(McCormick/Schilling)*, ¼ cup* 4.0
Pork liver, see "Liver"
Pork sandwich, barbecue, frozen *(Hormel Quick
Meal)*, 4.3 oz. 40.0
Pork seasoning and coating mix:
(French's Roasting Bag), ⅕ pkg. 6.0
all varieties *(Shake'n Bake)*, ⅛ packet 8.0
extra crispy *(Oven Fry)*, ⅛ packet 10.0
chop *(McCormick/Schilling* Bag'n Season), 1 pkg. 24.0
spare ribs *(McCormick/Schilling* Bag'n Season),
1 pkg. 42.0
Pork skins, fried:
(Baken-ets), 1 oz. 2.0
hot'n spicy *(Baken-ets)*, 1 oz. 1.0
Pork and beans, see "Baked beans" and specific
listings
Pot roast, see "Beef dinner" and "Beef entree"
Pot roast seasoning mix:
(French's Roasting Bag), ⅐ pkg. 4.0
(Lawry's Seasoning Blends), 1 pkg. 25.0
(McCormick/Schilling Bag'n Season), 1 pkg. 9.0

onion *(French's* Roasting Bag), 1/7 pkg. 4.0
Potato:
raw:
  unpeeled, 1 lb.. 61.2
  peeled, 1 medium, 2½″ diameter 20.1
  peeled, diced, ½ cup 13.5
baked:
  in skin, 1 medium, 4¾″ × 2⅓″ diameter...................... 51.0
  without skin, 4 oz. 24.4
  without skin, ½ cup 13.2
boiled in skin:
  baby *(Frieda's),* 4 oz.. 19.4
  peeled, 1 medium, 2½″ diameter 27.4
  peeled, 4 oz... 22.8
  peeled, ½ cup 15.7
  without skin, 1 medium, 2½″ diameter 27.0
microwaved:
  in skin, 1 medium, 4¾″ × 2⅓″ diameter...................... 48.7
  in skin, 4 oz. 27.4
  peeled, ½ cup 18.2
  skin only, 2 oz. 16.8
mashed, with whole milk, ½ cup 18.4
mashed, with butter or margarine, ½ cup 17.5
Potato, canned:
with liquid, 4 oz... 9.8
drained, 1.2-oz. potato 4.8
(Stokely), ½ cup 11.0
whole *(Allens/Butterfield),* ½ cup..................................... 10.0
whole, new *(Hunt's),* 4 oz. 15.0
sliced or diced *(Allens/Butterfield),* ½ cup....................... 9.0
Potato, freeze-dried*, hash brown *(Mountain
  House),* 1 cup 36.0
Potato, frozen (see also "Potato dishes, frozen"):
whole, white, boiled *(Seabrook),* 3.2 oz. 13.0
diced and hash shred *(Seabrook),* 4 oz. 19.0
fried or french-fried:
  (Ore-Ida), 3 oz.. 23.0

Potato, frozen, fried or french-fried *(cont.)*
(Ore-Ida Country Style Dinner Fries/Golden Fries),
  3 oz. 20.0
(Ore-Ida Crispers!), 3 oz. 24.0
(Ore-Ida Crispy Crowns), 3 oz. 21.0
(Ore-Ida Golden Twirls), 3 oz. 22.0
battered *(Ore-Ida Zesties!),* 3 oz. 21.0
cottage cut *(Ore-Ida),* 3 oz. 21.0
crinkle cut *(Micro-Magic),* 3 oz. 27.0
crinkle cut *(Ore-Ida Deep Fries),* 3 oz. 23.0
crinkle cut *(Ore-Ida Golden Crinkles),* 3 oz. 21.0
crinkle cut *(Ore-Ida Lites),* 3 oz. 17.0
crinkle cut *(Ore-Ida* Microwave), 3.5 oz. 27.0
crinkle cut *(Ore-Ida Pixie Crinkles),* 3 oz. 21.0
seasoned *(Ore-Ida Crispy Crunchers),* 3 oz. 23.0
shoestring *(Ore-Ida),* 3 oz. 23.0
sticks *(MicroMagic Tater Sticks),* 4 oz. 29.0
wedges *(Ore-Ida Home Style Potato Wedges),*
  3 oz. 19.0
hash brown:
(MicroMagic Okray), 3 oz. 14.0
(Ore-Ida Golden Patties), 2.5 oz. 16.0
(Ore-Ida Microwave), 2 oz. 13.0
(Ore-Ida Southern Style), 3 oz. 16.0
(Ore-Ida Toaster), 1.75 oz. 12.0
with cheddar *(Ore-Ida Cheddar Browns),* 3 oz. 14.0
shredded *(Ore-Ida),* 3 oz. 15.0
mashed *(Simplot Singles),* 4 oz. 21.0
O'Brien *(Ore-Ida),* 3 oz. 13.0
puffs, all varieties, except microwave *(Ore-Ida Tater
Tots),* 3 oz. 21.0
puffs, microwave *(Ore-Ida Tater Tots),* 4 oz. 28.0
Potato, stuffed, see "Potato dishes, frozen"
Potato, sweet, see "Sweet potato"
Potato chips and crisps:
(Lay's/Lay's Unsalted/*Lay's* Flamin' Hot), 1 oz. 15.0
(Lay's Crunch Tators/Crunch Tators Amazin' Cajun),
  1 oz. 17.0

(Munchos), 1 oz. 15.0
(No Fries), 1 oz. 24.0
(O'Boisies), 1 oz. 16.0
(Ripplin's Original/Barbecue Flavor), 1 oz. 16.0
(Ruffles Light), 1 oz. 19.0
all varieties *(Barbara's True Blues)*, 1 oz. 15.0
all varieties *(Kettle Chips)*, 1 oz. 15.0
all varieties *(Krunchers!)*, 1 oz. 16.0
all varieties *(Mr. Phipps)*, 1 oz. 20.0
all varieties *(Pringles/Pringles* Rippled/*Pringels*
   Cheezums), 1 oz. 14.0
all varieties *(Pringels* Light), 1 oz. 17.0
all varieties *(Ruffles)*, 1 oz. 15.0
all varieties, except vinegar and salt *(Tom's)*,
   1⅛-oz. pkg. 16.0
au gratin *(King Kold)*, 1 oz. 15.0
barbecue flavor, plain or Kansas City *(Lay's*
   Bar-B-Q)*, 1 oz. 15.0
Cajun *(Lay's Crunch Tators Amazin' Cajun)*, 1 oz. 17.0
cheddar *(Lay's)*, 1 oz. 14.0
cheddar *(O'Boisies)*, 1 oz. 15.0
dill *(King Kold)*, 1 oz. 16.0
jalapeño *(Lay's Crunch Tators Hoppin' Jalapeño)*,
   1 oz. 18.0
mesquite *(Lay's Crunch Tators Mighty Mesquite)*,
   1 oz. 17.0
ranch *(Lay's Tangy Ranch)*, 1 oz. 15.0
ranch *(Ripplin's)*, 1 oz. 13.0
salt and vinegar *(Lay's)*, 1 oz. 14.0
sea salt and vinegar *(Eagle Ripples)*, 1 oz. 16.0
sour cream and onion:
   (Lay's), 1 oz. 15.0
   (Lay's Crunch Tators Supreme Sour Cream), 1 oz. 16.0
   (O'Boisies), 1 oz. 15.0
   (Ruffles Light), 1 oz. 18.0
vinegar and salt *(Tom's)*, 1⅛-oz. pkg. 18.0
Potato dishes, frozen:
au gratin *(Stouffer's)*, 5.75 oz. 17.0

Potato dishes, frozen *(cont.)*
baked, with broccoli:
  and cheddar *(Lean Cuisine)*, 10⅜ oz.............................. 37.0
  and cheese *(The Budget Gourmet* Light and
    Healthy)*, 10.5 oz. 40.0
  and cheese *(Ore-Ida* Topped Baked)*, 5.63 oz. 25.0
  and cheese *(Weight Watchers)*, 10.5 oz. 43.0
  and ham *(Weight Watchers)*, 11.5 oz............................... 30.0
baked, butter or cheese *(Ore-Ida* Twice Baked)*, 5 oz....... 28.0
baked, chicken divan *(Weight Watchers)*, 11.25 oz. 38.0
baked, with sour cream *(Lean Cuisine)*, 10⅜ oz. 33.0
baked, with sour cream and chives *(Ore-Ida* Twice
  Baked)*, 5 oz. 27.0
baked, turkey, homestyle *(Weight Watchers)*,
  11.25 oz... 27.0
baked, vegetable primavera *(Ore-Ida* Topped Baked)*,
  6.13 oz.. 23.0
baked, vegetable primavera *(Weight Watchers)*,
  11.15 oz... 49.0
baked, wedges, with broccoli and cheese *(Healthy
  Choice)*, 9.5 oz. 41.0
and broccoli, with cheese sauce *(Green Giant* One
  Serving)*, 5.5 oz.. 19.0
casserole, garden *(Healthy Choice* Quick Meal)*,
  9.25 oz.. 23.0
cheddared *(The Budget Gourmet* Side Dish)*, 5.5 oz......... 22.0
cheddared, with broccoli *(The Budget Gourmet* Side
  Dish)*, 5 oz.. 14.0
pancake, see "Potato pancake"
scalloped *(Stouffer's)*, 5.75 oz. 16.0
stuffed, three cheese *(The Budget Gourmet* Side
  Dish)*, 5.75 oz... 23.0
Potato dishes, packaged, au gratin *(Green Giant*
  Pantry Express), ½ cup.. 17.0
Potato flakes *(Arrowhead Mills)*, 2 oz. 44.0
Potato flour, 1 cup 143.0
Potato mix*:
American cheese *(Betty Crocker* Homestyle)*, ½ cup........ 21.0

au gratin:
  (Betty Crocker), ½ cup 21.0
  (Fantastic Foods), ½ cup 24.0
  (Idahoan), ½ cup 18.0
  (Kraft Potatoes & Cheese), ½ cup.............................19.0
  broccoli *(Betty Crocker* Homestyle), ½ cup 19.0
  broccoli *(Kraft* Potatoes & Cheese), ½ cup...................20.0
  tangy *(Pillsbury)*, ½ cup 20.0
bacon and cheddar *(Betty Crocker* Twice Baked),
  ½ cup 21.0
cheddar:
  (Betty Crocker Homestyle), ½ cup 21.0
  'n bacon *(Betty Crocker)*, ½ cup 21.0
  and bacon *(Pillsbury)*, ½ cup...19.0
  classic *(Idahoan)*, ½ cup 21.0
  mild, with onion *(Betty Crocker* Twice Baked),
    ½ cup..20.0
  smokey *(Betty Crocker)*, ½ cup 21.0
cheese, two *(Kraft* Potatoes & Cheese), ½ cup 19.0
country style *(Fantastic Foods)*, ½ cup..............................19.0
hash brown *(Betty Crocker)*, ½ cup 24.0
hash brown *(Idahoan* Quick One-Pan), ½ cup 18.0
julienne *(Betty Crocker)*, ½ cup...19.0
mashed:
  (Hungry Jack Flakes), ½ cup 17.0
  (Idahoan Complete), ½ cup 17.0
  (Idahoan), ½ cup 16.0
  (Pillsbury Idaho Granules/*Pillsbury Idaho* Spuds),
    ½ cup..16.0
  (Potato Buds), ½ cup 17.0
pancake, see "Potato pancake"
ranch, creamy *(Idahoan)*, ½ cup...18.0
scalloped:
  (Betty Crocker), ½ cup..20.0
  (Idahoan), ½ cup 20.0
  cheesy *(Betty Crocker* Homestyle), ½ cup.....................20.0
  cheesy or creamy white sauce *(Pillsbury)*, ½ cup..........20.0
  with ham *(Betty Crocker Scalloped'N Ham)*, ½ cup......22.0

Potato mix, scalloped *(cont.)*
   regular or with ham *(Kraft* Potatoes & Cheese),
     ½ cup... 20.0
  sour cream, chives:
   (Betty Crocker), ½ cup.. 20.0
   (Betty Crocker Twice Baked), ½ cup........................... 19.0
   (Kraft Potatoes & Cheese), ½ cup............................... 20.0
   (Pillsbury), ½ cup... 20.0
  Western *(Idahoan),* ½ cup 18.0
Potato pancake:
frozen, regular or Mexican *(Golden),* 1 piece...................... 11.0
mix *(Pillsbury),* 3 cakes*, 3″ each 16.0
Potato planks, catsup flavor *(Durkee),* 1 oz. 14.0
Potato salad seasoning *(Tone's),* 1 tsp........................ .3
Potato sticks:
1 oz. 15.1
(Allens/Butterfield), ½ cup 16.0
(Durkee), 1 oz. 16.0
plain or cheddar *(Andy Capp's* Pub Fries), 1 oz............... 18.0
bacon and cheddar *(Tom's),* ⅞ oz. 15.0
hot *(Andy Capp's* Fries), 1 oz................................... 20.0
hot *(Tom's* Fries), 1 oz. 17.0
salt 'n vinegar *(Andy Capp's),* 1 oz. 17.0
Poultry, see specific listings
Poultry seasoning, 1 tsp....................................... 1.0
Pout, ocean, without added ingredients 0
Preserves, see "Jam and preserves"
Pretzel (see also "Crackers"):
(Andy Capp's Pub Pretzels), 1 oz................................. 23.0
(Barbara's Bavarian/9-Grain/Honeysweet), 1 oz.,
  2 pieces 21.0
(Mr. Salty Mini), 1 oz.. 21.0
cheddar *(Combos),* 1.8 oz. 34.0
chips, regular or sesame *(Mr. Phipps),* 1 oz. 20.0
chips, fat free or lightly salted *(Mr. Phipps)* 22.0
Dutch *(Mr. Salty),* 1 oz.. 22.0
hard, plain, 1 oz. 22.5
hard, sourdough *(Eagle* Bavarian), 1 oz. 24.0

mini *(Barbara's* Regular/No Salt Added), 1 oz.,
  17 pieces 21.0
nacho *(Combos)*, 1.8 oz. 34.0
pizza *(Combos)*, 1.8 oz. 35.0
sticks *(Eagle)*, 1 oz. 22.0
sticks *(Mr. Salty* Very Thin), 1 oz. 22.0
sticks or twists *(Mr. Salty* Fat Free), 1 oz. 23.0
twists *(Mr. Salty)*, 1 oz. 21.0
whole wheat, hard, 1 oz. 23.0
Pretzel, frozen *(Super-Pretzel)*, 1 piece 37.0
Prickly pear:
1 medium, 4.8 oz. 9.9
(Frieda's), 1 oz. 3.1
Prosciutto, boneless, *(Hormel* Deli), 1 oz. .... <2.0
Protein shake mix:
(Naturade Mega Protein), 1 oz. 0
(Naturade N-R-G Protein+), 1.1 oz. 2.0
carob or vanilla *(Naturade* N-R-G), 1 oz. 1.0
Prune:
canned, in heavy syrup:
  pitted, 4 oz. 31.5
  ½ cup 32.5
  5 medium and 2 tbsp. liquid 23.9
dehydrated, uncooked, ½ cup 58.8
dehydrated, cooked, ½ cup 41.6
dried:
  (Dole), 2 oz. 36.0
  with pits *(Sunsweet)*, 2 oz. 32.0
  with plts, ½ cup 50.5
  pitted, 10 prunes 52.7
  pitted *(Sunsweet)*, 2 oz. 36.0
  stewed, with pits, unsweetened, ½ cup 29.8
Prune juice:
6 fl. oz. 33.5
(R.W. Knudsen Organic), 8 fl. oz. 42.0
(Mott's All Natural), 6 fl. oz. 34.0
(Mott's Country Style), 6 fl. oz. 37.0
(Sunsweet), 6 fl. oz. 33.0

Pudding, ready-to-serve:

banana *(Hunt's Snack Pack)*, 4.25 oz. 22.0
butterscotch *(Hunt's Snack Pack)*, 4.25 oz. 27.0
butterscotch *(Swiss Miss)*, 4 oz. 29.0
butterscotch-chocolate-vanilla swirl *(Jell-O* Pudding
  Snacks), 4 oz. 28.0
chocolate:
  (Hershey's), 4 oz. 29.0
  (Hershey's Special Dark), 4 oz. 30.0
  (Hunt's Snack Pack), 4.25 oz. 26.0
  (Hunt's Snack Pack Light), 4 oz. 20.0
  (Jell-O Free Pudding Snacks), 4 oz. 24.0
  (Swiss Miss), 4 oz. 29.0
  fudge *(Hunt's Snack Pack)*, 4.25 oz. 27.0
  fudge *(Swiss Miss)*, 4 oz. 38.0
  parfait *(Swiss Miss)*, 4 oz. 27.0
  regular or fudge *(Jell-O* Pudding Snacks), 4 oz. 28.0
  regular or fudge *(Swiss Miss* Light), 4 oz. 20.0
  sundae *(Swiss Miss)*, 4 oz. 36.0
chocolate and almond *(Hershey's)*, 4 oz. 29.0
chocolate caramel *(Hershey's Caramello)*, 4 oz. 28.0
chocolate caramel swirl *(Jell-O* Pudding Snacks),
  4 oz. 28.0
chocolate marshmallow *(Hunt's Snack Pack)*,
  4.25 oz. 26.0
chocolate mint *(Hershey's York* Peppermint Pattie),
  4 oz. 29.0
chocolate/mint or chocolate/vanilla swirl *(Jell-O Free*
  Pudding Snacks), 4 oz. 24.0
chocolate and vanilla *(Hershey's Kisses)*, 4 oz. 29.0
chocolate-vanilla swirl *(Jell-O* Pudding Snacks), 4 oz. 28.0
lemon *(Hunt's Snack Pack)*, 4.25 oz. 30.0
tapioca:
  (Hunt's Snack Pack), 4.25 oz. 23.0
  (Hunt's Snack Pack Light), 4 oz. 18.0
  (Jell-O Pudding Snacks), 4 oz. 29.0
  (Swiss Miss), 4 oz. 27.0

vanilla:
    (Hunt's Snack Pack), 4.25 oz. 27.0
    (Jell-O Free Pudding Snacks), 4 oz. 23.0
    (Jell-O Pudding Snacks), 4 oz. 25.0
    (Swiss Miss), 4 oz. 30.0
    (Swiss Miss Light), 4 oz. 20.0
    parfait *(Swiss Miss)*, 4 oz. 29.0
    sundae *(Swiss Miss)*, 4 oz. 36.0
vanilla-chocolate parfait *(Swiss Miss Light)*, 4 oz. 20.0
vanilla-chocolate swirl *(Jell-O* Pudding Snacks), 4 oz. 28.0
Pudding, frozen:
almond *(Imagine Foods Dream)*, 4 oz. 31.0
banana, butterscotch, or lemon *(Imagine Foods
    Dream)*, 4 oz. 30.0
butterscotch *(Rich's)*, 3 oz. 18.0
carob *(Imagine Foods Dream)*, 4 oz. 31.0
chocolate *(Imagine Foods Dream)*, 4 oz. 39.0
chocolate *(Rich's)*, 3 oz. 19.0
coconut *(Imagine Foods Dream)*, 4 oz. 32.0
vanilla *(Rich's)*, 3 oz. 18.0
Pudding bar, frozen, all varieties *(Jell-O Pudding
    Pops)*, 1 bar 13.0
Pudding mix*:
banana cream *(Jell-O)*, ⅙ recipe 17.0
banana cream, butter pecan, or butterscotch *(Jell-O
    Instant)*, ½ cup 28.0
butterscotch *(Jell-O)*, ½ cup 30.0
caramel, creme *(Knorr* Dessert Mix), 1 serving mix
    and sauce 27.4
chocolate, milk chocolate, or chocolate fudge
    (Jell-O), ½ cup 28.0
chocolate, milk chocolate, or chocolate fudge *(Jell-O
    Instant)*, ½ cup 31.0
coconut cream *(Jell-O)*, ⅙ recipe 16.0
coconut cream *(Jell-O* Instant), ½ cup 27.0
custard, golden egg *(Jell-O Americana)*, ½ cup 24.0
flan *(Jell-O)*, ½ cup 26.0
lemon *(Jell-O)*, ⅙ recipe 38.0

Pudding mix *(cont.)*

lemon *(Jell-O* Instant), ½ cup 29.0
pistachio *(Jell-O* Instant), ½ cup 28.0
raspberry or strawberry *(Salada Danish Dessert),*
  ½ cup 32.0
rennet custard, chocolate *(Junket),* ½ cup 15.0
rennet custard, raspberry, strawberry, or vanilla
  (Junket), ½ cup 16.0
rice *(Jell-O Americana),* ½ cup 30.0
tapioca, vanilla *(Jell-O Americana),* ½ cup 26.0
tapioca, vanilla *(Royal),* ½ cup 27.0
vanilla:
  (Jell-O), ½ cup 27.0
  (Jell-O Instant), ½ cup 29.0
  French *(Jell-O),* ½ cup 30.0
  French *(Jell-O* Instant), ½ cup 28.0
Puff pastry, see "Pastry dough"
Pummelo:
1 medium, 5½" diameter 58.6
sections, ½ cup 9.1
trimmed *(Frieda's),* 1 oz. 2.7
Pumpkin:
fresh, pulp, raw, 1" cubes, ½ cup 3.8
fresh, boiled, drained, mashed, ½ cup 6.0
canned *(Libby's),* ½ cup 10.1
canned, with or without winter squash, ½ cup 9.9
Pumpkin butter *(Smucker's* Autumn Harvest), 1 tsp. 3.0
Pumpkin flower:
raw, ½ cup 5
boiled, drained, ½ cup 2.2
Pumpkin leaf:
raw, ½ cup 5
boiled, drained, ½ cup 1.2
Pumpkin pie spice, 1 tsp. 1.2
Pumpkin seeds:
roasted, in shell, 1 oz. or 85 seeds 15.3
roasted, in shell, 1 cup 34.4
roasted, shelled, 1 oz. 3.8

dried, shelled, 1 oz. or 142 kernels...5.1
Punch, see "Fruit punch" and specific fruit listings
Purslane:
raw, ½ cup..7
boiled, drained, ½ cup 2.1

Q

Food and Measure	Carbohydrate Grams
Quail, without added ingredients	0
Quince:	
1 medium, 5.3 oz.	14.1
peeled, seeded, 1 oz.	4.3
pineapple, peeled, seeded *(Frieda's)*, 1 oz.	4.3
Quinoa, dry:	
1 oz.	19.5
(Eden), 2 oz.	38.0

R

Food and Measure	Carbohydrate Grams

Rabbit, without added ingredients.. 0
Radicchio, fresh:
trimmed, 1 oz. 1.3
1 medium leaf, .3 oz. 4
shredded, ½ cup 9
Radish:
10 medium, ¾"–1" diameter.. 1.6
sliced, ½ cup 2.1
Radish, black, 1 oz. 1.0
Radish, Oriental:
raw, 1 medium, 7" × 2¼" diameter 13.9
raw, sliced, ½ cup 1.8
boiled, drained, sliced, ½ cup... 2.5
dried, 1 oz. 18.0
Radish, white-icicle:
1 medium, .6 oz. 5
sliced, ½ cup 1.3
Raisins:
seeded, not packed, ½ cup 56.9
seedless:
  not packed, ½ cup... 57.4
  (Cinderella Thompson), ½ cup..................................... 66.0
  (Dole/Dole Golden), ½ cup 66.0
  (Sun-Maid), ½ cup 69.0
  golden, not packed, ½ cup 57.7
Ranch dip mix, cracked pepper *(Knorr),* 1 serving
  dry.. .8
Raspberry, red:
fresh, 1 pint... 36.1

Raspberry *(cont.)*
fresh, ½ cup.. 7.1
frozen, sweetened, ½ cup................................... 32.7
frozen, in syrup *(Birds Eye)*, 5 oz. 25.0
Raspberry drink mix*:
(Kool-Aid), 8 fl. oz. 25.0
(Kool-Aid Presweetened), 8 fl. oz. 18.0
Raspberry float *(R.W. Knudsen)*, 8 fl. oz. 31.0
Raspberry juice:
(Chiquita Raspberry Passion), 6 fl. oz. 26.0
(Dole Pure & Light Country Raspberry), 6 fl. oz. 24.0
red *(Smucker's* Naturally 100%), 8 fl. oz............ 30.0
Raspberry nectar, red *(R.W. Knudsen)*, 8 fl. oz. 30.0
Raspberry-cranberry juice *(Master Choice)*, 6 fl. oz. 21.0
Raspberry-peach juice *(R.W. Knudsen)*, 8 fl. oz............. 28.0
Raspberry-tamarind dipping sauce *(Helen's Tropical Exotics)*, 2 tbsp... 11.0
Ravioli, canned or packaged:
beef:
   (Hormel Micro Cup), 7.5 oz............................... 34.0
   in meat sauce *(Franco-American* RavioliO's),
     7.5 oz. 35.0
   in sauce *(Libby's Diner)*, 7.5 oz...................... 35.0
mini *(Hormel Kid's Kitchen)*, 7.5 oz.................... 34.0
Ravioli, frozen or refrigerated:
(Celentano), 6.5 oz. 61.0
cheese *(Contadina)*, 3 oz..................................... 30.0
mini *(Celentano)*, 4 oz. 42.0
Ravioli entree, cheese, frozen:
(The Budget Gourmet Light and Healthy), 9.5 oz. 34.0
baked:
   (Healthy Choice), 9 oz..................................... 44.0
   (Weight Watchers), 9 oz.................................. 27.0
   with tomato sauce *(Lean Cuisine)*, 8.5 oz. 30.0
Rax, 1 serving:
sandwiches:
   beef, bacon'n cheddar...................................... 37.0
   chicken breast, country fried 49.0

chicken breast, grilled	26.0
Philly melt	40.0
Rax, regular	25.0
roast beef, deluxe	39.0
side dishes:	
french fries, 3.25 oz.	36.0
potato, baked, plain or with margarine	61.0
salads, without dressing:	
grilled chicken garden	14.0
gourmet garden	13.0
salad dressings, 2 oz.:	
French	20.0
Italian, light	8.0
sauces:	
barbecue, 1 packet	3.0
cheddar cheese, 1 oz.	4.0
mushroom, 1 oz.	1.0
chocolate chip cookie, 2 pieces	36.0
chocolate shake, 16 oz.	77.0
Colombo yogurt shakes:	
candy cane	62.0
blackberry	58.0
buckeye/peanut butter kiss	63.0
cherry, chocolate covered	72.0
chocolate, fat free	66.0
chocolate chip	57.0
mint chocolate chip	80.0
mocha	64.0
orange, cool	35.0
peach	60.0
strawberry, fat free	64.0
vanilla, fat free	44.0
Red bean mix*:	
and rice *(Fantastic* Cajun), 10 oz.	44.0
(Mahatma), ¾ cup	44.0
Red beans, canned:	
(Allens), ½ cup	17.0
(Green Giant/Joan of Arc), ½ cup	19.0

Red beans *(cont.)*
small *(Hunt's)*, 4 oz. 18.0
Red snapper, without added ingredients 0
Redfish, without added ingredients 0
Refried bean mix* *(Fantastic* Instant), ½ cup 23.0
Refried beans, canned:
4 oz. 21.0
½ cup 23.3
(Chi-Chi's), 7.5 oz. 29.0
(Gebhardt), 4 oz. 20.0
with bacon or nacho cheese *(Rosarita)*, 4 oz. 20.0
with green chilies *(Old El Paso)*, ¼ cup 8.0
jalapeño *(Gebhardt)*, 4 oz. 19.0
with onions *(Rosarita)*, 4 oz. 21.0
plain, vegetarian, or with green chilies *(Rosarita)*,
  4 oz. 18.0
plain or vegetarian *(Old El Paso)*, 4 oz. 15.0
with sausage *(Old El Paso)*, ¼ cup 8.0
spicy *(Rosarita)*, 4 oz. 19.0
vegetarian *(Hain)*, 4 oz. 15.0
Relish:
corn *(New Morning)*, 1 oz. 8.0
hamburger:
  1 cup 84.1
  1 tbsp. 5.2
  (Heinz), 1 oz. 7.0
  (Vlasic), 1 oz. 9.0
hot dog:
  1 cup 57.0
  1 tbsp. 3.5
  (Heinz), 1 oz. 8.0
  (Vlasic), 1 oz. 8.0
India *(Heinz)*, 1 oz. 9.0
India *(Vlasic)*, 1 oz. 8.0
jalapeño *(Old El Paso)*, 2 tbsp. 4.0
piccalilli:
  (Heinz), 1 oz. 7.0
  (New Morning), 1 oz. 6.0

green tomato or hot *(Vlasic)*, 1 oz. 8.0
pickle *(Claussen)*, 1 tbsp. 3.0
sweet:
   1 cup 85.5
   1 tbsp. 5.3
   (Heinz), 1 oz. 9.0
   (New Morning), 1 oz. 8.0
   (Vlasic), 1 oz. 8.0
Rennet *(Junket)*, 1 tablet 0
Rennet custard, see "Pudding mix"
Rhubarb:
fresh, diced, 1/2 cup 2.8
fresh, regular or hot house *(Frieda's)*, 1 oz. 1.0
frozen, cooked, sweetened, 1/2 cup 37.4
Rib sauce *(Dip n'Joy Saucey Rib)*, 1 oz. 14.0
Rice (see also "Rice dishes"), cooked, except as
  noted:
basmati:
   brown *(Arrowhead Mills)*, 2 oz. dry 44.0
   brown *(Arrowhead Mills* Indian), 2 oz. dry 43.0
   brown *(Fantastic Foods)*, 1/2 cup 23.0
   brown *(Master Choice Texmati)*, 1/2 cup 23.0
   white *(Arrowhead Mills* Indian), 2 oz. dry 44.0
   white *(Fantastic Foods)*, 1/2 cup 22.0
   white *(Master Choice Texmati)*, 1/2 cup 22.0
   white *(Texmati)*, 1/2 cup 31.0
   white and wild *(Master Choice Texmati)*, 1/2 cup 20.0
brown, all varieties *(Arrowhead Mills)*, 2 oz. dry 44.0
brown, long grain:
   (Carolina/Mahatma/River), 1/2 cup 23.0
   (Uncle Ben's Whole Grain), 1.3 oz. dry 27.6
   (Uncle Ben's Fast Cooking Whole Grain),
     .9 oz. dry 19.6
brown, instant *(Minute)*, 1/2 cup 26.0
glutinous or sweet, 1/2 cup 25.4
jasmine *(Fantastic Foods)*, 1/2 cup 22.0
jasmine, brown *(Fantastic Foods)*, 1/2 cup 23.0

Rice *(cont.)*
white, long grain:
½ cup 22.3
(Carolina/Mahatma/River/Water Maid), ½ cup 22.0
parboiled *(Success)*, ½ cup 20.0
parboiled *(Uncle Ben's Converted)*, 1.2 oz. dry 27.2
white, long grain, instant:
(Carolina/Mahatma), ½ cup 23.0
(Minute/Minute Premium), ⅔ cup 27.0
(Minute Boil-in-Bag), ½ cup 21.0
(Uncle Ben's Boil-in-Bag), 1 oz. dry 21.6
(Uncle Ben's Fast Cook), 1.1 oz. dry 25.1
white, medium grain, ½ cup 26.6
Rice, wild, see "Wild rice"
Rice beverage:
carob lite *(Rice Dream)*, 8 fl. oz. 32.0
chocolate *(Rice Dream)*, 8 fl. oz. 44.0
organic original lite *(Rice Dream)*, 8 fl. oz. 28.0
vanilla lite *(Rice Dream)*, 8 fl. oz. 30.0
Rice bran, crude, 1 cup 41.2
Rice cake:
plain *(Hain* Mini/*Hain* Mini No Salt), ½ oz. 12.0
plain, 5-grain, or with popcorn *(Hain/Hain* No Salt),
  1 piece 8.0
all varieties *(Crispy Cakes)*, 1 piece 7.0
apple cinnamon *(Hain* Mini), ½ oz. 12.0
apple cinnamon *(Hollywood* Mini), ½ oz. 12.0
apple spice *(Mini Crispys)*, 1.1 oz. 25.0
barbecue *(Hain* Mini), ½ oz. 10.0
barbecue *(Mini Crispys)*, 1.1 oz. 24.0
brown, .3-oz. piece 7.3
butter flavor, with popcorn *(Hain)*, 1 piece 8.0
cheese:
(Hollywood Mini), ½ oz. 10.0
regular or nacho *(Hain* Mini), ½ oz. 10.0
nacho or white cheddar, with popcorn *(Hain)*,
  1 piece 8.0
honey almond *(Mini Crispys)*, 1.1 oz. 26.0

honey nut *(Hain* Mini), ½ oz. 11.0
honey nut *(Hollywood* Mini), ½ oz. 11.0
popcorn *(Hain* Mini), ½ oz. 11.0
popcorn, butter flavor or mild cheddar *(Hain* Mini),
  ½ oz. 10.0
ranch *(Hain* Mini), ½ oz. 9.0
sesame *(Hain/Hain* No Salt), 1 piece 8.0
teriyaki *(Hain* Mini), ½ oz. 11.0
Rice chips, brown *(Eden)*, 1 oz. 19.0
Rice dishes, canned, fried *(La Choy)*, ¾ cup 41.0
Rice dishes, freeze-dried*, and chicken *(Mountain
  House)*, 1 cup 41.0
Rice dishes, frozen:
(Green Giant Rice Originals Rice Medley), ½ cup 19.0
and broccoli:
  au gratin *(Freezer Queen* Family), 4.5 oz. 21.0
  in cheese sauce *(Green Giant* One Serving),
    5.5 oz. 26.0
  in cheese sauce *(Green Giant Rice Originals)*,
    ½ cup 18.0
Florentine *(Green Giant Rice Originals)*, ½ cup 22.0
fried, with chicken *(Chun King)*, 8 oz. 41.0
fried, with pork *(Chun King)*, 8 oz. 44.0
Oriental, with vegetables *(The Budget Gourmet* Side
  Dish)*, 5.75 oz. 28.0
pilaf *(Green Giant Rice Originals)*, ½ cup 21.0
pilaf, with green beans *(The Budget Gourmet* Side
  Dish)*, 5.5 oz. 30.0
white and wild *(Green Giant Rice Originals)*, ½ cup 24.0
Rice dishes, mix, cooked, except as noted:
almondine *(Hain* 3-Grain Side Dish), ½ cup 17.0
au gratin, herbed *(Country Inn)*, 1.2 oz. dry 23.6
beef flavor:
  (Lipton Rice and Sauce), ½ cup 25.0
  (Rice-A-Roni), ½ cup 24.0
  almond *(Mahatma)*, ½ cup 20.0
  broccoli *(Lipton* Rice and Sauce), ½ cup 24.0
  Oriental *(Success)*, ½ cup 19.0

Rice dishes, mix *(cont.)*

beef and mushroom *(Rice-A-Roni)*, ½ cup 26.0
broccoli:
  almondine *(Country Inn)*, 1.2 oz. dry 24.5
  au gratin *(Country Inn)*, 1.1 oz. dry............................ 22.2
  au gratin *(Rice-A-Roni ⅓ Less Salt)*, ½ cup 24.0
  and cheddar, white *(Country Inn)*, 1.2 oz. dry................ 23.8
  and cheese *(Success)*, ½ cup 23.0
brown *(Arrowhead Mills Quick Brown Rice)*, 2 oz. dry 43.0
brown, Spanish or vegetable herb *(Arrowhead Mills*
  Quick Brown Rice), 2 oz. dry.. 30.0
brown and wild *(Success)*, ½ cup...................................... 23.0
brown and wild, herb *(Arrowhead Mills Quick Brown*
  Rice), 2 oz. dry 28.0
Cajun *(Lipton Rice and Sauce)*, ½ cup.............................. 26.0
cheddar broccoli *(Lipton Rice and Sauce)*, ½ cup............. 25.0
chicken flavor:
  (Lipton Rice and Sauce), ½ cup...................................... 25.0
  (Rice-A-Roni/Rice-A-Roni ⅓ Less Salt), ½ cup 24.0
  (Success Classic), ½ cup.. 19.0
  broccoli *(Golden Sauté)*, ½ cup 25.0
  broccoli *(Lipton Rice and Sauce)*, ½ cup 25.0
  broccoli *(Rice-A-Roni)*, ½ cup 25.0
  creamy *(Lipton Rice and Sauce)*, ½ cup 27.0
  creamy, and mushroom *(Country Inn)*, 1.3 oz. dry......... 24.5
  creamy, and wild rice *(Country Inn)*, 1.3 oz. dry 26.8
  drumstick *(Minute)*, ½ cup.. 25.0
  sesame *(Mahatma)*, ½ cup 20.0
  stock *(Country Inn)*, 1.2 oz. dry 23.9
  and vegetables *(Rice-A-Roni)*, ½ cup 24.0
  and vegetables, homestyle *(Country Inn)*, 1.3 oz.
    dry 24.1
Florentine *(Country Inn)*, 1.2 oz. dry................................ 23.9
fried:
  (Minute), ½ cup 25.0
  with almonds *(Rice-A-Roni)*, ½ cup................................ 26.0
  beef flavor *(Golden Sauté)*, ½ cup.................................. 22.0
  chicken flavor or Oriental *(Golden Sauté)*, ½ cup.......... 23.0

green bean almondine *(Country Inn)*, 1.2 oz. dry 24.8
herb and butter:
  (Golden Sauté), ½ cup 23.0
  (Lipton Rice and Sauce), ½ cup 24.0
  (Rice-A-Roni), ½ cup 22.0
long grain and wild:
  (Lipton Rice and Sauce Original), ½ cup 26.0
  (Minute), ½ cup 25.0
  (Near East), ½ cup 21.0
  (Uncle Ben's Original), 1 oz. dry 20.6
  (Uncle Ben's Original Fast Cook), 1 oz. dry 22.0
  chicken stock sauce *(Uncle Ben's)*, 1.3 oz. dry 25.4
  mushroom and herbs *(Lipton* Rice and Sauce),
    ½ cup.. 26.0
Mexican *(Old El Paso)*, ½ cup.. 28.0
mushroom, Oriental *(Hain* 3-Grain Goodness), ½ cup 15.0
pilaf:
  (Lipton Rice and Sauce), ½ cup...................................... 26.0
  (Mahatma Classic), ½ cup 20.0
  (Rice-A-Roni), ½ cup 26.0
  (Success), ½ cup... 24.0
  all varieties *(Near East)*, ½ cup 21.0
  basmati, tomato and herb *(Knorr* Pilafs), 1 serving
    dry 32.6
  brown, with miso *(Quick Pilaf)*, ½ cup............................. 22.0
  harvest, medley with carrots *(Knorr* Pilafs),
    1 serving dry 20.0
  jasmine, with lemon and herbs *(Knorr* Pilafs),
    1 serving dry 27.9
  Spanish, brown *(Quick Pilaf)*, ½ cup 22.0
  vegetable *(Country Inn)*, 1.2 oz. dry, ½ cup.................... 24.8
Spanish:
  (Lipton Rice and Sauce), ½ cup...................................... 25.0
  (Mahatma Authentic), ½ cup.. 20.0
  (Rice-A-Roni), 1/7 pkg. dry 22.0
  (Success), ½ cup... 23.0
  and beans *(Fantastic Only a Pinch)*, 10 oz. 48.0
vegetable blend, garden *(Uncle Ben's)*, 1.3 oz. dry........... 26.5

Rice dishes, mix *(cont.)*
yellow *(Rice-A-Roni)*, ½ cup.. 25.0
yellow, saffron *(Mahatma)*, ½ cup 21.0
wild *(Mahatma)*, ½ cup 20.0
Rice flour:
brown, 1 cup... 120.8
brown *(Arrowhead Mills)*, 2 oz.. 44.0
white, 1 cup 126.6
Rigatoni entree, frozen:
bake, with meat sauce and cheese *(Lean Cuisine)*,
  9 oz.. 29.0
with chicken and vegetables *(Healthy Choice Extra
  Portions)*, 12.5 oz. 50.0
in cream sauce, with broccoli and chicken *(The
  Budget Gourmet Light and Healthy)*, 10.8 oz. 44.0
in meat sauce *(Healthy Choice)*, 9.5 oz. 34.0
with meat sauce *(Stouffer's Homestyle)*, 12 oz. 49.0
Roast, vegetarian, frozen *(Worthington Dinner
  Roast)*, 2 oz. 5.0
Robert sauce *(Escoffier)*, 1 tbsp. 5.0
Rockfish, without added ingredients.................................... 0
Roe (see also "Caviar"):
raw, 1 oz. 4
raw, 1 tbsp.. .2
baked, broiled or microwaved, 4 oz............................... 2.2
carp *(Krinos Tarama)*, 1 tbsp. 0
Roll (see also "Roll, sweet"):
(Arnold Bakery Light), 1 piece 21.0
(Arnold Bran'nola Buns), 1 piece.................................. 20.0
(Francisco 8"), 1 piece.. 39.0
(Wonder Bakery Style), 1 piece 24.0
(Wonder Enriched Buns), 1 piece................................. 13.0
assorted *(Brownberry Hearth)*, 1 piece 20.0
brown and serve:
  (Pepperidge Farm Hearth), 1 piece............................. 10.0
  (Roman Meal), 1 piece 11.8
  Bavarian wheat *(Bread du Jour)*, 1 piece..................... 15.0
  plain or buttermilk *(Wonder)*, 1 piece 14.0

club *(Pepperidge Farm)*, 1 piece..................................... 19.0
Italian, crusty *(Bread du Jour)*, 1 piece 16.0
sourdough *(Francisco)*, 1 piece.................................... 19.0
crescent, butter *(Pepperidge Farm Heat & Serve)*,
  1 piece.. 13.0
croissant, see "Croissant"
dinner:
  (August Bros.), 1 piece.. 18.0
  (Pepperidge Farm Country Style), 1 piece 9.0
  (Pepperidge Farm Party), 1 piece 5.0
  (Roman Meal), 1 piece 11.8
  (Wonder), 1 piece 14.0
  parker house or sesame seed finger *(Pepperidge*
    Farm), 1 piece... 9.0
  plain or sesame *(Arnold)*, 1 piece 9.0
  poppy seed finger *(Pepperidge Farm)*, 1 piece.......... 8.0
  potato *(Pepperidge Farm Hearty)*, 1 piece 14.0
  wheat or white *(Home Pride)*, 1 piece 10.0
egg, Dutch *(Arnold)*, 1 piece... 21.0
French style:
  (Francisco 6"), 1 piece 39.0
  (Pepperidge Farm), 1 piece....................................... 20.0
  mini *(Francisco)*, 1 piece 24.0
  7-grain *(Pepperidge Farm)*, 1 piece 18.0
  sourdough *(Pepperidge Farm)*, 1 piece 19.0
hamburger:
  (Arnold), 1 piece 20.0
  (Pepperidge Farm), 1 piece....................................... 22.0
  (Roman Meal), 1 piece 19.2
  (Wonder Light), 1 piece 14.0
hoagie, soft *(Pepperidge Farm)*, 1 piece....................... 34.0
honey wheat *(Wonder Buns)*, 1 piece 22.0
hot dog:
  (Arnold, 12 oz.), 1 piece.. 21.0
  (Arnold Bran'nola), 1 piece.. 18.0
  (Arnold New England), 1 piece 20.0
  (Pepperidge Farm), 1 piece....................................... 24.0
  (Roman Meal), 1 piece 18.0

Roll, hot dog *(cont.)*
   (Wonder Light), 1 piece 14.0
   Dijon *(Pepperidge Farm)*, 1 piece 23.0
   sliced *(Brownberry)*, 1 piece 21.0
Italian *(Savoni 8")*, 1 piece 38.0
kaiser:
   (Arnold Deli), 1 piece 34.0
   (August Bros.), 1 piece 35.0
   (Brownberry Hearth), 1 piece 26.0
   (Francisco 6"), 1 piece 34.0
onion:
   (Arnold Deli), 1 piece 34.0
   (Arnold Premium), 1 piece 38.0
   (August Bros.), 1 piece 33.0
   soft *(Arnold)*, 1 piece 28.0
pan *(Wonder)*, 1 piece 14.0
pan Cubano *(Arnold Agusto)*, 1 piece 43.0
party, petite *(Arnold)*, 2 pieces 10.0
potato *(Arnold)*, 1 piece 25.0
sandwich:
   (Arnold), 1 piece 18.0
   (Roman Meal), 1 piece 31.4
   onion, with poppy seeds *(Pepperidge Farm)*,
     1 piece 26.0
   potato *(Pepperidge Farm)*, 1 piece 28.0
   sesame *(Arnold)*, 1 piece 23.0
   with sesame seeds *(Pepperidge Farm)*, 1 piece 23.0
   wheat or white *(Brownberry)*, 1 piece 23.0
sesame *(August Bros.)*, 1 piece 35.0
sourdough *(Francisco)*, 1 piece 19.0
sourdough *(Wonder* Bakery Style), 1 piece 25.0
sub *(Levy* Old country), 1 piece 34.0
twist, golden *(Pepperidge Farm* Heat & Serve),
   1 piece 14.0
wheat *(Wonder* Bakery Style), 1 piece 25.0
wheat or white *(Arnold* Old Fashioned), 2 pieces 11.0
Roll, frozen or refrigerated (see also "Roll, sweet"):
butterflake *(Pillsbury)*, 1 piece 20.0

crescent *(Pillsbury)*, 1 piece.. 11.0
homestyle *(Rich's)*, 1 piece... 13.0
Parkerhouse *(Bridgford)*, 1-oz. piece................................ 16.0
ranch, white *(Bridgford)*, 1.5-oz. piece............................. 24.0
Roll, sweet (see also "Bun, sweet"):
(Tastykake Tasty Twist), 1 piece... 3.0
apple cinnamon *(Aunt Fanny's Old Fashioned)*,
    1 piece... 34.0
caramel nut *(Aunt Fanny's)*, 1 piece................................. 33.0
cinnamon:
    (Aunt Fanny's), 2-oz. piece 34.0
    (Aunt Fanny's Duos), 1 piece...................................... 32.0
    (Awrey's Homestyle), 1 piece...................................... 40.0
    (Sara Lee Deluxe), 1 piece.. 31.0
    swirl *(Awrey's Grande)*, 1 piece 46.0
    twirl *(Aunt Fanny's)*, 1 piece.. 16.0
fruit roll *(Aunt Fanny's Dixie)*, 1 piece.............................. 34.0
pecan twirl *(Aunt Fanny's)*, 1 piece.................................. 16.5
pecan twirl *(Tastykake)*, 1 piece.. 17.0
Roll, sweet, frozen or refrigerated:
caramel with nuts, refrigerated *(Pillsbury)*, 1 piece............. 19.0
cinnamon:
    frozen *(Pepperidge Farm)*, 1 piece.............................. 34.0
    glazed, frozen *(Weight Watchers)*, 1 piece 31.0
    with icing, refrigerator *(Pillsbury)*, 1 piece................... 17.0
Roll mix*:
hot *(Dromedary)*, 1 piece 41.0
hot *(Pillsbury)*, 1 piece 21.0
Roseapple, trimmed, 1 oz. 1.6
Roselle, 1 oz. or ½ cup 3.2
Rosemary, dried, 1 tsp. 8
Rotini entree, frozen:
cheddar *(Green Giant Garden Gourmet Right for
    Lunch)*, 9.5 oz... 32.0
cheese, three *(Weight Watchers)*, 9 oz............................. 34.0
seafood *(Mrs. Paul's Light)*, 8 oz...................................... 34.0
Roughy, orange, without added ingredients 0

Roy Rogers, 1 serving:

breakfast items, see "*Hardee's*"

burgers:

cheeseburger 27.4

cheeseburger, bacon 25.0

hamburger 26.6

R Bar Burger 28.0

Roy's Roasters:

skin on, breast/wing 3.0

skin on, thigh/leg quarter 2.0

skin off, breast/wing 2.0

skin off, thigh/leg quarter 1.0

roast beef sandwich:

regular 29.1

regular, with cheese 29.9

large 29.6

large, with cheese 30.3

french fries, regular 32.0

baked topped potato:

plain or with margarine 47.9

broccoli & cheese 39.6

sour cream & chives 47.6

Rum runner mixer, frozen*, with rum *(Bacardi)*,

7 fl. oz. 33.0

Rutabaga:

fresh:

raw, cubed, ½ cup 5.7

boiled, drained, cubed, ½ cup 7.4

boiled, drained, mashed, ½ cup 10.5

canned, diced *(Allens/Sunshine)*, ½ cup 4.0

Rye, whole-grain:

1 cup 117.9

(Arrowhead Mills), 2 oz. 42.0

Rye flakes *(Arrowhead Mills)*, 2 oz. 42.0

Rye flour:

dark, 1 cup 88.0

light, 1 cup 81.8
medium, 1 cup 79.0
medium *(Pillsbury's Best)*, 1 cup 83.0
and wheat *(Pillsbury's Best* Bohemian Style), 1 cup 86.0

brine, drained, 1 cup 6.9
mesquite, 1 tsp 11.0
mesquite, with onion, 1 tbsp. 9.0
and sour cherry, in a sweet sauce, Nestlé cup 39.0

S

Food and Measure	Carbohydrate Grams

Sablefish, fresh or smoked, without added
  ingredients 0
Safflower seed kernels, dried, 1 oz. 9.7
Safflower seed meal, partially defatted, 1 oz. 13.8
Saffron, 1 tsp. 5
Sage, ground, 1 tsp. 4
Salad dip (Nasoya Vegi-Dip), 1 oz. 3.0
Salad dressing:
all varieties:
  (Hain Canola), 1 tbsp. 1.0
  (Nasoya Vegi-Dressing), 1 tbsp. 1.0
  except creamy Caesar (Hain), 1 tbsp. 0
bacon and tomato (Kraft), 1 tbsp. 1.0
blue cheese:
  (Cains Country), 1 tbsp. 2.0
  (La Martinique), 2 tbsp. 0
  (Marie's Lite & Luscious), 1 tbsp. 4.0
  (Roka Brand), 1 tbsp. 1.0
  chunky (Kraft), 1 tbsp. 2.0
  chunky (Marie's), 1 tbsp. 2.0
  chunky (Wish-Bone), 1 tbsp. .... <1.0
  creamy (Bernstein's Restaurant), 1 tbsp. 1.0
buttermilk:
  (Hain Old Fashioned), 1 tbsp. 0
  (Seven Seas Buttermilk Recipe), 1 tbsp. 1.0
  creamy (Kraft), 1 tbsp. 1.0
Caesar:
  (Lawry's Classic), 1 oz. 1.0

creamy *(Hain)*, 1 tbsp. 1.0
creamy *(Lawry's* Classic), 1 oz. 1.8
creamy *(Marie's)*, 1 tbsp. 2.0
golden *(Kraft)*, 1 tbsp. 1.0
with olive oil *(Wish-Bone)*, 1 tbsp. 5.0
Champagne *(Lawry's* Classic), 1 oz. 2.3
Chinese vinaigrette *(Lawry's* Classic), 1 oz. 2.4
coleslaw:
  (Kraft), 1 tbsp. 4.0
  (Marie's), 1.05 oz. 6.0
  (Miracle Whip), 1 tbsp. 3.0
cucumber, creamy *(Herb Magic)*, 2 tbsp. 4.0
cucumber, creamy *(Kraft)*, 1 tbsp. 1.0
Dijon, creamy *(Light Fantastic)*, 1 tbsp. 3.0
Dijon, golden *(Lawry's* Classic), 1 oz. 4.0
dill, creamy *(Light Fantastic)*, 1 tbsp. 3.0
French:
  (Cains Country), 1 tbsp. 3.0
  (Catalina), 1 tbsp. 4.0
  (Kraft), 1 tbsp. 2.0
  (Kraft Miracle), 1 tbsp. 3.0
  (Seven Seas French! Light), 1 tbsp. 2.0
  (Wish-Bone Deluxe), 1 tbsp. 2.0
  (Wish-Bone Sweet'n Spicy), 1 tbsp. 3.0
  creamy *(Marie's)*, 1 tbsp. 4.0
  creamy *(Seven Seas)*, 1 tbsp. 2.0
  vinaigrette, true *(La Martinique)*, 2 tbsp. .... <1.0
fruit salad *(Knott's)*, 1 tbsp. 3.0
garlic, creamy *(Kraft)*, 1 tbsp. 1.0
herb, classic *(Marie's* Zesty Fat Free), 1 tbsp. 4.0
herb, Italian, and Romano *(Marie's)*, 1 tbsp. 2.0
herb and spice *(Seven Seas Viva/Viva Herbs &*
  Spices! Light), 1 tbsp. 1.0
honey mustard:
  (Marie's), 1 tbsp. 4.0
  (PeggyJane's), 1 tbsp. 2.0
  vinaigrette *(Cain's* Country), 1 tbsp. 3.0

Salad dressing *(cont.)*
Italian:
  (Herb Magic), 1 tbsp. 2.0
  (Kraft House/*Kraft Presto)*, 1 tbsp. 1.0
  (Light Fantastic Classico), 1 tbsp.................................... 3.0
  (Marie's), 1 tbsp... 2.0
  (Marie's Zesty Fat Free), 1 tbsp...................................... 4.0
  (Ott's), 1.1 oz. 1.0
  (Seven Seas Viva/Seven Seas Free Viva/Viva
    Italian! Light), 1 tbsp. 1.0
  (Wish-Bone/Wish-Bone Robusto), 1 tbsp...................... 2.0
  blended or creamy *(Wish-Bone)*, 1 tbsp.......................... 1.0
  with bleu cheese *(Lawry's* Classic), 1 oz..................... 1.9
  cheese and garlic *(Bernstein's)*, 1 tbsp. 1.0
  with cheese *(Bernstein's* Reduced Calorie/Cheese
    Fantastico!)*, 1 tbsp.. 1.0
  creamy *(Seven Seas/Seven Seas Viva Creamy*
    Italian Light), 1 tbsp. 1.0
  creamy *(Weight Watchers)*, 1 tbsp................................. 2.0
  creamy, with basil *(Cains* Country), 1 tbsp.................... 1.0
  creamy, with real sour cream *(Kraft)*, 1 tbsp. 1.0
  garlic or herb and Romano *(Marie's)*, 1 tbsp. 2.0
  garlic *(Marie's Lite & Luscious)*, 1 tbsp......................... 3.0
  olive oil *(Wish-Bone* Classic), 1 tbsp. 2.0
  olive oil blend *(Cains* Country), 1 tbsp. 2.0
  with Parmesan *(Lawry's* Classic), 1 oz. 4.5
  zesty *(Kraft)*, 1 tbsp.. 1.0
lemon pepper *(Lawry's* Classic), 1 oz. 3.0
mayonnaise type (see also "Mayonnaise"):
  (Kraft Free), 1 tbsp. 3.0
  (Miracle Whip/Miracle Whip Light), 1 tbsp..................... 2.0
  (Miracle Whip Free), 1 tbsp.. 5.0
  (Spin Blend), 1 tbsp. 3.0
  (Spin Blend Cholesterol Free), 1 tbsp............................ 2.0
  (Weight Watchers Fat Free), 1 tbsp. 4.0
  (Weight Watchers Light/Low Sodium), 1 tbsp.................. 1.0
  whipped *(Cains)*, 1 tbsp. 2.0
  whipped *(Cains* Fat Free), 1 tbsp.................................... 3.0

whipped *(Weight Watchers Fat Free)*, 1 tbsp. 4.0
oil and vinegar *(Kraft)*, 1 tbsp. 1.0
olive oil vinaigrette *(Wish-Bone)*, 1 tbsp. 2.0
Oriental *(Light Fantastic)*, 1 tbsp. 5.0
Oriental chicken salad *(PeggyJane's)*, 1 tbsp. 2.0
(Ott's Famous/Ott's Fat Free/Reduced Calorie),
    1.1 oz. 8.0
peppercorn, ground *(PeggyJane's)*, 1 tbsp. 1.0
peppercorn, with Parmesan *(Cains Country)*, 1 tbsp. 1.0
poppyseed:
    (La Martinique Original), 2 tbsp. 8.0
    (Marie's), 1 tbsp. 4.0
    (Ott's Reduced Calorie), 1 tbsp. 8.0
    (PeggyJane's), 1 tbsp. 4.0
ranch:
    (Cains Country), 1 tbsp. 1.0
    (Herb Magic), 2 tbsp. 4.0
    (Kraft Free), 1 tbsp. 3.0
    (Light Fantastic), 1 tbsp. 3.0
    (Marie's), 1 tbsp. 1.0
    (Marie's Lite & Luscious), 1 tbsp. 4.0
    (Ott's), 1.1 oz. 2.0
    (Seven Seas Buttermilk Recipe Ranch! Light/Viva),
        1 tbsp. 1.0
    (Seven Seas Free), 1 tbsp. 4.0
    (Seven Seas Viva Ranch! Light), 1 tbsp. 2.0
    (Wish-Bone), 1 tbsp. .... <1.0
    buttermilk spice *(Marie's)*, 1 tbsp. 2.0
    creamy *(Marie's)*, 1 tbsp. 1.0
    creamy *(Rancher's Choice)*, 1 tbsp. 1.0
    Italian *(Bernstein's)*, 1 tbsp. 2.0
    Parmesan garlic *(Light Fantastic)*, 1 tbsp. 2.0
red wine vinaigrette:
    (Cains Country), 1 tbsp. 2.0
    (Lawry's Classic), 1 oz. 4.9
    (Marie's Zesty Fat Free), 1 tbsp. 5.0
red wine vinegar *(Seven Seas Free)*, 1 tbsp. 1.0

Salad dressing (cont.)
red wine vinegar and oil:
  (Kraft), 1 tbsp... 4.0
  (Seven Seas Viva/Viva Red Wine! Vinegar & Oil
    Light), 1 tbsp.. 1.0
  olive oil (Wish-Bone), 1 tbsp. 2.0
rice wine vinaigrette (Lawry's Classic), 1 oz. 6.0
Russian:
  (Kraft Reduced Calorie), 1 tbsp. 4.0
  (Weight Watchers), 1 tbsp.. 2.0
  (Wish-Bone), 1 tbsp... 7.0
  creamy (Kraft), 1 tbsp.. 2.0
  with honey (Kraft), 1 tbsp.. 4.0
San Francisco, with Romano (Lawry's Classic), 1 oz. 2.0
Santa Fe (Wish-Bone), 1 tbsp. 1.0
sour (Friendship Sour Treat), 1 oz. 2.0
sour cream and dill (Marie's), 1 tbsp.................................. 10.0
sour cream and dill (Marie's Lite & Luscious), 1 tbsp. 4.0
sun-dried tomato vinaigrette (PeggyJane's), 1 tbsp. 1.0
sweet and sour (Old Dutch), 1 tbsp. 6.5
Thousand Island:
  (Herb Magic), 2 tbsp. 4.0
  (Kraft), 1 tbsp.. 2.0
  (Marie's), 1 tbsp.. 3.0
  (Seven Seas Thousand Island! Light), 1 tbsp. 3.0
  (Weight Watchers), 1 tbsp.. 2.0
  (Wish Bone), 1 tbsp... 3.0
  and bacon (Kraft), 1 tbsp. 2.0
  creamy (Seven Seas), 1 tbsp. 2.0
vinaigrette (Herb Magic), 1 tbsp. 1.5
vintage, with sherry wine (Lawry's Classic), 1 oz. 2.5
white wine vinaigrette (Lawry's Classic), 1 oz...................... 2.7
white wine vinaigrette (Marie's Zesty Fat Free),
  1 tbsp. 5.0
Salad dressing mix*:
all varieties, except honey mustard, fat free creamy
  Italian, and lite ranch (Good Seasons), 1 tbsp. 1.0

honey mustard, fat free creamy Italian, or lite ranch
  (Good Seasons), 1 tbsp. 2.0
Salad mix*:
(Kraft Light Rancher's Choice), 1/2 cup 23.0
(Kraft Rancher's Choice), 1/2 cup 21.0
Caesar *(Suddenly Salad)*, 1/2 cup 22.0
pasta:
  (McCormick/Schilling Pasta Prima), 1/2 cup 41.0
  bacon vinaigrette *(Country Recipe)*, 1/2 cup 24.0
  broccoli, creamy *(Lipton)*, 1/2 cup 23.0
  broccoli and vegetables *(Kraft)*, 1/2 cup 15.0
  classic *(Suddenly Salad)*, 1/2 cup 23.0
  Dijon, creamy *(Country Recipe)*, 1/2 cup 24.0
  garden primavera or homestyle *(Kraft)*, 1/2 cup 21.0
  Italian *(Kraft)*, 1/2 cup 20.0
  Italian *(Suddenly Salad)*, 1/2 cup 22.0
  Italian, creamy *(Country Recipe)*, 1/2 cup 22.0
  Italian, herb *(Fantastic)*, 1/2 cup 21.0
  Italian, robust *(Lipton)*, 1/2 cup 25.0
  Oriental, spicy *(Fantastic)*, 1/2 cup 20.0
  ranch *(Country Recipe)*, 1/2 cup 19.0
primavera *(Suddenly Salad)*, 1/2 cup 20.0
ranch and bacon *(Suddenly Salad)*, 1/2 cup 24.0
Salad Savoy *(Frieda's)*, 1 cup 6.0
Salad seasoning *(McCormick/Schilling* Salad
  Supreme), 1 tsp. 5
Salami:
beer *(Oscar Mayer* Salami for Beer), 2 slices .... <1.0
all varieties *(Kahn's/Kahn's* Family Pack), 1 slice 1.0
beef *(Hebrew National)*, 1 oz. .... <1.0
beef *(Oscar Mayer* Machiaeh), 2 slices 1.0
cotto, regular or beef *(Oscar Mayer)*, 2 slices .... <1.0
dry or hard *(Hormel Homeland)*, 1 oz. .... <2.0
dry, hard, or Genoa *(Oscar Mayer)*, 3 slices 0
Genoa *(Hormel DiLusso)*, 1 oz. 1.0
Genoa *(Hormel San Remo Brand)*, 1 oz. .... <2.0
"Salami," vegetarian, frozen *(Worthington)*, 2 slices 2.0

Salisbury steak, see "Beef dinner" and "Beef entree"

Salmon, fresh, smoked, or canned, without added ingredients 0

Salmon seasoning mix (*Old Bay Salmon Classic*), 1 pkg. 21.0

Salsa:

(*La Victoria* Suprema), 2 tbsp. 2.0

all varieties (*Tio Sancho*), ¼ cup 4.0

green chili (*La Victoria*), 2 tbsp. 2.0

green chili (*Old El Paso* Thick'n Chunky), 2 tbsp. 1.0

hot or medium (*Hain* Thick & Chunky), 2 tbsp. 1.0

hot, medium, or mild:

  (*Chi-Chi's*), 1 oz. 2.0

  (*Frito-Lay's* Chunky), 1 oz. 2.0

  (*Master Choice*), 1 oz. 2.0

  (*Old El Paso* Thick'n Chunky), 2 tbsp. 1.0

  (*Rosarita*), 3 tbsp. 6.0

hot or mild (*Hain*), ¼ cup 4.0

mild (*Hain* Thick & Chunky), 2 tbsp. .... <1.0

picante (see also "Picante sauce"):

  all varieties (*Old El Paso*), 2 tbsp. 2.0

  medium or ranchera (*La Victoria*), 2 tbsp. 1.0

  mild (*La Victoria*), 2 tbsp. 2.0

taco (see also "Taco sauce"), medium or mild (*Rosarita*), 3 tbsp. 6.0

Texas (*Hot Cha Cha*), 1 oz. 2.5

verde (*Old El Paso* Thick'n Chunky), 2 tbsp. 2.0

Victoria (*La Victoria*), 2 tbsp. 1.0

Salsa seasoning mix (*Lawry's* Seasoning Blends), 1 pkg. 20.5

Salsify:

raw, untrimmed, 1 lb. 73.4

raw, sliced, ½ cup 12.5

boiled, drained, sliced, ½ cup 10.5

black, raw (*Frieda's*), 1 oz. 5.3

Salt, 1 tbsp. 0

Salt, seasoned (see also specific listings):
(Lawry's), 1 tsp...6
(Lawry's Lite), 1 tsp.. 1.7
(McCormick/Shilling/McCormick/Shilling Salt'n
  Spice), 1 tsp. 6
(Morton/Morton Nature's Seasons), 1 tsp. ....<1.0
hot'n spicy *(Lawry's* Spice Blends), 1 tsp...................... 1.5
Salt, substitute:
(Lawry's Salt-Free 17), 1 tsp....................................... 1.8
(Morton), 1 tsp. 1
seasoned *(Lawry's Salt-Free)*, 1 tsp. 6
Salt pork
Sandwich, see specific listings
Sandwich sauce (see also specific listings):
(Hunt's Manwich Extra Thick & Chunky), 2.5 oz............... 15.0
(Hunt's Manwich Extra Thick & Chunky), 1 sandwich*...... 36.0
Mexican *(Hunt's Manwich)*, 2.5 oz. 9.0
Mexican *(Hunt's Manwich)*, 1 sandwich*........................... 30.0
sloppy Joe (see also "Barbecue sauce"):
  (Hormel Not-So-Sloppy Joe Sauce), 2.24 oz. 16.0
  (Hunt's Manwich), 2.5 oz.. 10.0
  (Hunt's Manwich), 1 sandwich*................................... 31.0
  (Libby's), 2.5 oz. 10.0
Sandwich seasoning mix:
(Hunt's Manwich), ¼ oz... 5.0
(Hunt's Manwich), 1 sandwich* 31.0
sloppy Joe:
  (Lawry's Seasoning Blends), 1 pkg............................ 27.7
  (Tone's), 1 tsp. 3.1
  (French's), ⅛ pkg. 3.0
  (McCormick/Schilling), ¼ pkg. 6.0
Sandwich spread:
meatless:
  (Blue Plate), 1 tbsp.. 3.0
  (Hellman's/Best Foods), 1 tbsp..................................... 2.0
  (Kraft), 1 tbsp... 3.0
  (LaLoma), 3 tbsp. 4.0
meat *(Oscar Mayer)*, 2 oz. 9.0

Sapodilla:
1 medium, 3″ × 2½″ 33.9
½ cup 24.1
Sapote:
1 medium, 11.2 oz. 76.0
trimmed, 1 oz. 9.6
white *(Frieda's)*, 1 oz. 9.0
Sardine, fresh, see "Herring"
Sardine, canned:
Atlantic, in oil 0
Norwegian, in oil, drained *(Empress)*, 3.75 oz. 1.0
Portugese, skinless and boneless, in oil *(Empress)*,
　4.375-oz. can 2.0
kippered *(Brunswick Kippered Snacks)*, 3.53-oz. can 1.0
in mustard or tomato sauce *(Underwood)*, 3.75 oz. 2.0
in soya oil, drained *(Underwood)*, 3.75 oz. 1.0
Sauce, see specific listings
Sauerkraut:
with liquid, ½ cup 5.1
(Claussen), 3 oz. 4.0
*(New Morning Kozmic Kraut/Kozmic Kraut Low
　Sodium)*, 1 oz. 1.0
(Stokely), ½ cup 4.0
(Vlasic Old Fashioned), 1 oz. 1.0
Sausage (see also "Sausage stick" and specific
　listings):
all varieties, except Golden Brown Light *(Jones Dairy
　Farm)*, 2 oz. ....tr.
beef and cheddar *(Hillshire Farm Flavorseal)*, 2 oz. 1.0
brown and serve, country recipe *(Hillshire Farm
　Flavorseal)*, 2 oz. 2.0
Italian, hot or mild *(Hillshire Farm Links)*, 2 oz. 1.0
Italian, pork, cooked, 1 oz. 4
pork:
　fresh, cooked, ½ oz. (yield from 1 oz. raw link) 1
　(Hormel Little Sizzlers), 1 oz. .... <2.0
　(Jones Dairy Farm Golden Brown Light), 1 link 1.0
　(Oscar Mayer Little Friers), 2 links 1.0

patty, plain, extra mild, or sage, cooked *(Jimmy Dean)*, 1 patty .... <1.0
patty, fresh, cooked, 1 oz. (yield from 2 oz. raw patty) 3
smoked:
   (Hillshire Farm Bun Size), 2 oz. 2.0
   (Hillshire Farm Flavorseal/Flavorseal Lite/Links), 2 oz. 1.0
   (Oscar Mayer Little Smokies), 6 links 1.0
   (Oscar Mayer Smokie Links), 1 link .... <1.0
   beef *(Hillshire Farm* Bun Size/Flavorseal), 2 oz. 2.0
   beef or cheese *(Oscar Mayer* Cheese/Beef Smokies), 1 link .... <1.0
   hot *(Hillshire Farm* Flavorseal), 2 oz. 2.0
   Italian seasoned *(Hillshire Farm* Flavorseal), 2 oz. 1.0
turkey, see "Turkey sausage"
Sausage, freeze-dried, patty *(Mountain House)*, ½ pkg. 0
"Sausage," vegetarian:
.9-oz. link 2.5
1.3-oz. patty 3.7
canned *(LaLoma* Little Links), 2 links 2.0
canned *(Worthington Saucettes)*, 2 pieces 3.0
frozen:
   (Morningstar Farms Breakfast Links), 2 links 3.0
   (Morningstar Farms Breakfast Patties), 2 patties 6.0
   (Worthington Prosage Links), 2 links 3.0
   (Worthington Prosage Patties), 2 patties 4.0
   roll *(Worthington Prosage)*, 2.5 oz. 4.0
Sausage breakfast biscuit, frozen:
(Hormel Quick Meal), 3.7 oz. 29.0
(Swanson), 3.2 oz. 23.0
(Weight Watchers), 3 oz. 19.0
and cheese *(Hormel Quick Meal)*, 4.3 oz. 31.0
"Sausage" breakfast biscuit, vegetarian, frozen *(Morningstar Farms)*, 3.5 oz. 31.0
Sausage seasoning, pork *(Tone's)*, 1 tsp. 2.7

Sausage stick (see also "Beef jerky"):
beef:
   pepperoni *(Pemmican)*, 1.64-oz. piece 3.0
   Tabasco (Pemmican), 1.64-oz. piece 4.0
   teriyaki *(Pemmican)*, 1.64-oz. piece 7.0
pickled, all varieties *(Penrose Firecracker/Penrose
   Giant Firecracker)*, 1 piece 1.0
smoked:
   (Slim Jim Big Slim), 1 piece 1.0
   (Slim Jim Giant Slim), 1 piece 2.0
   all varieties *(Slim Jim Handi-Paks)*, 1 piece 1.0
   plain, nacho, or *Tabasco (Slim Jim Super Slim)*,
     1 piece 1.0
   beef'n cheese *(Slim Jim)*, 1 pkg. 2.0
summer sausage, plain or Teriyaki *(Slim Jim)*, 1 piece 1.0
Savory, ground, 1 tsp 1.0
Scallion, see "Onion, green"
Scallop, meat only:
raw, 4 oz. 2.7
raw, 2 large or 5 small, 1.1 oz. 7
"Scallop," imitation, made from surimi, 4 oz. 12.1
"Scallop," vegetarian, canned, *(Worthington
   Vegetable Skallops/Worthington Vegetable Skallops
   No Salt)*, ½ cup 4.0
Scallop entree, fried, frozen *(Mrs. Paul's)*, 3.5 oz. 18.0
Scallop squash:
raw, sliced, ½ cup 2.5
boiled, drained, sliced, ½ cup 3.0
boiled, drained, mashed, ½ cup 4.0
Scrapple *(Jones Dairy Farm)*, 1.5-oz. slice 5.0
Scrod, without added ingredients 0
Scup, without added ingredients 0
Sea bass, without added ingredients 0
Sea trout, without added ingredients 0
Seafood, see specific listings
Seafood entree, frozen:
combination platter, breaded *(Mrs. Paul's)*, 9 oz. 55.0
Creole, with rice *(Swanson Homestyle)*, 9 oz. 40.0

Newburg *(Healthy Choice)*, 8 oz. 30.0
Seafood sauce (see also "Cocktail sauce"):
barbecue, Cajun style *(Golden Dipt)*, 2 tbsp. 5.0
cooking sauce:
   Creole style or Dijonnaise *(Golden Dipt)*, 2 tbsp. 2.0
   French white *(Golden Dipt)*, 2 tbsp. 3.0
   lemon butter dill *(Golden Dipt)*, 2 tbsp. 4.0
marinade, lemon herb *(Golden Dipt)*, 2 tbsp. 2.0
marinade, ginger teriyaki *(Golden Dipt)*, 2 tbsp. 12.0
Seafood seasoning, see "Fish seasoning and
   coating mix"
Seasoning and coating mix (see also specific
   listings):
country mild *(Shake'n Bake)*, 1/4 packet 10.0
Italian herb *(Shake'n Bake)*, 1.4 packet 14.0
Seaweed:
agar, raw, 1 oz. 1.9
agar, dried, 1 oz. 22.9
Irish moss, raw, 1 oz. 3.5
kelp, raw, 1 oz. 2.7
laver, raw, 1 oz. 1.4
spirulina, raw, 1 oz. 7
spirulina, dried, 1 oz. 6.8
wakame, raw, 1 oz. 2.6
Seitan mix *(Arrowhead Mills)*, 2.5 oz. 14.0
Semolina, whole-grain, 1 cup 121.6
Sesame butter (see also "Sesame paste"):
(Roaster Fresh), 1 oz. 6.0
(Erewhon), 2 tbsp. 3.0
Sesame flour, 1 oz.:
high fat, 1 oz. 7.6
partially defatted, 1 oz. 10.0
lowfat, 1 oz. 10.1
Sesame meal, partially defatted, 1 oz. 7.4
Sesame paste (see also "Tahini"), from whole
   sesame seeds, 1 tbsp. 4.1
Sesame seasoning, all-purpose *(McCormick/
Schilling Parsley Patch)*, 1/2 tsp. 5

Sesame seeds:
(Spice Islands), 1 tsp. 9
whole *(Arrowhead Mills)*, 1 oz. 6.0
whole, roasted and toasted, 1 oz. 7.3
kernels, decorticated:
  (Arrowhead Mills), 2 oz. 4.0
  dried, 1 tsp. 3
  toasted, 1 oz. 7.4
Sesbania flower:
raw, 1 cup 1.4
steamed, ½ cup 2.7
Shad, without added ingredients 0
Shallot:
fresh, peeled, 1 oz. 4.8
fresh, chopped, 1 tbsp. 1.7
freeze-dried, 1 tbsp. 7
Shark, without added ingredients 0
Sheepshead, without added ingredients 0
Shellie bean, canned, with liquid, ½ cup 7.6
Shells, pasta, entree, stuffed, frozen:
(Celentano), 6.25 oz. 32.0
(Celentano Great Choice), 10 oz. 41.0
broccoli *(Celentano Great Choice)*, 10 oz. 31.0
cheese, with tomato sauce *(Stouffer's)*, 9.25 oz. 28.0
with sauce *(Celentano)*, 10 oz. 34.0
with tomato sauce *(Healthy Choice Extra Portion)*,
  12 oz. 53.0
Shells, pasta, mix*, and curry, with tofu *(Tofu*
  Classics), ½ cup 16.0
Sherbet (see also "Sorbet"):
all flavors *(Sealtest)*, ½ cup 28.0
orange:
  ½ cup 29.2
  (Blue Bell), ½ cup 29.0
  bar, 2.75-fl.-oz. bar 20.1
Shoney's:
breakfast, kitchen ordered:
  bacon, 3 strips 1
  biscuit, 1 piece 21.6

blueberry muffin, 2 pieces...................................35.4
country gravy, 3 oz. 5.7
croissant, 1 piece 22.0
egg, fried, 1 egg 6
grits, 3 oz...6.2
ham, breakfast, 2 slices 6
hash browns, 3 oz...14.1
home fries, 3 oz. 18.7
honey bun, 1 piece 32.0
pancakes, 1 piece 19.9
sausage patty, 1 patty 2
sirloin steak, charbroiled 0
syrup, low-cal, 2.2 oz..24.4
toast, buttered, 2 slices 24.6

soups, 6 oz.:
bean...9.8
beef cabbage...9.4
broccoli, cream of 10.5
broccoli/cauliflower...11.9
cheddar chowder 14.4
cheese Florentine ham 11.8
chicken, cream of...13.5
chicken gumbo 7.0
chicken noodle 9.2
chicken rice 13.3
chicken vegetable, cream of...............................13.4
clam chowder..9.6
corn chowder 22.1
onion...1.5
potato 16.8
tomato Florentine 11.0
tomato vegetable..9.8
vegetable beef..14.1

entrees, 1 serving[1]:
beef patty, light 0
chicken tenders 16.6

---

[1] *Does not include potato, bread, or salad bar.*

Shoney's, entrees, 1 serving *(cont.)*

fish, baked	2.4
fish, fried, light	21.5
Fish N'Chips, with fries	50.4
Fish N'Shrimp	36.5
Italian feast	43.8
lasagna	44.9
Liver N'Onions	15.4
seafood platter	45.7
shrimp, bite size	24.7
shrimp, boiled	0
shrimp, charbroiled	3.0
shrimp sampler	26.1
Shrimper's Feast	29.9
Shrimper's Feast, large	44.9
spaghetti	63.4
steak, country fried	33.9
steak, rib eye, 8 oz.	0
steak, sirloin, 6 oz.	0
Steak N'Shrimp (with fried shrimp)	15.0
Steak N'Shrimp (with charbroiled shrimp)	1.0

burgers, 1 serving:

All-American	26.8
bacon	28.6
mushroom/Swiss	28.8
Old Fashioned	25.6
Shoney	22.2

sandwiches, 1 serving:

bacon & cheese, grilled	27.9
cheese, grilled	25.1
chicken, charbroiled	28.1
chicken fillet	38.9
country fried	67.0
fish	41.0
ham, baked	28.2
ham club, whole wheat	45.2
Patty Melt	29.5
Philly steak	37.2

Reuben 31.5
Slim Jim 40.4
turkey club, whole wheat 44.1
side dishes, 1 serving:
Grecian bread 13.2
mushrooms, sauteed 4.3
onion rings, 1 piece 5.0
onions, sauteed 4.3
potato, baked, 10 oz. 61.1
french fries, 3 oz. 28.9
french fries, 4 oz. 38.6
rice 23.1
salads, prepared, ¼ cup:
Ambrosia 11.5
apple grape surprise 4.9
beet onion 3.0
broccoli/cauliflower 4.0
broccoli/cauliflower/carrot 2.7
broccoli/cauliflower/ranch 1.6
carrot apple 4.2
coleslaw 5.1
cucumber lite 2.7
fruit, glacé 12.9
fruit, mixed 9.3
fruit delight 10.1
kidney bean 6.8
macaroni 17.0
Oriental 13.3
pea 3.5
pistachio pineapple 19.6
pasta, Don's 8.6
pasta, rotelli 8.9
Seigan 8.1
snow 9.0
spaghetti 8.7
spring 2.4
squash, mixed 2.3
summer 2.2

Shoney's, salads, prepared, ¼ cup *(cont.)*
three bean.. 11.9
vegetable, Italian 2.5
Waldorf... 8.5
dressings, 2 tbsp.:
Biscayne, lo-cal 1.0
blue cheese or ranch 0
French or French rue... 2.0
honey mustard.. 2.4
Italian, creamy or golden... 1.0
Italian, W.W. 2.4
Thousand Island 2.0
sauces, 1 soufflé cup:
BBQ 8.2
cocktail 8.7
Sweet N'Sour 14.7
tartar 3.6
desserts, 1 serving:
apple pie à la mode 67.0
carrot cake.. 56.0
hot fudge cake 81.9
hot fudge sundae 60.0
strawberry pie... 44.5
strawberry sundae.. 47.7
walnut brownie à la mode... 60.6
Shortening, all varieties 0
Shrimp, meat only:
raw, 4 oz. 1.0
raw, 4 large, 1 oz. 3
Shrimp, canned, drained, 1 cup 1.3
"Shrimp," imitation, made from surimi, 4 oz................... 10.4
Shrimp cocktail:
(Sau-Sea), 4-oz. jar 17.0
(Sau-Sea), 6-oz. jar 26.0
Shrimp dinner, frozen:
Creole *(Armour Classics Lite),* 11.25 oz. 53.0
marinara *(Healthy Choice),* 10.5 oz. 51.0
Shrimp dinner mix, Creole *(Luzianne),* ⅕ pkg.................. 34.0

Shrimp entree, canned, chow mein:
(La Choy), ¾ cup 4.0
(La Choy Bi-Pack), ¾ cup 6.0
Shrimp entree, frozen:
breaded:
   (Gorton's Original), 5 pieces 17.0
   (Gorton's Microwave), 2 oz. 14.0
   (Mrs. Paul's Special Recipe), 5.5 oz. 34.0
   butter flavor *(Mrs. Paul's)*, 5.5 oz. 26.0
   garlic and herb *(Mrs. Paul's)*, 5.5 oz. 11.0
   Oriental seasoned *(Gorton's)*, 5 pieces 16.0
   popcorn style *(Gorton's)*, 2.7 oz. 18.0
   scampi seasoned *(Gorton's)*, 5 pieces 17.0
marinara, with linguini *(Weight Watchers Smart*
   Ones), 8 oz. 26.0
and okra gumbo *(Bodin's)*, 4 oz. 8.0
Shrimp spice *(Tone's Craboil)*, 1 tsp. 1.2
Skipper's:
thick cut cod:
   3 piece, with fries 68.0
   4 piece, with fries 74.0
   5 piece, with fries 80.0
famous fish fillets:
   1 fish, with fries 51.0
   2 fish, with fries 71.0
   3 fish, with fries 82.0
seafood combo, 1 fish:
   shrimp, with fries 77.0
   jumbo shrimp, with fries 75.0
   clam strips, with fries 81.0
   oysters, with fries 95.0
seafood basket:
   shrimp, with fries 82.0
   jumbo shrimp, with fries 79.0
   clam strips, with fries 90.0
   oysters, with fries 118.0
Skipper's Platter 97.0

Skipper's (cont.)

chicken tenderloin strips:

    5 piece, with fries 69.0

    3 piece, 1 fish, with fries 72.0

    3 piece, shrimp, with fries 77.0

salads & lite catch:

    2 fish, with small salad 27.0

    3 chicken, with small salad 17.0

    1 fish, 2 chicken, with small salad 24.0

    small salad 6.0

    shrimp and seafood salad 15.0

Create A Catch:

    chicken sandwich 44.0

    chicken strip 4.0

    fish sandwich 43.0

    fish sandwich, double 54.0

    fish fillet 11.0

    fries 50.0

    clam chowder cup 14.0

    clam chowder pint 19.0

    coleslaw, 5 oz. 10.0

condiments, 1 tbsp.:

    barbecue or cocktail sauce 5.0

    tartar sauce 0

salad dressing, 1 packet:

    blue cheese, premium 4.0

    Italian, gourmet or lo-cal 2.0

    ranch house 2.0

    Thousand Island 8.0

Sloppy Joe sauce, see "Sandwich sauce"

Smelt, without added ingredients 0

Snack bars (see also "Granola and Cereal bars"):

all varieties *(Health Valley Fat Free Bakes),* 1 bar 17.0

all varieties *(Health Valley* Fat Free Fruit Bars), 1 bar 33.0

Snack chips (see also specific listings):

cheddar:

    (Pepperidge Farm Swirl), ½ oz. 7.0

    (Sunchips Harvest Cheddar), 1 oz. 18.0

and jack *(Supremos)*, 1 oz. 17.0
onion *(Supremos Cool Onion)*, 1 oz. 17.0
original or French onion *(Sunchips)*, 1 oz. 18.0
Snack mix:
(Doo Dads Original), 1 oz. 17.0
(Flavor House Party Mix), 1 oz. 11.0
(Pepperidge Farm Classic), 1 oz. 14.0
(Pepperidge Farm Goldfish Party Mix), 1 oz. 16.0
(Ritz Traditional), 1 oz. 18.0
cheddar, super *(Pepperidge Farm* Goldfish Party
  Mix), 1 oz. 15.0
cheese *(Ritz)*, 1 oz. 18.0
nutty *(Pepperidge Farm)*, 1 oz. 15.0
smoked, lightly *(Pepperidge Farm)*, 1 oz. 13.0
spicy or zesty herb *(Pepperidge Farm)*, 1 oz. 14.0
Snail, sea, see "Whelk"
Snapper, without added ingredients 0
Snow peas, see "Peas, edible-podded"
Soft drinks and mixers (see also specific listings):
all varieties, except diet and vanilla cream *(Crush)*,
  12 fl. oz. 52.0
apple *(Slice)*, 12 fl. oz. 46.3
apple *(Welch's* Sparkling), 12 fl. oz. 56.0
cherry *(Sundrop)*, 12 fl. oz. 46.0
cherry, black *(Shasta)*, 12 fl. oz. 40.0
cherry cola *(Coca-Cola)*, 12 fl. oz. 40.0
cherry cola *(Shasta)*, 12 fl. oz. 37.0
cherry-lime *(Spree)*, 12 fl. oz. 44.0
citrus mist *(Shasta)*, 12 fl. oz. 48.0
club soda, 12 fl. oz. 0
cola:
  (Coca-Cola Classic), 12 fl. oz. 38.0
  (Coke II), 12 fl. oz. 40.0
  (R. W. Knudsen), 12 fl. oz. 33.0
  (Pepsi Regular/Free), 12 fl. oz. 40.8
  (Shasta/Shasta Caffeine Free), 12 fl. oz. 40.0
  (Shasta Low Sodium), 12 fl. oz. 26.0
  (Spree), 12 fl. oz. 44.0

Soft drinks and mixers *(cont.)*

collins mixer *(Schweppes)*, 12 fl. oz. 36.0
cream:
    (A&W), 1 fl. oz. 3.8
    (Hires), 12 fl. oz. 48.0
    (I.B.C.), 12 fl. oz. 42.0
    (Mug), 12 fl. oz. 47.3
    (Shasta Creme), 12 fl. oz. 41.0
    vanilla *(Crush)*, 12 fl. oz. 44.0
(Dr. Diablo), 12 fl. oz. 39.0
(Dr. Pepper Regular/Free), 12 fl. oz. 39.6
fruit punch *(Minute Maid)*, 12 fl. oz. 44.0
fruit punch *(Welch's Sparkling)*, 12 fl. oz. 53.0
ginger ale:
    (Fanta), 12 fl. oz. 32.0
    (R. W. Knudsen), 12 fl. oz. 37.0
    (R. W. Knudsen Organic), 12 fl. oz. 36.0
    (Schweppes), 12 fl. oz. 34.0
    (Shasta), 12 fl. oz. 33.0
    (Shasta Low Sodium), 12 fl. oz. 22.0
    (Spree), 12 fl. oz. 33.0
    raspberry *(R. W. Knudsen)*, 12 fl. oz. 32.0
    raspberry *(Schweppes)*, 12 fl. oz. 38.0
ginger beer *(Schweppes)*, 12 fl. oz. 36.0
grape:
    (Fanta), 12 fl. oz. 44.0
    (Minute Maid), 12 fl. oz. 46.0
    (Schweppes), 12 fl. oz. 48.0
    (Shasta), 12 fl. oz. 44.0
    (Welch's Sparkling), 12 fl. oz. 51.0
grapefruit:
    (Schweppes), 12 fl. oz. 40.0
    (Spree), 12 fl. oz. 44.0
    (Wink), 8 fl. oz. 30.0
kiwi-strawberry *(Shasta)*, 12 fl. oz. 44.0
lemon, bitter *(Schweppes)*, 12 fl. oz. 42.0
lemon sour or lemon-lime *(Schweppes)*, 12 fl. oz. 38.0

lemon-lime:
  (Shasta), 12 fl. oz..37.0
  (Shasta Low Sodium), 12 fl. oz. 24.0
  (Slice), 12 fl. oz...38.6
  (Spree), 12 fl. oz..43.0
lemon tangerine *(Spree)*, 12 fl. oz. 47.0
lime, mandarin *(Spree)*, 12 fl. oz. 44.0
lime, tropical *(R. W. Knudsen)*, 12 fl. oz......................40.0
(Mello Yello), 12 fl. oz..44.0
mineral water, sparkling, all flavors *(à Santé)*,
  10 fl. oz...0
(Mountain Dew), 12 fl. oz...44.4
(Mr. Pibb), 12 fl. oz. 38.0
orange:
  (Fanta), 12 fl. oz..46.0
  (Minute Maid), 12 fl. oz. 44.0
  (Shasta), 12 fl. oz...46.0
  (Welch's Sparkling), 12 fl. oz................................51.0
  mandarin *(Slice)*, 12 fl. oz. 50.0
peach *(Shasta)*, 12 fl. oz. 44.0
peach *(Welch's* Sparkling), 12 fl. oz. 52.0
pineapple *(Shasta)*, 12 fl. oz. 53.0
pineapple *(Welch's* Sparkling), 12 fl. oz. 53.0
pineapple-orange *(Shasta)*, 12 fl. oz............................47.0
pop, red *(Shasta)*, 12 fl. oz. 44.0
raspberry creme *(Shasta)*, 12 fl. oz. 45.0
root beer:
  (A&W), 1 fl. oz...3.8
  (Fanta), 12 fl. oz..40.0
  (Hires), 12 fl. oz. 46.0
  (I.B.C.), 12 fl. oz..42.0
  (Mug), 12 fl. oz. 42.8
  (Ramblin'), 12 fl. oz. 46.0
  (Shasta), 12 fl. oz...40.0
  (Spree), 12 fl. oz...43.0
seltzer, plain or flavored *(Schweppes)*, 12 fl. oz. 0
(7Up), 12 fl. oz. 36.3
(7Up Cherry), 12 fl. oz. 38.7

Soft drinks and mixers *(cont.)*

(Slice Red), 12 fl. oz. 49.8
(Sprite), 12 fl. oz. 36.0
spritzer:
  apple *(R. W. Knudsen)*, 12 fl. oz. 42.0
  boysenberry *(R. W. Knudsen)*, 12 fl. oz. 41.0
  cherry, black *(R. W. Knudsen)*, 12 fl. oz. 31.0
  cranberry *(R. W. Knudsen)*, 12 fl. oz. 25.0
  grape *(R. W. Knudsen)*, 12 fl. oz. 28.0
  grape, Concord *(R. W. Knudsen)*, 12 fl. oz. 35.0
  lemon-lime *(R. W. Knudsen)*, 12 fl. oz. 30.0
  lemonade, Jamaican *(R. W. Knudsen)*, 12 fl. oz. 36.0
  lime, mandarin *(R. W. Knudsen)*, 12 fl. oz. 31.0
  orange *(R. W. Knudsen)*, 12 fl. oz. 37.0
  orange-passionfruit *(R. W. Knudsen)*, 12 fl. oz. 36.0
  peach *(R. W. Knudsen)*, 12 fl. oz. 38.0
  raspberry, red *(R. W. Knudsen)*, 12 fl. oz. 37.0
  strawberry *(R. W. Knudsen)*, 12 fl. oz. 30.0
  tangerine *(R. W. Knudsen)*, 12 fl. oz. 34.0
  tangerine-orange *(R. W. Knudsen)*, 12 fl. oz. 39.0
  tango mango *(R. W. Knudsen)*, 12 fl. oz. 24.0
(Squirt), 1 fl. oz. 3.2
strawberry:
  (Minute Maid), 12 fl. oz. 46.0
  (Shasta), 12 fl. oz. 38.0
  (Welch's Sparkling), 12 fl. oz. 51.0
strawberry-peach *(Shasta)*, 12 fl. oz. 43.0
(Sundrop), 12 fl. oz. 46.0
tonic *(Schweppes)*, 12 fl. oz. 34.0
tonic *(Shasta)*, 12 fl. oz. 32.0
tropical blend *(Spree)*, 12 fl. oz. 40.0
(Vernors), 1 fl. oz. 2.8
Sole, without added ingredients 0
Sole dinner, au gratin, frozen *(Healthy Choice)*,
  11 oz. 40.0
Sole entree, frozen:
breaded *(Mrs. Paul's Light)*, 4.25 oz. 20.0
breaded *(Van de Kamp's Light)*, 1 piece 18.0

country herb *(Gorton's)*, 2 pieces..................................... <1.0
with lemon butter sauce *(Healthy Choice)*, 8.25 oz. 33.0
seafood stuffed *(Gorton's)*, 1 piece..................................... 17.0
Sorbet (see also "Sherbet" and "Ice"):
all varieties *(Dole)*, 4 oz... 28.0
orange, and vanilla ice cream *(Häagen-Dazs)*, ½ cup 30.0
raspberry *(Frusen Glädjé)*, ½ cup..................................... 36.0
raspberry and vanilla ice cream *(Häagen-Dazs)*,
    ½ cup 26.0
bar, orange, and cream *(Häagen-Dazs)*, 1 bar.................. 18.0
Sorghum, whole-grain, 1 cup 143.3
Sorghum syrup:
½ cup... 123.7
1 tbsp. 15.7
Sorrel, see "Dock"
Soufflé, see specific listings
Soup, canned, ready-to-serve:
bean:
    (Grandma Brown's), 1 cup 30.9
    with bacon'n ham *(Campbell's* Microwave), 8 oz. 31.0
    with ham *(Campbell's* Chunky Old Fashioned),
        9.65 oz. 33.0
    and ham *(Campbell's* Home Cookin')*, 9.5 oz.................. 26.0
    and ham *(Healthy Choice)*, 7.5 oz................................. 35.0
    and ham *(Hormel* Hearty), 7.5 oz.................................. 29.0
bean, black:
    (Hain 99% Fat Free). 9.5 oz. 29.0
    (Progresso Hearty), 9.5 oz... 33.0
    and carrots *(Health Valley* Fat Free), 7.5 oz.................... 9.0
beef:
    (Campbell's Chunky), 9.5 oz. 21.0
    (Progresso), 9.5 oz. 15.0
    hearty *(Healthy Choice)*, 7.5 oz. 17.0
beef barley *(Progresso)*, 9.5 oz... 15.0
beef broth *(Health Valley* Natural Fat Free), 6.9 oz. 2.0
beef broth *(Swanson)*, 7.25 oz... 1.0
beef minestrone *(Progresso)*, 9.5 oz................................... 16.0
beef noodle *(Campbell's* Chunky), 9.5 oz. 8.0

Soup, canned, ready-to-serve *(cont.)*
beef noodle *(Progresso)*, 9.5 oz. 17.0
beef Stroganoff style *(Campbell's* Chunky),
   10.75-oz. can.. 28.0
beef vegetable:
   (Hormel Hearty), 7.5 oz. 15.0
   (Progresso), 9.5 oz. 14.0
   chunky *(Healthy Choice)*, 7.5 oz. 14.0
   and pasta *(Campbell's* Home Cookin'), 9.5 oz.............. 15.0
borscht:
   (Gold's), 1 cup 21.0
   with beets *(Manischewitz)*, 1 cup............................ 20.0
   low calorie *(Gold's)*, 1 cup 5.0
   low calorie *(Manischewitz)*, 1 cup 4.0
chickarina *(Progresso)*, 9.5 oz. 13.0
chicken:
   (Campbell's Chunky Old Fashioned), 9.5 oz. 18.0
   (Progresso Homestyle), 9.5 oz. 11.0
   hearty *(Healthy Choice)*, 7.5 oz. 17.0
   hearty *(Progresso)*, 9.5 oz. 11.0
chicken barley *(Progresso)*, 9.25 oz. 14.0
chicken broth:
   (Campbell's Low Sodium), 10.5 oz. 2.0
   (Hain), 9 oz. 0
   (Hain No Salt), 9 oz. 2.0
   (Health Valley Fat Free), 7.5 oz. 1.0
   (Swanson), 7.25 oz. 2.0
   clear *(Swanson* Natural Goodness), 7.25 oz. 1.0
chicken corn chowder *(Campbell's* Chunky), 9.5 oz. 19.0
chicken gumbo, with sausage *(Campbell's* Home
   Cookin')*, 9.5 oz. 13.0
chicken minestrone *(Campbell's* Home Cookin'),
   9.5 oz.. 14.0
chicken minestrone *(Progresso)*, 9.5 oz. 13.0
chicken mushroom, creamy *(Campbell's* Chunky),
   9.4 oz.. 12.0
chicken noodle:
   (Campbell's Chunky), 9.5 oz. 16.0

(Campbell's Chunky Classic), 9.5 oz. 17.0
(Campbell's Home Cookin'), 9.5 oz. 10.0
(Campbell's Low Sodium), 10.75 oz. 17.0
(Campbell's Microwave), 7.75 oz. 10.0
(Hain), 8 oz. 11.0
(Hain No Salt), 8 oz. 9.0
(Healthy Choice Old Fashioned), 7.5 oz. 9.0
(Hormel Hearty), 7.5 oz. 14.0
(Progresso), 9.5 oz. 9.0
(Progresso Healthy Classics), 8 oz. 10.0
hearty *(Campbell's* Healthy Request), 8 oz. 7.0
and vegetable *(Healthy Choice),* 7.5 oz. 18.0
chicken nuggets with vegetables and noodles
  (Campbell's Chunky), 9.5 oz. 22.0
chicken with rice:
  (Campbell's Chunky), 9.5 oz. 16.0
  (Campbell's Home Cookin'), 9.5 oz. 21.0
  (Campbell's Microwave), 7.75 oz. 15.0
  (Healthy Choice), 7.5 oz. 18.0
  (Hormel Hearty), 7.5 oz. 17.0
  (Progresso), 9.5 oz. 14.0
  hearty *(Campbell's* Healthy Request), 8 oz. 15.0
  with vegetables *(Progresso Healthy Classics),* 8 oz. 11.0
  wild rice *(Progresso),* 9.5 oz. 17.0
chicken vegetable:
  (Campbell's Chunky), 9.5 oz. 20.0
  (Campbell's Home Cookin'), 9.5 oz. 22.0
  (Hain), 8 oz. 13.0
  (Hain No Salt), 8 oz. 12.0
  (Progresso), 9.5 oz. 16.0
  hearty *(Campbell's* Healthy Request), 8 oz. 16.0
chili beef *(Campbell's* Chunky), 9.75 oz. 33.0
chili beef *(Campbell's* Microwave), 8 oz. 32.0
clam chowder, Manhattan *(Campbell's* Chunky),
  9.5 oz. 22.0
clam chowder, Manhattan *(Progresso),* 9.5 oz. 13.0
clam chowder, New England:
  (Campbell's Chunky), 9.5 oz. 23.0

Soup, canned, ready-to-serve, clam chowder, New England
(cont.)

    (Campbell's Home Cookin'), 9.5 oz. 13.0
    (Campbell's Microwave), 7.75 oz. 15.0
    (Hormel Hearty), 7.5 oz. 16.0
    (Progresso), 9.25 oz. 18.0
    hearty *(Campbell's* Healthy Request), 8 oz. 14.0
corn chowder *(Progresso)*, 9.25 oz. 22.0
corn and vegetable, country *(Health Valley* Fat Free),
    7.5 oz. 13.0
Creole style *(Campbell's* Chunky), 9.5 oz. 29.0
escarole in chicken broth *(Progresso)*, 9.25 oz. 2.0
ham and bean *(Progresso)*, 9.5 oz. 26.0
ham and butter bean *(Campbell's* Chunky),
    10.75-oz. can 34.0
lentil:
    (Progresso), 9.5 oz. 24.0
    (Progresso Healthy Classics), 8 oz. 19.0
    and carrots *(Health Valley* Fat Free), 7.5 oz. 10.0
    hearty *(Campbell's* Home Cookin'), 9.5 oz. 25.0
    with sausage *(Progresso)*, 9.5 oz. 21.0
    vegetarian *(Hain* 99% Fat Free), 9.5 oz. 25.0
    vegetarian *(Hain* 99% Fat Free No Salt), 9.5 oz. 22.0
macaroni and bean *(Progresso)*, 9.5 oz. 25.0
minestrone:
    (Campbell's Chunky), 9.5 oz. 24.0
    (Campbell's Home Cookin'), 9.5 oz. 21.0
    (Hain/Hain No Salt), 9.5 oz. 26.0
    (Health Valley), 7.5 oz. 18.0
    (Healthy Choice), 7.5 oz. 30.0
    (Hormel Hearty), 7.5 oz. 17.0
    (Progresso), 9.5 oz. 21.0
    (Progresso Healthy Classics), 8 oz. 19.0
    hearty *(Campbell's* Healthy Request), 8 oz. 13.0
    hearty *(Progresso)*, 9.25 oz. 16.0
    real Italian *(Health Valley* Fat Free), 7.5 oz. 12.0
    zesty *(Progresso)*, 9.5 oz. 19.0

mushroom, cream of *(Campbell's* Low Sodium),
    10.5 oz. 18.0
mushroom, cream of *(Progresso)*, 9.25 oz. 14.0
mushroom barley *(Hain* 99% Fat Free), 9.5 oz. 14.0
pea, split:
    (Campbell's Low Sodium), 10.75 oz. 37.0
    (Grandma Brown's), 1 cup 31.0
    and carrots *(Health Valley* Fat Free), 7.5 oz. 17.0
    green *(Progresso)*, 9.5 oz. 27.0
    with ham *(Campbell's* Chunky/Home Cookin')*,
        9.5 oz. 29.0
    and ham *(Healthy Choice)*, 7.5 oz. 25.0
    with ham *(Progresso)*, 9.5 oz. 22.0
    vegetarian *(Hain* 99% Fat Free), 9.5 oz. 30.0
    vegetarian *(Hain* 99% Fat Free No Salt), 9.5 oz. 27.0
pepper steak *(Campbell's* Chunky), 9.5 oz. 21.0
schav *(Gold's)*, 8 oz. 4.0
sirloin burger or steak and potato *(Campbell's*
    Chunky), 9.5 oz. 21.0
tomato:
    (Progresso), 9.5 oz. 18.0
    garden *(Campbell's* Home Cookin')*, 9.5 oz. 24.0
    garden *(Healthy Choice)*, 7.5 oz. 22.0
    with tomato pieces *(Campbell's* Low Sodium),
        10.5 oz. 30.0
tomato beef, with rotini *(Progresso)*, 9.5 oz. 17.0
tomato tortellini *(Progresso)*, 9.25 oz. 16.0
tomato vegetable *(Health Valley* Fat Free), 7.5 oz. 8.0
tortellini *(Progresso)*, 9.5 oz. 12.0
tortellini, creamy *(Progresso)*, 9.25 oz. 17.0
turkey rice *(Hain)*, 8 oz. 8.0
turkey rice *(Hain* No Salt), 8 oz. 11.0
turkey vegetable *(Campbell's* Chunky), 9.4 oz. 16.0
vegetable:
    (Campbell's Chunky), 9.5 oz. 25.0
    (Campbell's Microwave), 7.75 oz. 17.0
    (Progresso), 9.5 oz. 19.0
    (Progresso Healthy Classics), 8 oz. 13.0

Soup, canned, ready-to-serve, vegetable *(cont.)*
country *(Campbell's* Home Cookin'), 9.5 oz............... 25.0
country *(Healthy Choice)*, 7.5 oz.............................. 23.0
country *(Hormel* Hearty), 7.5 oz............................... 14.0
14 garden *(Health Valley* Fat Free), 7.5 oz.............. 9.0
5 bean *(Health Valley* Fat Free), 7.5 oz.................. 14.0
hearty *(Campbell's* Healthy Request), 8 oz. 17.0
Mediterranean *(Campbell's* Chunky), 9.5 oz............. 24.0
vegetarian *(Hain)*, 9.5 oz. 22.0
vegetarian *(Hain* No Salt), 9.5 oz. 23.0
vegetable barley *(Health Valley* Fat Free), 7.5 oz. 11.0
vegetable beef:
(Campbell's* Chunky Old Fashioned), 9.5 oz. 18.0
(Campbell's* Home Cookin'), 9.5 oz. 15.0
(Campbell's* Microwave), 7.75 oz. 14.0
(Healthy Choice)*, 7.5 oz. 21.0
chunky *(Campbell's* Low Sodium), 10.75 oz. 19.0
hearty *(Campbell's* Healthy Request), 8 oz. 17.0
vegetable broth, vegetarian *(Hain* 99% Fat Free).
9.25 oz.. 8.0
vegetable broth, vegetarian *(Hain* 99% Fat Free No
Salt), 9.25 oz. 9.0
vegetable with pasta *(Progresso* Hearty), 9.5 oz. 22.0
wild rice *(Hain* 99% Fat Free), 9.5 oz.................... 16.0
Soup, canned, condensed[1]:
asparagus, cream of *(Campbell's)*, 8 oz.................... 10.0
asparagus, cream of *(Campbell's)*, 8 oz.[2] 15.0
barley and bean *(Rokeach)*, 1 cup 15.0
bean *(Campbell's* Homestyle), 8 oz........................ 25.0
bean, with bacon *(Campbell's/Campbell's* Healthy
Request), 8 oz. 22.0
beef:
(Campbell's)*, 8 oz... 10.0
broth or bouillon *(Campbell's)*, 8 oz....................... 1.0
consomme *(Campbell's)*, 8 oz. 2.0

---

[1] *Prepared with water, except as noted.*
[2] *Prepared with 2% lowfat milk.*

beef noodle *(Campbell's)*, 8 oz.. 7.0
beef noodle *(Campbell's* Homestyle), 8 oz. 8.0
broccoli, cream of *(Campbell's)*, 8 oz................................... 8.0
broccoli, cream of *(Campbell's)*, 8 oz.[1] 14.0
broccoli cheese *(Campbell's)*, 8 oz. 9.0
celery, cream of *(Campbell's)*, 8 oz..................................... 8.0
cheese:
  cheddar *(Campbell's)*, 8 oz. 10.0
  nacho *(Campbell's)*, 8 oz. 8.0
  nacho *(Campbell's)*, 8 oz.[2] 11.0
chicken, cream of *(Campbell's)*, 8 oz................................... 9.0
chicken, cream of *(Campbell's* Healthy Request),
  8 oz.. 11.0
chicken alphabet or barley *(Campbell's)*, 8 oz.................. 10.0
chicken broth *(Campbell's)*, 8 oz... 2.0
chicken broth and noodles *(Campbell's)*, 8 oz. 8.0
chicken'n dumplings *(Campbell's)*, 8 oz............................. 9.0
chicken gumbo *(Campbell's)*, 8 oz. 8.0
chicken mushroom, creamy *(Campbell's)*, 8 oz. 10.0
chicken noodle:
  (Campbell's/Campbell's Healthy Request/
    Homestyle), 8 oz.. 8.0
  (Campbell's Noodle-O's), 8 oz. 9.0
  double noodle *(Campbell's)*, 8 oz. 13.0
chicken with pasta *(Campbell's* Souperstars), 8 oz........... 11.0
chicken with rice *(Campbell's)*, 8 oz.................................... 8.0
chicken with rice *(Campbell's* Healthy Request),
  8 oz.. 7.0
chicken and stars *(Campbell's)*, 8 oz. 9.0
chicken vegetable *(Campbell's)*, 8 oz................................ 11.0
chili beef *(Campbell's)*, 8 oz. 21.0
clam chowder, Manhattan *(Campbell's)*, 8 oz................... 11.0
clam chowder, Manhattan *(Doxsee/Snow's)*, 7.5 oz.......... 11.0
clam chowder, New England:
  (Campbell's), 8 oz.. 11.0

---

[1] *Prepared with 2% lowfat milk.*
[2] *Prepared with whole milk.*

Soup, canned, condensed, clam chowder, New England *(cont.)*

(Campbell's), 8 oz.[1] 17.0
(Gorton's), ¼ can[2] 17.0
(Doxsee/Snow's), 7.5 oz. 8.0
corn, golden (Campbell's), 8 oz. 18.0
corn, golden (Campbell's), 8 oz.[1] 23.0
minestrone (Campbell's), 8 oz. 13.0
mushroom, beefy (Campbell's), 8 oz. 5.0
mushroom, golden (Campbell's), 8 oz. 9.0
mushroom, cream of (Campbell's/Campbell's Healthy
  Request), 8 oz. 9.0
noodles, curly, with chicken (Campbell's), 8 oz. 11.0
noodles and ground beef (Campbell's), 8 oz. 10.0
onion, French (Campbell's), 8 oz. 9.0
onion, cream of (Campbell's), 8 oz. 12.0
onion, cream of (Campbell's), 8 oz.[3] 15.0
oyster stew (Campbell's), 8 oz. 6.0
oyster stew (Campbell's), 8 oz.[3] 10.0
pea, green (Campbell's), 8 oz. 25.0
pea, split (Rokeach), 1 cup 13.0
pea, split, with ham and bacon (Campbell's), 8 oz. 24.0
pepper pot (Campbell's), 8 oz. 9.0
potato, cream of (Campbell's), 8 oz. 12.0
potato, cream of (Campbell's), 8 oz.[3] 15.0
Scotch broth (Campbell's), 8 oz. 9.0
shrimp, cream of (Campbell's), 8 oz. 8.0
shrimp, cream of (Campbell's), 8 oz.[1] 13.0
tomato:
  (Campbell's/Campbell's Healthy Request), 8 oz. 17.0
  (Campbell's/Campbell's Healthy Request), 8 oz.[1] 22.0
  (Rokeach), 1 cup 9.0
  bisque (Campbell's), 8 oz. 22.0
  Italian or zesty (Campbell's), 8 oz. 21.0

---

[1] *Prepared with 2% lowfat milk.*
[2] *Prepared with whole milk.*
[3] *Prepared with equal parts 2% lowfat milk and water.*

tomato, cream of *(Campbell's* Homestyle), 8 oz.............. 19.0
tomato, cream of *(Campbell's* Homestyle), 8 oz.[1] 25.0
tomato rice *(Campbell's* Old Fashioned), 8 oz................... 22.0
tomato rice *(Rokeach)*, 1 cup 21.0
turkey noodle *(Campbell's)*, 8 oz...................................... 9.0
turkey vegetable *(Campbell's)*, 8 oz. 9.0
vegetable:
  (Campbell's), 8 oz... 14.0
  (Campbell's Dinosaur), 8 oz. 18.0
  (Campbell's Healthy Request), 8 oz............................... 14.0
  (Campbell's Homestyle/Old Fashioned), 8 oz. 9.0
  (Rokeach), 1 cup 13.0
vegetable beef *(Campbell's/Campbell's* Healthy
  Request), 8 oz. 9.0
vegetable, vegetarian *(Campbell's)*, 8 oz. 13.0
won ton *(Campbell's)*, 8 oz.. 5.0
Soup, frozen:
barley and bean *(Tabatchnick)*, 7.5 oz.............................. 22.0
bean, northern *(Tabatchnick)*, 7.5 oz. 29.0
broccoli, cream of *(Tabatchnick)*, 7.5 oz. 10.0
cabbage *(Tabatchnick)*, 7.5 oz... 21.0
chicken *(Tabatchnick)*, 7.5 oz. 10.0
lentil *(Tabatchnick)*, 7.5 oz. 27.0
minestrone *(Tabatchnick)*, 7.5 oz. 24.0
mushroom, cream of *(Tabatchnick)*, 6 oz. 11.0
mushroom barley *(Tabatchnick)*, 7.5 oz.............................. 16.0
mushroom barley *(Tabatchnick* No Salt), 7.5 oz. 14.0
New England chowder *(Tabatchnick)*, 7.5 oz. 14.0
pea *(Tabatchnick)*, 7.5 oz... 31.0
potato *(Tabatchnick)*, 7.5 oz. 19.0
spinach, cream of *(Tabatchnick)*, 7.5 oz............................. 12.0
tomato rice *(Tabatchnick)*, 6 oz. 14.0
vegetable *(Tabatchnick)*, 7.5 oz. 18.0
vegetable *(Tabatchnick No Salt)*, 7.5 oz. 16.0
zucchini, cream of *(Tabatchnick)*, 6 oz. 12.0

---

[1] *Prepared with whole milk.*

Soup base, mix:
beef barley *(Soup Starter),* ⅛ mix 17.0
beef vegetable *(Soup Starter),* ⅛ mix 18.0
chicken noodle or chicken and rice *(Soup Starter),*
  ⅛ mix... 14.0
Soup mix[1]:
barley *(Aunt Patsy's* Pantry Better Barley), 8 oz. 46.0
barley vegetable *(Fantastic Bouncin' Barley*
  Vegetable), 10 oz... 38.0
bean:
  black *(Fantastic Jumpin' Black Beans),* 10 oz. 40.0
  black *(Knorr* Cup-A-Soup), 1 serving.............................. 37.8
  many bean or navy bean *(Aunt Patsy's* Pantry),
    8 oz. 24.0
  navy *(Knorr* Cup-A-Soup), 1 serving............................. 26.9
  7, and barley *(Arrowhead Mills),* 1 oz. dry..................... 19.0
broccoli, in cheddar *(Fantastic Dancin' Broccoli),*
  10 oz.. 18.0
broccoli and cheese *(Lipton Cup-a-Soup),* 6 fl. oz............ 10.0
cheddar, creamy, with noodles *(Fantastic Noodles),*
  7 oz... 21.0
chicken flavor:
  creamy *(Lipton Cup-a-Soup),* 6 fl. oz. 12.0
  supreme *(Lipton Cup-a-Soup* Hearty), 6 fl. oz. 12.0
  thyme *(Aunt Patsy's* Pantry), 8 oz................................. 17.0
chicken noodle:
  (Campbell's Quality Soup & Recipe), 1 cup 16.0
  (Lipton Hearty), 1 cup 14.0
  (Lipton Cup-a-Soup Hearty), 6 fl. oz. 12.0
  (Mrs. Grass Homestyle), 1 cup...................................... 11.0
  with white meat *(Campbell's* Cup 2 Minute Soup),
    .7 oz. dry... 11.0
chicken with pasta *(Knorr* Chick'N Pasta), 1 cup 16.0
chicken rice *(Lipton Cup-a-Soup),* 6 fl. oz. 8.0
chicken rice *(Mrs. Grass),* 1 cup...................................... 12.0
chicken vegetable *(Lipton Cup-a-Soup),* 6 fl. oz. 10.0

---
[1] *Prepared with water, except as noted.*

chicken vegetable, creamy *(Lipton Cup-a-Soup)*,
  1 pouch.. 12.0
clam chowder, Manhattan *(Golden Dipt)*, ¼ pkg. dry 13.0
clam chowder, New England *(Golden Dipt)*, ¼ pkg.
  dry.. 12.0
corn and potato chowder *(Fantastic Jammin')*, 10 oz. 34.0
herb, savory, with garlic *(Lipton Recipe Secrets)*,
  1 cup.. 7.0
lentil:
  (Fantastic Laughin' Lentils), 10 oz..................................... 42.0
  (Knorr Cup-A-Soup), 1 serving 40.4
  red *(Aunt Patsy's* Pantry), 8 oz. 19.0
lobster bisque *(Golden Dipt)*, ¼ pkg. dry 5.0
minestrone *(Manischewitz)*, 6 fl. oz. 9.0
minestrone, with pasta *(Fantastic Serandin'*
  Minestrone), 10 oz.. 38.0
mushroom:
  beef *(Lipton Recipe Secrets)*, 1 cup 7.0
  cream of *(Fantastic Marchin' Cream of Mushroom)*,
    10 oz. 14.0
  creamy *(Lipton Cup-a-Soup)*, 6 fl. oz. 10.0
noodle:
  (Campbell's Quality Soup & Recipe), 1 cup 20.0
  (Lipton), 1 cup 12.0
  (Lipton Cup-a-Soup Ring Noodle), 6 fl. oz..................... 10.0
  double *(Campbell's* Quality Soup & Recipe), 1 cup 36.0
  hearty *(Campbell's* Quality Soup & Recipe), 1 cup........ 15.0
  hearty, with vegetables *(Campbell's* Cup
    Microwave), 1.7 oz. dry 32.0
  hearty, with vegetables *(Lipton)*, 1 cup 12.0
  whole wheat *(Fantastic Rockin' ABC's)*, 10 oz.............. 24.0
noodle, beef:
  (Campbell's Cup Microwave), 1.35 oz. dry..................... 25.0
  (Campbell's Ramen), 1.25 oz. dry................................. 27.0
  (Campbell's Ramen Block), 1.5 oz. dry 32.0
  (La Choy), 1 cup... 33.0
  (Maruchan Instant Lunch/Instant Picante),
    2.25 oz. dry... 37.0

Soup mix, noodle, beef *(cont.)*
  (Maruchan Ramen Supreme), 1.5 oz. dry 26.0
  with vegetables *(Campbell's* Cup-a-Ramen), 1 cup 38.0
noodle, cheddar, creamy *(Fantastic Noodles)*, 7 oz. 18.0
noodle, chicken:
  (Campbell's Cup Microwave), 1.35 oz. dry 24.0
  (Campbell's Ramen), 1.25 oz. dry 27.0
  (Campbell's Ramen Block), 1.5 oz. dry 32.0
  (La Choy), 1 cup 29.0
  (Maruchan Instant Lunch), 2.25 oz. dry 35.0
  (Maruchan Instant Picante), 2.25 oz. dry 38.0
  (Maruchan Ramen Supreme), 1.5 oz. dry 25.0
  with vegetables *(Campbell's* Cup-a-Ramen),
    2.2 oz. dry 38.0
noodle, with chicken broth:
  (Campbell's Cup Microwave), 1.35 oz. dry 25.0
  (Campbell's Cup 2 Minute Soup), 1.35 oz. dry 15.0
  (Lipton), 1 cup 10.0
  (Mrs. Grass), 1 cup 10.0
  real *(Lipton Ring-O-Noodle)*, 1 cup 11.0
noodle, chili *(Maruchan* Ramen Supreme), 1.5 oz. dry 26.0
noodle, curry vegetable *(Fantastic Noodles)*, 7 oz. 22.0
noodle, miso vegetable *(Fantastic Noodles)*, 7 oz. 20.0
noodle, mushroom *(Maruchan* Instant Lunch),
  2.25 oz. dry 37.0
noodle, mushroom *(Maruchan* Ramen Supreme),
  1.5 oz. dry 25.0
noodle, Oriental:
  (Campbell's Ramen), 1.25 oz. dry 27.0
  (Campbell's Ramen Block), 1.5 oz. dry 31.0
  (Maruchan Ramen Supreme), 1.5 oz. dry 26.0
  with vegetables *(Campbell's* Cup-a-Ramen),
    2.2 oz. dry 38.0
noodle, pork:
  (Campbell's Ramen), 1.25 oz. dry 27.0
  (Campbell's Ramen Block), 1.5 oz. dry 27.0
  (Maruchan Instant Lunch), 2.25 oz. dry 37.0
  (Maruchan Ramen Supreme), 1.5 oz. dry 25.0

noodle, shrimp:
  (Maruchan Instant Lunch/Instant Picante),
    2.25 oz. dry.. 36.0
  (Maruchan Ramen Supreme), 1.5 oz. dry...................... 26.0
  with vegetables *(Campbell's* Cup-a-Ramen),
    2.2 oz. dry... 40.0
noodle, tomato vegetable *(Fantastic Noodles)*, 7 oz. 24.0
noodle, vegetable, California, or vegetable beef
  (Maruchan Instant Picante/Instant Lunch),
    2.25 oz. dry 37.0
noodle, vegetable curry *(Fantastic Noodles)*, 7 oz............. 18.0
onion:
  (Campbell's Quality Soup & Recipe), 1 cup 7.0
  (Lipton Recipe Secrets), 1 cup 4.0
  (Mrs. Grass Soup & Dip Mix), .4 oz. dry......................... 6.0
  beefy *(Lipton Recipe Secrets)*, 1 cup 5.0
  golden or mushroom *(Lipton Recipe Secrets)*,
    1 cup... 11.0
  mushroom *(Mrs. Grass* Soup & Dip Mix), .6 oz. dry 10.0
pea:
  green *(Lipton Cup-a-Soup)*, 6 fl. oz. 17.0
  plentiful *(Aunt Patsy's* Pantry), 8 oz............................... 24.0
  split *(Fantastic Splittin' Peas)*, 10 oz.............................. 31.0
  split *(Manischewitz)*, 6 fl. oz. 9.0
  Virginia *(Lipton Cup-a-Soup)*, 6 fl. oz. 21.0
potato leek *(Knorr* Cup-A-Soup), 1 serving...................... 24.2
seafood chowder *(Golden Dipt)*, ¼ pkg. dry 12.0
shrimp bisque *(Golden Dipt)*, ¼ pkg. dry........................... 5.0
tomato:
  (Lipton Cup-a-Soup), 6 fl. oz. 21.0
  basil *(Knorr)*, 1 serving 14.1
  herb *(Lipton Recipe Secrets)*, 1 cup............................... 12.0
vegetable:
  (Campbell's Quality Soup & Recipe), 1 cup 8.0
  (Lipton Recipe Secrets), 1 cup 7.0
  (Manischewitz), 6 fl. oz. 9.0
  (Mrs. Grass Soup & Dip Mix), .4 oz. dry......................... 7.0
  country *(Lipton* Cook Up), 1 cup 13.0

Soup mix, vegetable *(cont.)*
　harvest *(Lipton Cup-a-Soup Hearty)*, 6 fl. oz. 19.0
　miso, with noodles *(Fantastic Noodles)*, 7 oz. 19.0
　spring *(Lipton Cup-a-Soup)*, 6 fl. oz. 9.0
　tomato, with noodles *(Fantastic Noodles)*, 7 oz. 20.0
vegetable beef *(Mrs. Grass)*, 1 cup 10.0
wonton:
　beef or chicken *(Maruchan)*, .68 oz. dry 8.0
　chicken, pork, shrimp, or Oriental *(Maruchan*
　　Instant), 1.49 oz. dry 19.0
　pork *(Maruchan)*, .68 oz. dry 9.0
　vegetable *(Maruchan)*, .7 oz. dry 9.0
Sour cream, see "Cream, sour"
Sour cream sauce mix *(McCormick/Schilling)*,
　¼ pkg. 4.0
Soursop, ½ cup 18.9
Souse loaf:
(Jesse Jones), 2 oz. 2.0
(Kahn's), 1 slice 1.0
Soy beverage:
(EdenSoy Original), 8.45 fl. oz. 14.0
(Soy Moo Fat Free), 8 fl. oz. 19.0
carob *(EdenSoy)*, 8.45 fl. oz. 30.0
vanilla *(EdenSoy)*, 8.45 fl. oz. 25.0
mix*, all purpose or no sucrose *(Soyagen)*, ¼ cup 14.0
mix*, carob *(Soyagen)*, ¼ cup 16.0
Soy flour:
(Arrowhead Mills), 2 oz. 18.0
stirred:
　full fat, raw, 1 cup 29.9
　full fat, roasted, 1 cup 28.6
　defatted, 1 cup 38.4
　lowfat, 1 cup 33.4
Soy meal, defatted, raw, 1 cup 49.0
Soy milk:
fluid, 8 fl. oz. 4.3
powder *(Soyamel)*, 1 oz. 11.0
Soy nuggets *(Love Natural Foods)*, 2 oz. 20.0

Soy protein, concentrate, 1 oz. 8.8
Soy sauce:
(La Choy/La Choy Lite), ½ tsp. .... <1.0
tamari, 1 tbsp. 1.0
shoyu, 1 tbsp. 1.5
Soybean:
green, raw, shelled, ½ cup 14.1
green, boiled, drained, ½ cup 10.0
dried:
  raw, ½ cup 28.1
  raw *(Arrowhead Mills),* 2 oz. 19.0
  boiled, ½ cup 8.5
  dry-roasted, ½ cup 28.1
  roasted, ½ cup 28.9
Soybean, fermented, see "Miso" and "Natto"
Soybean, sprouted:
raw, ½ cup 3.9
steamed, ½ cup 3.1
Soybean cake or curd, see "Tofu"
Soybean flakes *(Arrowhead Mills),* 2 oz. 18.0
Soybean kernels, roasted, toasted:
1 oz. or 95 kernels 8.7
whole, 1 cup 33.0
Spaghetti, see "Pasta"
Spaghetti dinner, and meatballs, frozen *(Swanson),*
  12.5 oz. 35.0
Spaghetti dishes, mix*:
(Kraft American Style Dinner), 1 cup 50.0
with meat sauce *(Kraft* Dinner), 1 cup 47.0
tangy *(Kraft* Italian Style Dinner), 1 cup 49.0
whole wheat *(Fantastic All-O-Round),* 10 oz. 40.0
Spaghetti entree, canned or packaged:
in tomato sauce, with cheese *(Franco-American),*
  7.35 oz. 35.0
in tomato and cheese sauce *(Franco-American*
  SpaghettiO's), 7.5 oz. 31.0
with franks *(Franco-American* SpaghettiO's), 7.35 oz. 26.0
with meat sauce *(Healthy Choice),* 7.5 oz. 21.0

Spaghetti entree, canned or packaged *(cont.)*
with meat sauce *(Hormel Top Shelf),* 10 oz. 37.0
with meatballs:
  (Franco-American), 7.35 oz. 28.0
  (Franco-American SpaghettiO's*),* 7.35 oz. 25.0
  (Hormel Micro Cup), 7.5 oz. 27.0
  (Libby's Diner), 7.75 oz. 31.0
rings *(Healthy Choice),* 7.5 oz. 30.0
Spaghetti entree, freeze-dried*, with meat and
  sauce (Mountain House), 1 cup 27.0
Spaghetti entree, frozen:
(Dining Lite), 9 oz. 25.0
with meat sauce:
  (Banquet Entree Express), 8.5 oz. 35.0
  (Healthy Choice Quick Meal*),* 10 oz. 42.0
  (Lean Cuisine), 11.5 oz. 45.0
  (Stouffer's), 12⅞ oz. 38.0
  (Weight Watchers), 10 oz. 28.0
with meatballs *(Stouffer's),* 12⅝ oz. 53.0
with meatballs and sauce *(Lean Cuisine),* 9.5 oz. 36.0
with tomato and meat sauce *(The Budget Gourmet*
  Light and Healthy*),* 10 oz. 44.0
Spaghetti sauce, see "Pasta sauce"
Spaghetti sauce seasoning mix:
Italian *(French's),* ⅕ pkg. 5.0
mushroom *(French's),* ⅕ pkg. 4.0
thick *(French's),* ⅙ pkg. 4.0
Spaghetti squash:
raw, strands *(Frieda's),* 1 oz. 2.8
baked or boiled, drained, ½ cup 5.0
Spareribs, without added ingredients 0
Spelt:
flakes *(Arrowhead Mills),* 1 oz. 21.0
flour *(Arrowhead Mills),* 2 oz. 40.0
Spice loaf:
regular or beef *(Kahn's* Family Pack*),* 1 slice 1.0
Spices, see specific listings

Spinach:
fresh, raw, chopped, ½ cup 1.0
fresh, boiled, drained, ½ cup 3.4
canned:
  with liquid, ½ cup 3.4
  (Allens/Popeye/Allens Low Sodium), ½ cup 3.0
  (Stokely), ½ cup 3.0
  chopped *(Allens/Popeye)* ½ cup 2.0
frozen:
  (Green Giant), ½ cup 6.0
  (Green Giant Harvest Fresh), ½ cup 5.0
  whole *(Frosty Acres),* 3.3 oz. 4.0
  creamed *(Birds Eye),* 3 oz. 5.0
  creamed *(Green Giant),* ½ cup 10.0
  creamed *(Stouffer's),* 4.5 oz. 8.0
  in butter sauce, cut *(Green Giant),* ½ cup 6.0
Spinach, New Zealand, see "New Zealand spinach"
Spinach au gratin, frozen *(The Budget Gourmet
  Side Dish),* 5.5 oz. 9.0
Spinach soufflé, frozen *(Stouffer's),* 6 oz. 11.0
Spiny lobster, meat only:
raw, 4 oz. 2.8
boiled or steamed, 2-lb. lobster 5.1
boiled or steamed, 4 oz. 3.5
Split peas, dry:
green *(Arrowhead Mills),* 2 oz. 35.0
boiled, ½ cup 20.7
Spot, without added ingredients 0
Spring onion, see "Onion, green"
Sprouts (see also specific listings):
bean:
  fresh, *(Frieda's),* 1 oz. 1.9
  stir-fry *(Frieda's* Sprout Munchies), 1 oz. 1.9
  canned *(La Choy),* ⅔ cup 1.0
mixed *(Shaw's* Premium), 2 oz. 0
Squab, without added ingredients 0
Squash, fresh, see specific listings

Squash, frozen (see also specific listings) *(Frosty Acres)*, 3.3 oz. 4.0
Squid, meat only, raw, 4 oz. 3.5
Star fruit, see "Carambola"
Steak biscuit sandwich, frozen *(Hormel Quick Meal)*, 4.2 oz. 36.0
Steak sauce:
(A.1.), 1 tbsp. 3.0
(French's), 1 tbsp. 6.0
(Heinz Traditional), 1 tbsp. 3.0
(Lea & Perrins), 1 tbsp. 6.0
(Maull's), 1 tbsp. 5.0
regular or hickory smoke *(Heinz 57)*, 1 tbsp. 4.0
sweet & mild *(Maull's)*, 1 tbsp. 4.0
Steak seasoning:
(McCormick/Schilling Grillmates), 1 tsp. 1.0
blackened *(Tone's)*, 1 tsp. 1.6
broiled *(McCormick/Schilling* Spice Blends), ¼ tsp. 1
Stir-fry entree mix:
(Tyson Stir-Fry Kit):
    meat/vegetable mix, 9 oz. 15.0
    Yoshida sauce, 1.6 oz. 22.0
Stir-fry seasoning *(Gilroy)*, 1 tsp. 1.0
Strawberry:
fresh, 1 pint 22.5
fresh, ½ cup 5.2
canned in heavy syrup, ½ cup 29.9
freeze-dried *(Mountain House Fruit Crisps)*, ¼ cup 13.0
frozen, unsweetened, ½ cup 6.8
frozen, in syrup *(Birds Eye Lite)*, 5 oz. 25.0
Strawberry colada mixer, frozen*, with rum *(Bacardi)*, 7 fl. oz. 34.0
Strawberry flavor drink mix*:
(Kool-Aid), 8 fl. oz. 25.0
(Kool-Aid Presweetened), 8 fl. oz. 18.0
(Wyler's), 8 fl. oz. 21.0
split *(Wyler's)*, 8 fl. oz. 20.0

Strawberry flavor milk drink:
chilled *(Nestlé Quik)*, 1 cup 32.0
chilled, lowfat *(Nestlé Quik)*, 1 cup 33.0
mix, powder:
  1 oz. 28.1
  (Carnation Instant Breakfast), 1 packet 29.0
  (Nestlé Quik), ¾ oz. or 1⅔ heaping tsp. 24.0
  (Pillsbury Instant Breakfast), 1 packet 27.0
Strawberry float *(R. W. Knudsen)*, 8 fl. oz. 32.0
Strawberry fruit roll, see "Fruit snack"
Strawberry nectar:
(Kern's), 6 fl. oz. 28.0
(R. W. Knudsen), 8 fl. oz. 29.0
(Libby's), 6 fl. oz. 27.0
(Libby's Ripe), 8 fl. oz. 36.0
Strawberry topping:
(Kraft), 1 tbsp. 14.0
(Smucker's), 2 tbsp. 30.0
Strawberry-banana nectar:
(Kern's), 6 fl. oz. 28.0
(Libby's Ripe), 8 fl. oz. 37.0
Strawberry-guava juice *(R. W. Knudsen)*, 8 fl. oz. 26.0
Strawberry-guava nectar *(Santa Cruz Natural)*,
  8 fl. oz. 24.0
String beans, see "Green beans"
Stroganoff entree, vegetarian, mix*:
(Natural Touch), 4 oz. 10.0
creamy, with tofu *(Tofu Classics)*, ½ cup 13.0
Stroganoff sauce mix:
(Lawry's), 1 pkg. 25.5
(Natural Touch), 4 oz.* 10.0
Stroganoff seasoning *(French's)*, ¼ pkg. 6.0
Stuffing:
apple and raisin *(Pepperidge Farm* Distinctive), 1 oz. 21.0
chicken, classic *(Pepperidge Farm* Distinctive), 1 oz. 20.0
corn *(Arnold)*, 1 oz. 18.0
cornbread:
  (Brownberry), 1 oz. 18.0

Stuffing, cornbread *(cont.)*
 (Pepperidge Farm), 1 oz. 22.0
 honey pecan *(Pepperidge Farm* Distinctive), 1 oz. 19.0
country style *(Pepperidge Farm)*, 1 oz. 21.0
cube *(Pepperidge Farm)*, 1 oz. 22.0
cube, unspiced *(Arnold)*, ½ oz. 9.0
herb, country garden *(Pepperidge Farm* Distinctive),
 1 oz. 18.0
herb seasoned *(Arnold/Brownberry)*, ½ oz. 10.0
herb seasoned *(Pepperidge Farm)*, 1 oz. 22.0
sage and onion *(Arnold/Brownberry)*, ½ oz. 9.0
sage and onion *(Pepperidge Farm* Distinctive), 1 oz. 21.0
seasoned *(Arnold)*, ½ oz. 9.0
vegetable, harvest, and almond *(Pepperidge Farm*
 Distinctive), 1 oz. 19.0
wild rice and mushroom *(Pepperidge Farm*
 Distinctive), 1 oz. 17.0
Stuffing mix*:
(Stove Top Americana San Francisco), ½ cup 20.0
beef *(Stove Top)*, ½ cup 21.0
broccoli and cheese *(Stove Top* Microwave), ½ cup 20.0
chicken:
 (Betty Crocker), ½ cup 21.0
 (Stove Top/Stove Top Flexible Serving/Microwave),
  ½ cup 20.0
 with rice *(Stove Top)*, ½ cup 22.0
cornbread:
 (Stove Top), ½ cup 21.0
 (Stove Top Flexible Serving), ½ cup 22.0
 homestyle *(Stove Top* Microwave), ½ cup 20.0
herb:
 homestyle *(Stove Top* Flexible Serving), ½ cup 20.0
 savory *(Stove Top)*, ½ cup 20.0
 traditional *(Betty Crocker)*, ½ cup 22.0
long grain and wild rice *(Stove Top)*, ½ cup 22.0
mushroom and onion *(Stove Top)*, ½ cup 20.0
mushroom and onion *(Stove Top* Microwave), ½ cup 21.0
pork *(Stove Top/Stove Top* Flexible Serving), ½ cup 20.0

turkey *(Stove Top)*, 1/2 cup 20.0
Sturgeon, fresh or smoked, without added
  ingredients 0
Succotash:
fresh, boiled, drained, 1/2 cup 23.4
canned, with whole kernel corn, 1/2 cup 17.9
canned, with cream-style corn, 1/2 cup 23.4
frozen, boiled, drained, 1/2 cup 17.0
frozen *(Frosty Acres)*, 3.3 oz. 19.0
Sucker, without added ingredients 0
Sugar, beet or cane:
brown:
  1 oz. 27.6
  1 cup, not packed 141.0
  1 cup, packed 214.0
cane baton *(Frieda's)*, 1 oz. 49.9
granulated:
  1 oz. 28.3
  1 cup 199.8
  1 tbsp. 12.0
  1 tsp. 4.0
powdered or confectioner's:
  1 oz. 28.2
  1 cup, sifted 99.5
  1 tbsp., unsifted 8.0
Sugar, maple, 1 oz. 25.5
"Sugar," substitute:
(Equal), 1 packet .... <1.0
(NutraSweet), 1 tsp. .... <1.0
(Sweet 'n Low), 1 packet 1.0
Sugar apple:
1 medium, 9.9 oz. 36.6
1/2 cup 29.6
Sugar snap peas, see "Peas, edible-podded"
Summer sausage (see also "Thuringer cervelat"):
(Oscar Mayer), 2 slices 0
beef *(Oscar Mayer)*, 2 slices .... <1.0
regular, beef, or with cheese *(Hillshire Farm)*, 2 oz. 1.0

Sunburst squash, raw *(Frieda's)*, 1 oz. 9
Sunfish, pumpkinseed, without added ingredients 0
Sunflower seed butter:
1 oz. 7.8
1 tbsp. 4.4
(Erewhon), 2 tbsp. 3.0
(Roaster Fresh), 1 oz. 5.0
Sunflower seed flour, partially defatted, 1 cup 28.7
Sunflower seeds, 1 oz.:
(Arrowhead Mills), 1 oz. 6.0
(Frito-Lay's), 1 oz. 6.0
dried, kernels, 1 oz. 5.3
dry-roasted:
   (Flavor House), 1 oz. 8.0
   in shell or kernels *(Fisher)*, 1 oz. 6.0
   kernels, 1 oz. 6.8
oil roasted *(Fisher)*, 1 oz. 4.0
oil-roasted, kernels, 1 oz. 4.2
salted, in shell *(Fisher)*, 1 oz. 6.0
toasted, kernels, 1 oz. 5.9
unsalted *(Fisher)*, 1 oz. 6.0
Surimi[1], 4 oz. 7.8
Swamp cabbage:
raw, .6-oz. shoot 4
boiled, drained, chopped, 1/2 cup 1.8
Sweet potato:
raw, 1 medium, 5" × 2" diameter 31.6
baked in skin, 1 medium 27.7
baked in skin, mashed, 1/2 cup 24.3
boiled without skin, 4 oz. 27.5
boiled without skin, mashed, 1/2 cup 39.8
Sweet potato, canned:
whole *(Pride of Louisiana Yams)*, 1/2 cup 20.0
cut *(Allens Yams)*, 1/2 cup 20.0
in syrup, with liquid, 1/2 cup 23.9
in syrup, drained, 1/2 cup 24.9

---

[1] *Processed from walleye (Alaska) pollock.*

vacuum pack, pieces, ½ cup 21.1
vacuum pack, mashed, ½ cup 26.9
Sweet potato, frozen:
baked, cubed, ½ cup 20.6
candied *(Mrs. Paul's)*, 4 oz. 46.0
candied, with apples *(Mrs. Paul's Sweets 'N Apples)*,
    4 oz. 38.0
patty *(Stilwell Yam Patties)*, 2 pieces 33.0
Sweet potato leaf:
raw, chopped, ½ cup 1.1
steamed, ½ cup 2.3
Sweet and sour drink mixer, bottled *(Holland
    House)*, 3 fl. oz. 24.0
Sweet and sour sauce:
(Bennett's), 1 tbsp. 7.0
(Contadina), ½ cup 32.0
(La Choy/La Choy Duck Sauce), 1 tbsp. 7.0
(Sauceworks), 1 tbsp. 5.0
(Woody's), 2 tbsp. 17.0
Sweetbreads, without added ingredients 0
Swiss chard, fresh:
raw, chopped, ½ cup 7
boiled, drained, chopped, ½ cup 3.6
Swiss steak, see "Beef dinner"
Swiss steak seasoning mix:
(French's Roasting Bag), ⅕ pkg. 5.0
(McCormick/Schilling Bag'n Season), 1 pkg. 17.0
Swordfish, without added ingredients 0
Syrup, see specific listings
Szechwan sauce *(La Choy)*, 1 oz. 12.0

T

Food and Measure	Carbohydrate Grams

Tabbouleh mix*, with or without oil *(Fantastic Tabouli)*, ½ cup 17.0
Taco dip:
(Wise), 2 tbsp. 3.0
and sauce *(Hain),* 4 tbsp. 5.0
Taco John's, 1 serving:
apple grande 44.0
beans, refried 79.0
burrito:
    bean 36.0
    beef 25.0
    combo 30.0
    super 66.0
    with green chili 38.0
    with Texas chili 48.0
chili, Texas 35.0
chimi 54.0
churro 12.0
enchilada 33.0
nachos 42.0
nachos, super 57.0
Potato Olé Large 96.0
taco:
    burger 31.0
    Bravo, super 51.0
    regular 15.0
    soft shell 23.0
taco salad, super 48.0

tostada 15.0
Taco mix:
(Old El Paso), 1 taco* 8.0
(Tio Sancho Dinner Kit):
   sauce, 2 oz. 13.4
   seasoning, 1.25 oz. 20.9
   shell 8.1
vegetarian *(Natural Touch)*, 2 tbsp. 6.0
Taco sauce:
(Chi-Chi's Thick & Chunky), 1 oz. 3.0
(Lawry's Sauce'n Seasoner), 1/4 cup 7.6
(Old El Paso), 2 tbsp. 3.0
chunky *(Lawry's)*, 1/4 cup 4.0
hot *(Chi-Chi's)*, 1 oz. 4.0
hot or mild *(Ortega)*, 1 oz. 3.0
red *(La Victoria)*, 1 tbsp. 1.0
red, mild *(El Molino)*, 2 tbsp. 2.0
western style *(Ortega)*, 1 oz. 2.0
Taco seasoning mix:
(French's), 1/12 pkg. 2.0
(Hain), 1/10 pkg. 2.0
(Lawry's Seasoning Blends), 1.25 oz. 23.6
(McCormick/Schilling), 1/4 pkg. 6.0
(Old El Paso), 1/12 pkg. 2.0
(Tio Sancho), 1.51 oz. 26.0
onion, real *(French's)*, 1/12 pkg. 3.0
salad *(Lawry's* Seasoning Blends), 1 pkg. 24.7
Taco shell:
(Chi-Chi's), 1 piece 17.0
(Gebhardt), 1 piece 7.0
(Lawry's), 1 piece 8.0
(Lawry's Super), 1 piece 13.0
(Old El Paso), 1 piece 6.0
(Old El Paso Super), 1 piece 11.0
(Ortega), 1 piece 8.0
(Rosarita), 1 piece 7.0
(Tio Sancho), 1 piece 8.1
(Tio Sancho Super), 1 piece 11.3

Taco shell *(cont.)*
corn *(Azteca)*, 1 piece 7.0
mini *(Old El Paso)*, 3 pieces... 7.0
salad, flour *(Azteca)*, 1 piece 18.0
Tahini:
from unroasted kernels, 1 tbsp. 2.5
from roasted, toasted kernels, 1 tbsp....................................... 3.2
(Arrowhead Mills), 1 oz. 4.0
(Erewhon), 2 tbsp. 3.0
(Joyva), 1 oz. 3.0
(Krinos), 1 oz. 2.0
Tamale, canned:
(Derby), 2 pieces 15.0
(Gebhardt), 2 pieces 19.0
(Gebhardt Jumbo), 2 pieces 26.0
(Old El Paso), 2 pieces 16.0
beef, regular or hot *(Hormel)*, 7.5 oz. 19.0
Tamalito, in chili gravy, canned *(Dennison's)*, 7.5 oz. 37.0
Tamari, see "Soy sauce"
Tamarind:
1 medium, 3″ × 1″ 1.3
pulp, ½ cup.. 37.5
pulp *(Frieda's* Tamarindo), 1 oz. 17.7
Tangerine:
fresh, 1 medium, 2⅜″ diameter.. 9.4
fresh, sections without membrane, ½ cup 10.9
canned:
    (Dole mandarin), ½ cup 19.0
    in juice, ½ cup 11.9
    in light syrup, ½ cup... 20.4
Tangerine juice:
fresh, 6 fl. oz. 18.7
chilled or frozen* *(Minute Maid)*, 6 fl. oz. 22.0
Tapioca, pearl, dry, 1 oz. 25.1
Taramosalata *(Krinos)*, 1 tbsp. 0
Taro:
raw, sliced, ½ cup 13.8
cooked, sliced, ½ cup.. 22.8

cooked *(Frieda's)*, 5 oz. 36.0
Taro chips:
1 oz. 19.3
½ cup 8.1
Taro leaf:
raw, ½ cup 9
steamed, ½ cup 3.0
Taro shoots:
raw, sliced, ½ cup 1.0
cooked, sliced, ½ cup 2.2
Taro, Tahitian:
raw, sliced, ½ cup 4.3
cooked, sliced, ½ cup 4.7
Tarragon, ground, 1 tsp. 8
Tart shell, see "Pastry dough"
Tartar sauce:
(Bennett's), 1 tbsp. .... <1.0
(Golden Dipt), 1 tbsp. 2.0
(Golden Dipt Lite), 1 tbsp. 4.0
(Heinz), 1 tbsp. 2.0
(Hellmann's/Best Foods), 1 tbsp. 0
(Lyon), 1 tbsp. 3.0
(Lyon Lite), 1 tbsp. 2.0
(Sauceworks), 1 tbsp. 2.0
natural lemon and herb flavor *(Sauceworks)*, 1 tbsp. 0
Tea*:
caffeine-free *(Celestial Seasonings)*, 1 cup 1
instant, 1 cup *(Nestea 100%)*, 1 cup 0
instant, lemon flavor *(Nestea)*, 1 cup 1.0
Tea, flavored*:
all flavors *(Celestial Seasonings Distinctive)*, 1 cup .... <.2
blackberry, peach, or raspberry *(Lipton)*, 1 cup 0
lemon, orange, or cinnamon, with honey *(Lipton)*,
    1 cup .... <1.0
Tea, herbal*:
all flavors *(Lipton)*, 1 cup 0
all flavors, except lemon and mint *(Celestial
    Seasonings)*, 1 cup .... <2.0

Tea, herbal *(cont.)*
lemon *(Celestial Seasonings Lemon Zinger)*, 1 cup...........<1.0
mint *(Celestial Seasonings Mint Magic)*, 1 cup 4
Tea, iced:
brewed, herbal *(Celestial Seasonings Iced Delight)*,
  8 fl. oz. .... <.7
boxed, lemon or orange *(Boku)*, 12 fl. oz. 44.0
canned *(Lipton Brisk)*, 12 fl. oz. 39.0
canned *(Shasta)*, 12 fl. oz. 34.0
canned, with fruit juice:
  cherry spice *(Fruit Teazers)*, 12 fl. oz. 25.0
  ginger peach *(Fruit Teazers)*, 12 fl. oz. 27.0
  hibiscus blossom or raspberry rose *(Fruit Teazers)*,
    12 fl. oz. 26.0
chilled, with or without lemon *(Lipton)*, 8 fl. oz. 20.0
mix*:
  all flavors *(Nestea Ice Teasers)*, 8 fl. oz. 1.0
  citrus or lemon-lime, with sugar *(Lipton)*, 8 fl. oz. 14.0
  lemon flavor *(Lipton Multi Pack)*, 6 fl. oz. 14.0
  with lemon *(Nestea Presweetened)*, 8 fl. oz. 19.0
Teff seed or flour *(Arrowhead Mills)*, 2 oz. 41.0
Tempeh:
1 oz. 4.8
½ cup 14.1
quinoa-sesame *(Lightlife)*, 4 oz. 14.0
Tempura batter mix *(Golden Dipt)*, 1 oz. 22.0
Teriyaki marinade:
(Lawry's), 2 tbsp. 11.0
barbecue *(Lawry's)*, ¼ cup 27.4
seafood, see "Seafood sauce"
Teriyaki sauce:
(La Choy/La Choy Lite), ½ tsp. 1.0
basting *(La Choy)*, ½ tsp. .... <1.0
Thirst quencher drink:
all flavors *(PowerAde)*, 6 fl. oz. 14.0
all flavors *(10-K)*, 8 fl. oz. 15.0
lemon *(Recharge)*, 8 fl. oz. 14.0

lemon *(Recharge Organic)*, 8 fl. oz. 11.0
orange or tropical *(Recharge)*, 8 fl. oz. 13.0
Thuringer cervelat (see also "Summer sausage")
  (Hillshire Farm), 2 oz. 1.0
Thyme, ground, 1 tsp. 9
Thymus, beef or veal, without added ingredients 0
Tilefish, without added ingredients 0
Toaster muffins and pastries, 1 piece:
all fruit varieties *(Kellogg's Pop-Tarts)*, 1 piece 37.0
apple:
  (Pillsbury Toaster Strudel), 1 piece 26.0
  cinnamon *(Pepperidge Farm* Croissant Toaster
    Tarts), 1 piece 25.0
  spice *(Toaster Muffins)*, 1 piece 21.0
banana nut *(Thomas' Toast-r-Cakes)*, 1 piece 17.0
banana nut *(Toaster Muffins)*, 1 piece 19.0
blueberry:
  (Pillsbury Toaster Strudel), 1 piece 26.0
  (Thomas' Toast-r-Cakes), 1 piece 17.0
  wild Maine *(Toaster Muffins)*, 1 piece 23.0
brown sugar-cinnamon *(Kellogg's Pop-Tarts)*, 1 piece 33.0
brown sugar-cinnamon, frosted *(Kellogg's Pop-Tarts)*,
  1 piece 34.0
cheese *(Pepperidge Farm* Croissant Toaster Tarts),
  1 piece 22.0
chocolate chip *(Thomas' Toast-r-Cakes)*, 1 piece 15.0
chocolate fudge, graham, or vanilla creme *(Kellogg's
  Pop-Tarts)*, 1 piece 37.0
cinnamon *(Pillsbury Toaster Strudel)*, 1 piece 23.0
corn *(Thomas' Toast-r-Cakes)*, 1 piece 20.0
corn, old fashioned *(Toaster Muffins)*, 1 piece 17.0
oat bran with raisins *(Awrey's* Toastums), 1 piece 17.0
raisin bran *(Toaster Muffins)*, 1 piece 16.0
raisin bran *(Thomas' Toast-r-Cakes)*, 1 piece 18.0
strawberry *(Pepperidge Farm* Croissant Toaster
  Tarts), 1 piece 28.0
strawberry *(Pillsbury Toaster Strudel)*, 1 piece 26.0

Tofu:
raw:
1 oz.	.5
½ cup	2.3
extra firm *(Nasoya)*, 4 oz.	1.1
firm, 1 oz.	1.2
firm, ½ cup	5.4
pasteurized *(Frieda's)*, 4.2 oz.	2.9
silken *(Nasoya)*, 4 oz.	2.3
soft *(Nasoya)*, 4 oz.	1.7
dried-frozen (koyadofu), 1 oz.	4.1
flavored, Chinese 5-spice *(Nasoya)*, 4 oz.	2.0
flavored, French country herb *(Nasoya)*, 4 oz.	1.0
fried, 1 oz.	3.0
okara, 1 oz.	3.6
okara, ½ cup	7.7
salted and fermented (fuyu), 1 oz.	1.5

Tofu dishes, see specific listings
Tofu patty, frozen:
(Natural Touch Okara), 1 patty	7.0
garden *(Natural Touch)*, 1 patty	8.0

Tofu "yogurt," see " 'Yogurt,' tofu"
Tom collins mixer:
bottled *(Holland House)*, 3 fl. oz.	33.0
instant *(Holland House)*, .56 oz. dry	16.0

Tomatillo:
1 medium, 1⅝" diameter	2.0
chopped, ½ cup	3.8

Tomato:
fresh:
raw, 1 medium, 2⅗"-diameter	5.7
raw, chopped, ½ cup	4.2
boiled, ½ cup	7.0

dried, see "Tomato, sun-dried"
Tomato, canned (see also "Tomato sauce"):
whole:
(Contadina/Contadina Recipe Ready), ½ cup	5.0
(Contadina Pasta Ready), ½ cup	8.0

(Del Monte), ½ cup 6.0
(Hunt's/Hunt's No Salt), 4 oz. 5.0
Italian, pear *(Contadina)*, ½ cup 5.0
Italian flavored *(Hunt's)*, 4 oz. 6.0
chunky:
    chili style *(Del Monte)*, ½ cup 6.0
    pasta style *(Del Monte)*, ½ cup 9.0
    pizza style *(Del Monte)*, ½ cup 8.0
cut, peeled *(Hunt's Choice-Cut)*, 4 oz. 5.0
diced, in tomato juice *(Del Monte)*, ½ cup 6.0
diced, with olive oil, herbs *(Master Choice)*, ½ cup 20.0
crushed:
    (Contadina), ½ cup 6.0
    (Eden No Salt Added), ½ cup 6.0
    (Hunt's Angela Mia), 4 oz. 7.0
    with basil *(Master Choice)*, ½ cup 9.0
    Italian flavored *(Hunt's)*, 4 oz. 9.0
with green chilies *(Old El Paso)*, ¼ cup 3.0
with jalapeños *(Old El Paso)*, ¼ cup 2.0
with jalapeños *(Ortega)*, 1 oz. 1.0
paste, see "Tomato paste"
puree:
    ½ cup 12.5
    (Contadina), ½ cup 8.0
    (Del Monte), ¼ cup 7.0
    (Hunt's), 4 oz. 10.0
    (Progresso), ½ cup 10.0
    heavy concentrate *(Progresso)*, ½ cup 11.0
stewed:
    ½ cup 8.3
    (Contadina), ½ cup 8.0
    (Del Monte/Del Monte No Salt), ½ cup 9.0
    (Hunt's/Hunt's No Salt), 4 oz. 8.0
    Italian flavored *(Hunt's)*, 4 oz. 9.0
    Italian recipe *(Del Monte)*, ½ cup 7.0
    Italian style *(Del Monte)*, ½ cup 8.0
    Italian or Mexican style *(Contadina)*, ½ cup 8.0
    Mexican or pizza style *(Del Monte)*, ½ cup 9.0

Tomato, canned, stewed *(cont.)*
  sliced *(Libby's)*, ½ cup 9.0
  sliced *(Master Choice)*, ½ cup 9.0
  wedges *(Del Monte)*, ½ cup 9.0
  wedges, in tomato juice, ½ cup................................... 8.3
Tomato, green, 1 medium, 2⅗"-diameter........................ 6.3
Tomato, pickled *(Claussen)*, 3 oz. 3.0
Tomato, sun-dried:
1 oz. 15.8
1 piece (32 per cup).. 1.1
½ cup 15.1
(Frieda's), 1 oz. 21.2
Tomato juice:
regular or low-sodium, 6 fl. oz. 7.7
(Campbell's), 6 fl. oz. 8.0
(Hunt's), 6 fl. oz... 7.0
(Hunt's No Salt Added), 6 fl. oz. 8.0
(R. W. Knudsen Organic), 6 fl. oz. 10.0
(Libby's), 6 fl. oz... 8.0
(Welch's), 6 fl. oz. 7.0
Tomato paste, canned:
1 oz. 5.3
(Contadina), 2 oz... 11.0
(Del Monte), 2 tbsp. 7.0
all varieties *(Hunt's)*, 2 oz... 11.0
Italian *(Contadina)*, 2 oz. 12.0
Tomato sauce, canned (see also "Tomato, canned"
  and "Pasta sauce"):
½ cup 8.8
(Contadina), ½ cup 7.0
(Contadina Thick & Zesty), ½ cup.................................. 8.0
(Del Monte/Del Monte No Salt), ¼ cup........................ 4.0
(Hunt's), 4 oz. 7.0
(Hunt's No Salt/Special), 4 oz. 8.0
(Progresso), ½ cup 9.0
with garlic *(Hunt's)*, 4 oz. 10.0
herb flavored *(Hunt's)*, 4 oz. 12.0

Italian style:

   (Contadina), ½ cup.. 7.0

   (Hunt's), 4 oz. 10.0

   (Rokeach), 3 oz.. 8.0

marinara, see "Pasta sauce"

for meat loaf *(Hunt's Meatloaf Fixin's)*, 2 oz. 5.0

with mushrooms:

   ½ cup 10.3

   (Hunt's), 4 oz. 6.0

   (Rokeach), 1 cup 16.0

with onions, ½ cup 12.1

with onions *(Hunt's)*, 4 oz.. 9.0

with tomato bits *(Hunt's)*, 4 oz..................................... 7.0

with tomato bits, low-sodium, ½ cup 8.7

Tomato-beef cocktail *(Beefamato)*, 6 fl. oz. 19.0

Tomato-chili cocktail *(Snap-E-Tom)*, 6 fl. oz..................... 7.0

Tomato-clam juice cocktail *(Clamato)*, 6 fl. oz............... 17.9

Tongue, braised:

beef, 4 oz. 4

lamb, pork, or veal (calf), 4 oz..................................... 0

Tortellini, refrigerated:

cheese and herb *(Contadina)*, 3 oz. 37.0

chicken *(Contadina)*, 3 oz. 39.0

chicken and proscuitto *(Contadina)*, 3 oz. 36.0

Tortellini dishes, cheese, frozen *(The Budget*

   Gourmet Side Dish), 5.5 oz.................................... 25.0

Tortellini entree, frozen:

(Weight Watchers), 9 oz.. 50.0

in Alfredo sauce *(Stouffer's)*, 8⅞ oz.............................. 35.0

with tomato sauce *(Stouffer's)*, 9¼ oz. 39.0

Provençale *(Green Giant Garden Gourmet Right for*

   Lunch), 9.5 oz.. 44.0

Tortilla:

corn, enchilada style *(Tyson)*, 1 piece 11.0

flour:

   (Old El Paso), 1 piece... 27.0

   burrito style *(Tyson)*, 1 piece................................. 29.0

   burrito style, hand stretched *(Tyson)*, 1 piece 19.0

Tortilla, flour *(cont.)*
    burrito style, heat pressed *(Tyson)*, 1 piece 33.0
    fajita style *(Tyson)*, 1 piece 18.0
    soft taco or whole wheat *(Tyson)*, 1 piece 20.0
Tortilla chips:
corn:
    (Barbara's Organic Yellow), 1 oz. 18.0
    (Doritos), 1 oz. 19.0
    (Doritos Jumpin' Jack/Cool Ranch/Salsa Rio), 1 oz. 18.0
    (Hain Taco Style), 1 oz. 15.0
    (Lafamous), 1 oz. 18.0
    (NaChips), 1 oz. 18.0
    all varieties *(Tyson)*, 1 oz. 17.0
    all varieties, except white *(Tostitos)*, 1 oz. 18.0
    blue *(Kettle Tias* Lightly Salted/No Salt), 1 oz. 18.0
    nacho *(Tom's)*, 1¼-oz. pkg. 22.0
    nacho or ranch *(Eagle* Thins), 1 oz. 17.0
    nacho or taco flavor *(Doritos)*, 1 oz. 18.0
    sesame *(Hain/Hain* No Salt), 1 oz. 19.0
    sesame cheese *(Hain)*, 1 oz. 20.0
    white, restaurant style *(Tostitos)*, 1 oz. 20.0
    white, round *(NaChips* Low Sodium), 1 oz. 17.0
flour:
    original *(Chacho's)*, 1 oz. 18.0
    cheesy quesadilla *(Chacho's)*, 1 oz. 17.0
    cinnamon crispana *(Chacho's)*, 1 oz. 19.0
Tortilla mix, corn *(Albers Ricamasa)*, ⅓ cup dry 28.0
Tostaco shell *(Old El Paso)*, 1 piece 11.0
Tostada shell:
(Lawry's), 1 piece 9.5
(Old El Paso), 1 piece 6.0
(Ortega), 1 piece 8.0
(Pancho Villa), 1 piece 6.0
(Rosarita), 1 piece 8.0
(Tio Sancho), 1 piece 8.4
Tree fern, cooked, chopped, ½ cup, 1 piece 7.8
Triticale, whole-grain, 1 cup 138.5
Triticale flour, whole-grain, 1 cup 95.1

Tropical nectar (Kern's), 6 fl. oz. 27.0
Tropical punch, see "Fruit punch"
Trout, without added ingredients 0
Tuna, fresh or smoked, without added ingredients 0
Tuna, canned, drained:
all varieties, in oil or water (Bumble Bee), 2 oz. 0
all varieties, in oil or water (Star-Kist/Star-Kist Diet/
  Prime Catch/Select), 2 oz. .... <1.0
all varieties, in water (Weight Watchers), 2 oz. .... <1.0
solid light, in oil (Progresso), 1/3 cup .... <1.0
solid light, in water (Empress), 2 oz. 0
solid white, albacore, in water (Master Choice Line
  Caught), 2 oz. .... <1.0
"Tuna," vegetarian, frozen (Worthington Tuno), 2 oz. 3.0
Tuna entree, frozen, noodle casserole:
(Stouffer's), 10 oz. 33.0
(Weight Watchers), 9 oz. 27.0
Tuna entree, packaged, noodle casserole (Dinty
  Moore American Classics), 10 oz. 28.0
Tuna entree mix*:
au gratin (Tuna Helper), 6 oz. 30.0
fettucini Alfredo (Tuna Helper), 7 oz. 28.0
garden and herb, zesty tomato, or classic Italian
  (Bumble Bee Tuna Mix-Ins), 1 oz. dry 5.0
lemon herb (Bumble Bee Tuna Mix-Ins), 1 oz. dry 6.0
mushroom, creamy (Tuna Helper), 7 oz. 28.0
noodles, cheesy (Tuna Helper), 7.75 oz. 27.0
noodles, creamy (Tuna Helper), 8 oz. 29.0
pot pie (Tuna Helper), 5.1 oz. 31.0
rice, buttery (Tuna Helper), 6 oz. 32.0
Romanoff (Tuna Helper), 8 oz. 38.0
salad (Tuna Helper), 5.5 oz. 29.0
tetrazzini (Tuna Helper), 6 oz. 26.0
Tuna salad:
(Longacre), 1 oz. 4.1
spread (Libby's Spreadables), 1.9 oz. 5.0
Tuna seasoning mix (Old Bay Tuna Classic), 1 pkg. 15.0
Turbot, without added ingredients 0

Turkey, without added ingredients 0
Turkey, boneless and luncheon meat (see also
   "Turkey bologna," "Turkey ham," etc.):
all varieties, except tan label *(Norbest)*, 1 oz. .... <1.0
breast:
   (Healthy Deli Gourmet), 1 oz. 6
   (Hormel Bread Ready), 1 oz. 1.0
   (Hormel Deli No Salt/No Salt), 1 oz. .... <2.0
   (Tyson), 1 slice 3
   Black Forest *(Healthy Deli)*, 1 oz. 5
   browned, glazed *(Longacre* Gourmet), 1 oz. 5
   browned, roasted *(Longacre* Gourmet), 1 oz. 7
   cooked *(Healthy Deli* Lessalt), 1 oz. 7
   honey *(Healthy Deli)*, 1 oz. 2.0
   honey roasted *(Louis Rich)*, 1 oz. 1.2
   mini *(Longacre* Gourmet), 1 oz. 6
   oven cooked *(Healthy Deli)*, 1 oz. 1.2
   oven roasted *(Hillshire Farm* Deli Select), 1 oz. .... <1.0
   oven roasted *(Longacre* Lean-Lite), 1 oz. 0
   oven roasted *(Louis Rich)*, .4-oz. slice 4
   oven roasted *(Louis Rich)*, 1 oz. 1.0
   oven roasted *(Weight Watchers)*, 1 oz. .... <1.0
   roast *(Oscar Mayer Deli-Thin)*, 5 slices 2.0
   roll *(Longacre* Sliced), 1 oz. 6
breast, skinless:
   (Hormel Deli Premium), 1 oz. .... <2.0
   (Longacre Gourmet/Premium), 1 oz. 7
   (Longacre Lean-Lite/No Salt/Salt Watchers), 1 oz. 0
   (Norbest Extra Tan Label), 1 oz. 1.1
   (Norbest Tan Label), 1 oz. 7
breast, smoked:
   (Healthy Deli Gourmet), 1 oz. 6
   (Hillshire Farm Deli Select), 1 oz. .... <1.0
   (Longacre Gourmet), 1 oz. 6
   (Longacre Lean-Lite), 1 oz. 0
   (Longacre Sliced), 1 oz. 9
   (Louis Rich), .7-oz. slice 1
   (Louis Rich), 1 oz. 2

(Oscar Mayer), 1 oz. 0
(Oscar Mayer Deli-Thin), 5 slices 0
(Oscar Mayer Healthy Favorites), 5 slices..................... <1.0
(Weight Watchers), 1 oz. .... <1.0
breast and white, skinless *(Longacre Deli Chef)*,
 1 oz.. .8
dark, smoked, cured *(Longacre/Longacre Chunk)*,
 1 oz.. .4
luncheon loaf *(Louis Rich)*, 1 oz. 4
roll, combination *(Longacre)*, 1 oz. 5
roll, white *(Longacre)*, 1 oz. 7
smoked *(Louis Rich)*, 1 oz. 3
Turkey, canned, chunk:
(Hormel), 2.5 oz.. 1.0
(Swanson Premium), 2.5 oz. 2.0
white *(Swanson* Premium), 2.5 oz. 1.0
Turkey, frozen or refrigerated:
all varieties *(Norbest)*, 1 oz. .... <1.0
breast, raw *(Longacre Cook-In-The-Bag)*, 1 oz. 4
breast, cooked:
 barbecued *(Louis Rich)*, 1 oz. 7
 hen, without wing *(Louis Rich)*, 1 oz........................ 0
 hickory smoked *(Louis Rich)*, 1 oz. 6
 honey roasted *(Louis Rich)*, 1 oz. 1.2
 oven roasted *(Louis Rich)*, 1 oz. 3
 roast *(Louis Rich)*, 1 oz. 2
 slices, steaks, or tenderloins *(Louis Rich)*, 1 oz. 0
dark meat, roast, raw *(Longacre)*, 1 oz. 0
drumstick or thigh, cooked *(Louis Rich)*, 1 oz. 0
ground, see "Turkey, ground"
whole, browned and roasted or smoked *(Longacre)*,
 1 oz... 0
whole, cooked, without giblets *(Louis Rich)*, 1 oz. 0
wing, cooked *(Louis Rich/Louis Rich* Drumettes/
 Portions), 1 oz. 0
Turkey, ground (see also "Turkey patties"):
raw or cooked, without added ingredients 0
(Norbest), 1 oz.. <1.0

Turkey, ground *(cont.)*
cooked *(Louis Rich/Louis Rich 90% Fat Free)*, 1 oz. 0
cooked *(Perdue)*, 1 oz. 0
"Turkey," vegetarian:
canned *(Worthington Turkee)*, 2 slices 3.0
frozen, smoked *(Worthington)*, 4 slices 5.0
Turkey bacon, 1 slice 0
Turkey bologna:
(Longacre), 1 oz. 0
(Louis Rich), 1 oz. 6
mild *(Louis Rich)*, 1 oz. 7
Turkey burger, see "Turkey patty"
Turkey and corned beef *(Healthy Deli*
Doubledecker)*, 1 oz. 6
Turkey dinner, frozen:
(Banquet Extra Helping), 17 oz. 64.0
(Swanson), 11.5 oz. 43.0
(Swanson Hungry Man), 16.5 oz. 59.0
breast of *(Healthy Choice)*, 10.5 oz. 41.0
breast, stuffed *(The Budget Gourmet Light and*
Healthy)*, 11 oz. 31.0
breast, stuffed *(Weight Watchers)*, 8.5 oz. 31.0
with dressing and gravy *(Armour Classics)*, 11.5 oz. 34.0
with gravy *(Tyson Premium)*, 9.5 oz. 34.0
sliced *(Freezer Queen)*, 9.25 oz. 24.0
tetrazzini *(Healthy Choice)*, 12.6 oz. 49.0
Turkey entree, canned, and dressing, with gravy
(Libby's Diner), 7 oz. 15.0
Turkey entree, freeze-dried*, tetrazzini *(Mountain*
House)*, 1 cup 21.0
Turkey entree, frozen or refrigerated:
breast:
nuggets *(Perdue Done It!)*, 1 piece 3.0
roast, with mushrooms, in gravy *(Healthy Choice)*,
8.5 oz. 26.0
roast, with stuffing *(Stouffer's Homestyle)*, 7⅞ oz. 27.0
sliced, with dressing *(Lean Cuisine)*, 7⅞ oz. 22.0

sliced, in mushroom sauce, with rice pilaf *(Lean
  Cuisine)*, 8 oz. 24.0
croquettes *(On-Cor)*, 8 oz. 23.0
croquettes, gravy and *(Freezer Queen* Family), 7 oz. 19.0
Dijon *(Lean Cuisine)*, 9.5 oz. 20.0
with dressing *(Freezer Queen)*, 9 oz. 27.0
with dressing *(On-Cor)*, 8 oz. 24.0
glazed *(The Budget Gourmet* Light and Healthy),
  9 oz. 38.0
and gravy:
  (Banquet Meals), 9.25 oz. 31.0
  (On-Cor), 8 oz. 10.0
  with dressing *(Banquet Healthy Balance)*, 11.25 oz. 40.0
  with dressing *(Freezer Queen* Family), 7 oz. 14.0
  with dressing *(Swanson)*, 9 oz. 29.0
  with dressing, sliced *(Healthy Choice Homestyle
    Classic)*, 10 oz. 30.0
gravy and:
  (Banquet Cookin' Bag), 5 oz. 5.0
  (Banquet Family), 6 oz. 6.0
  (Freezer Queen Family), 7 oz. 8.0
  with dressing *(Banquet Entree Express)*, 7 oz. 26.0
medallions, roast *(Weight Watchers Smart Ones)*,
  8.5 oz. 35.0
pie:
  (Stouffer's), 10 oz. 33.0
  (Swanson), 7 oz. 38.0
  (Swanson Hungry Man), 14 oz. 58.0
tetrazzini *(Stouffer's)*, 10 oz. 26.0
with vegetables, homestyle *(Healthy Choice)*, 9.5 oz. 28.0
with vegetables and pasta, homestyle *(Lean Cuisine)*,
  9³/₈ oz. 25.0
Turkey entree, packaged, with dressing and gravy
  (Dinty Moore American Classics), 10 oz. 33.0
Turkey entree, refrigerated:
hickory barbecue *(Turkey By George)*, 5 oz. 8.0
lemon pepper *(Turkey By George)*, 5 oz. 4.0

Turkey entree, refrigerated *(cont.)*
mustard tarragon or Italian Parmesan *(Turkey By*
  George), 5 oz... 3.0
Turkey fat 0
Turkey frankfurter:
(Longacre), 1 oz. 0
(Louis Rich), 1 link.. 1.3
(Louis Rich Bun Length), 1 link................................... 1.7
(Perdue), 1.6-oz. link.. 2.0
cheese *(Louis Rich)*, 1 link... 1.3
Turkey giblets:
simmered, 4 oz. 2.4
simmered, chopped or diced, 1 cup............................... 3.0
Turkey gravy:
canned:
  (Franco-American), ¼ cup 3.0
  (Heinz HomeStyle), ¼ cup 3.0
  seasoned *(Pepperidge Farm)*, ¼ cup 4.0
mix:
  (French's), ¼ pkg. 5.0
  (Lawry's), 1 cup*.. 14.9
  (McCormick/Schilling), ¼ cup*................................ 4.0
Turkey ham:
(Healthy Deli), 1 oz. 7
(Longacre Sliced), 1 oz. 0
(Louis Rich), 1 oz. 3
(Louis Rich Round), 1 oz. 4
(Louis Rich Square), .7-oz. slice..................................2
(Louis Rich Thin Sliced), 1 slice...................................1
(Norbest/Norbest Sliced/Canadian Style/Gourmet/
  Tavern Ham), 1 oz. .... <1.0
(Tyson), 1 slice... 1.0
baked *(Longacre, 12% Water Added)*, 1 oz............... 0
baked *(Longacre, 20% Water Added)*, 1 oz.............. 1.5
chopped *(Louis Rich)*, 1 oz...3
honey cured *(Louis Rich)*, .7-oz. slice 5
roll *(Norbest)*, 1 oz. 5
Turkey ham salad *(Longacre)*, 1 oz. 2.9

Turkey luncheon meat, see "Turkey, boneless and luncheon meat"

Turkey nuggets, breaded, heated *(Louis Rich)*,
  1 piece... 4.0

Turkey pastrami:
(Healthy Deli), 1 oz... 1.4
(Longacre Sliced), 1 oz... 0
(Norbest Sliced), 1 oz... <1.0

Turkey patty:
breaded, heated *(Louis Rich)*, 1 patty 13.3
frozen *(Longacre)*, 1 oz.. 0
frozen, barbecued *(Longacre)*, 1 oz......................... 1.0

Turkey pie, see "Turkey entree"

Turkey salad:
(Longacre), 1 oz... 3.0
spread *(Libby's Spreadables)*, 1.9 oz....................... 6.0

Turkey salami:
(Longacre), 1 oz.. .6
(Louis Rich), 1 oz.. 0
cooked, 1 oz.. .2
cotto *(Louis Rich)*, 1 oz... .1

Turkey sandwich, pocket, frozen:
with broccoli'n cheese *(Lean Pockets)*, 4.5 oz.......... 31.0
with ham'n cheese *(Hot Pockets)*, 4.5 oz. 40.0

Turkey sausage:
(Longacre Chub or Patties), 1 oz................................ 0
(Norbest Chub/Links), 1 oz.................................... <1.0
breakfast, cooked:
  (Louis Rich), 1 oz.. 0
  (Louis Rich), 1 link.. .3
  (Perdue), 1 link or patty...................................... <1.0
Italian, hot or sweet, cooked *(Perdue)*, 2-oz. link 0
Polish *(Louis Rich Polska)*, 1 oz................................. .5
smoked *(Louis Rich)*, 1 oz.. .8
smoked, with cheese *(Louis Rich)*, 1 oz. 7

Turkey and pork sausage, cooked, all varieties
  (Jimmy Dean Light), 1 oz..................................... <1.0

Turkey seasoning and coating mix, roast
(McCormick/Schilling Bag'n Season), 1 pkg. 20.0
Turkey spread, canned, chunky (Underwood Light),
2⅛ oz. 2.0
Turkey sticks, breaded, heated* (Louis Rich),
1 piece 4.5
Turkey summer sausage (Louis Rich), 1 oz. 4
Turmeric:
ground, 1 tsp. 1.4
(Spice Islands), 1 tsp. 1.3
Turnip:
fresh:
  raw, cubed, ½ cup 4.1
  boiled, drained, cubed, ½ cup 3.8
  boiled, drained, mashed, ½ cup 5.6
frozen, boiled, drained, 4 oz. 4.9
Turnip greens:
fresh:
  raw, untrimmed, 1 lb. 18.2
  raw, chopped, ½ cup 1.6
  boiled, drained, chopped, ½ cup 3.1
canned:
  with liquid, ½ cup 2.8
  (Allens/Sunshine), ½ cup 3.0
  chopped, with diced turnips (Allens/Sunshine),
    ½ cup 1.0
frozen:
  boiled, drained, with turnips, 4 oz. 3.3
  chopped (Frosty Acres), 3.3 oz. 4.0
  chopped, with diced turnips (Seabrook), 3.3 oz. 3.0
Turnover, frozen or refrigerated:
apple or cherry (Pepperidge Farm), 1 piece 33.0
apple, flaky (Pillsbury), 1 piece 23.0
blueberry (Pepperidge Farm), 1 piece 32.0
cherry, flaky (Pillsbury), 1 piece 24.0
peach (Pepperidge Farm), 1 piece 34.0
raspberry (Pepperidge Farm), 1 piece 36.0

V

Food and Measure	Carbohydrate Grams
Vanilla extract *(Virginia Dare)*, 1 tsp.	.3
Vanilla flavor drink:	
canned *(Sego* Very Vanilla), 10 fl. oz.	34.0
mix *(Carnation* Instant Breakfast), 1 packet	28.0
mix *(Pillsbury* Instant Breakfast), 1 packet	28.0
Veal, without added ingredients	0
"Veal," vegetarian, frozen *(Worthington Veelets)*, 1 patty	12.0
Veal parmigiana dinner, frozen:	
(Armour Classics), 11.25 oz.	34.0
(Freezer Queen), 9 oz.	44.0
(Swanson), 11.5 oz.	40.0
(Swanson Hungry Man), 18.25 oz.	57.0
Veal parmigiana entree, frozen:	
(Banquet Meals), 9 oz.	35.0
(On-Cor), 8 oz.	29.0
(Swanson), 10 oz.	33.0
with pasta Alfredo *(Stouffer's* Homestyle), 9.25 oz.	26.0
patty *(Banquet Family)*, 7 oz.	29.0
patty *(Weight Watchers Ultimate 200)*, 8.2 oz.	5.0
Vegetable chips:	
exotic *(Terra)*, 1 oz.	18.0
sea *(Eden)*, 1 oz.	22.0
Vegetable entree, canned:	
chow mein, meatless *(La Choy)*, ¾ cup	5.0
stew *(Dinty Moore)*, 8 oz.	20.0
Vegetable entree, freeze-dried*, stew, with beef *(Mountain House)*, 1 cup	27.0

Vegetable entree, frozen:
Chinese, and chicken (*The Budget Gourmet* Light
and Healthy), 10 oz. 47.0
Italian, and chicken (*The Budget Gourmet* Light and
Healthy), 10.25 oz. 50.0
and pasta mornay, with ham (*Lean Cuisine*), 9⅜ oz. 29.0
pot pie, with beef, chicken, or turkey (*Banquet*),
7 oz. 39.0
pot pie, with beef, chicken, or turkey (*Morton*), 7 oz. 27.0
Vegetable juice cocktail:
all varieties (*R. W. Knudsen Very Veggie*), 8 fl. oz. 8.0
all varieties (*"V-8"*), 6 fl. oz. 8.0
all varieties (*Smucker's*), 8 fl. oz. 13.0
Vegetable oyster, see "Salsify"
Vegetable pie, see "Vegetable entree"
Vegetable pocket sandwich, frozen:
Bar-B-Q (*Veggie Pockets*), 5 oz. 50.0
broccoli cheddar (*Veggie Pockets*), 5 oz. 37.0
Greek (*Veggie Pockets*), 5 oz. 35.0
Indian (*Veggie Pockets*), 5 oz. 41.0
Oriental (*Veggie Pockets*), 5 oz. 40.8
pizza (*Veggie Pockets*), 5 oz. 42.0
Tex-Mex (*Veggie Pockets*), 5 oz. 43.0
Vegetable protein:
original or chocolate (*Naturade*), 1 oz. 1.0
soy free (*Naturade*), 1 oz. 3.0
Vegetable sticks, breaded, frozen (*Stilwell*), 5 pieces 24.0
Vegetables, see specific listings
Vegetables, mixed, canned or packaged:
(*Green Giant* Garden Medley), ½ cup 9.0
(*Green Giant Pantry Express*), ½ cup 8.0
(*La Choy* Chop Suey/Fancy Mix), ½ cup 2.0
(*Stokely*), ½ cup 8.0
Dijon (*Del Monte Vegetable Classics*), ½ cup 8.0
Vegetables, mixed, frozen:
(*Frosty Acres*), 3.3 oz. 13.0
(*Green Giant/Green Giant Harvest Fresh*), ½ cup 9.0
(*Seabrook*), 3.3 oz. 13.0

(Southern), 3.5 oz.. 13.9
Austrian style *(Birds Eye* International), ½ cup.................... 6.0
Bavarian style *(Birds Eye* International), ½ cup.................. 10.0
for beef, without added ingredients:
  Burgundy *(Bird's Eye* Easy Recipe), 7 oz. 17.0
  Italiano *(Bird's Eye* Easy Recipe), 7 oz. 28.0
in butter sauce *(Green Giant)*, ½ cup 11.0
California style *(Green Giant)*, ½ cup................................. 6.0
for chicken, without added ingredients:
  Alfredo *(Bird's Eye* Easy Recipe), 7 oz. 22.0
  glazed *(Bird's Eye* Easy Recipe), 7 oz. 30.0
  primavera *(Bird's Eye* Easy Recipe), 7 oz...................... 14.0
  teriyaki *(Bird's Eye* Easy Recipe), 7 oz. 28.0
Dutch style *(Frosty Acres)*, 3.2 oz. 5.0
heartland style *(Green Giant)*, ½ cup................................ 6.0
Japanese style *(Birds Eye* Stir-Fry), ½ cup........................ 6.0
mandarin *(The Budget Gourmet* Side Dish), 5.25 oz......... 13.0
Manhattan style *(Green Giant)*, ½ cup............................... 5.0
medley, breaded *(Ore-Ida)*, 3 oz...................................... 16.0
New England:
  recipe *(The Budget Gourmet* Side Dish), 5.5 oz. 21.0
  style *(Birds Eye* International), ½ cup.............................. 12.0
  style *(Green Giant)*, ½ cup.. 14.0
San Francisco or Seattle style *(Green Giant)*, ½ cup.......... 7.0
Santa Fe style *(Green Giant)*, ½ cup................................. 16.0
soup mix *(Frosty Acres)*, 3 oz.. 11.0
spring, cheese sauce *(The Budget Gourmet* Side
  Dish), 5 oz.. 9.0
stew:
  (Frosty Acres), 3 oz. 10.0
  (Kohl's), 3.3 oz.. 10.0
  (Ore-Ida), 3 oz.. 11.0
Western style *(Green Giant)*, ½ cup................................. 12.0
Vegetables, mixed, pickled, hot and spicy *(Vlasic
  Garden Mix)*, 1 oz.. 1.0
Vegetarian burger, see " 'Hamburger,' vegetarian"
Vegetarian entree (see also specific listings):
frozen *(Natural Touch* Dinner Entree), 3-oz. patty.............. 6.0

Vegetarian entree (cont.)

mix*, chow mein, Mandarin, with tofu (Tofu Classics),
½ cup 17.0

mix*, loaf (Natural Touch), 4 oz. 12.0

Vegetarian foods, see specific listings

Venison, without added ingredients 0

Vienna sausage, canned:

(Hormel), 1 oz. .... <2.0

in barbecue sauce (Libby's), 2.5 oz. 2.0

in beef broth (Libby's 5 oz.), 2. oz. 1.0

beef and pork, 2″ link, .6 oz. 3

chicken (Hormel), 1 oz. 1.0

chicken, in beef broth (Libby's), 2 oz. 3.0

Vine spinach, raw, untrimmed, 1 lb. 15.4

Vinegar:

all varieties (Heinz/Heinz Gourmet), 1 tbsp. 0

apple cider (White House), 1 fl. oz. 2.0

apple cider, raw unpasturized (Hain), 1 tbsp. .... <1.0

wine, all varieties (Regina), 1 fl. oz. 0

W

Food and Measure	Carbohydrate Grams

Waffle, frozen:

(*Aunt Jemima* Low Fat), 1 piece... 16.0
(*Downyflake*), 1 piece.. 10.0
(*Downyflake* Hot-N-Buttery), 1 piece.................................. 13.5
(*Downyflake* Jumbo), 1 piece... 15.0
(*Eggo* Homestyle), 1 piece.. 16.0
(*Eggo* Minis), 4 pieces 14.0
(*Eggo* Nutri-Grain), 1 piece 18.0
(*Kellogg's Special K*), 1 piece.. 16.0
plain or apple cinnamon (*Downyflake* Crisp &
   Healthy), 1 piece.. 16.0
apple cinnamon (*Eggo*), 1 piece.. 18.0
Belgian (*Belgian Chef*), 1 piece 11.0
blueberry (*Downyflake*), 1 piece... 16.0
blueberry (*Eggo*), 1 piece.. 18.0
buttermilk:
   (*Downyflake* Jumbo), 1 piece.. 15.0
   (*Eggo*), 1 piece 16.0
   or cinnamon (*Aunt Jemima*), 1 piece............................... 16.0
multibran (*Eggo Nutri-Grain*), 1 piece................................. 17.0
nut and honey (*Eggo*), 1 piece 17.0
oat bran (*Eggo Common Sense*), 1 piece.......................... 16.0
oat bran, with fruit and nut (*Eggo Common Sense*),
   1 piece.. 17.0
raisin and bran (*Eggo Nutri-Grain*), 1 piece 18.0
sticks (*Swanson Breakfast Blast*), 2.75 oz. 34.0
strawberry (*Eggo*), 1 piece.. 18.0
whole grain (*Roman Meal*), 1 piece.................................... 16.5

Waffle breakfast, frozen, with sausage *(Swanson Budget),* 2.25 oz. 21.0
Waffle mix, see "Pancake and waffle mix"
Walnut, dried:
black:
  shelled, 1 oz. 3.4
  chopped, 1 cup 15.1
  (Fisher), 1 oz. 3.0
English or Persian:
  shelled, 1 oz. 5.2
  pieces, 1 cup 22.0
  halves, 1 cup 18.3
  raw, chopped or ground *(Fisher),* 1 oz. 5.0
Walnut topping, in syrup *(Smucker's),* 2 tbsp. 27.0
Waterchestnut, Chinese:
fresh:
  4 medium, 2″ diameter 8.6
  sliced, ½ cup 14.8
  (Frieda's), 1 oz. 5.4
canned:
  4 medium or 1 oz. 3.5
  with liquid, sliced, ½ cup 8.7
  whole *(La Choy),* 4 medium 4.0
  sliced *(La Choy),* ¼ cup 4.0
Watercress. fresh:
10 sprigs, 11¼″ long 3
chopped, ½ cup 2
Watermelon, fresh:
1 slice, 10″ diameter × 1″ thick 34.6
diced, ½ cup 5.7
seedless *(Frieda's),* 1 oz. 1.8
Watermelon seeds, dried, 1 oz. 4.4
Wax beans: fresh, see "Green beans"
canned, golden, all cuts *(Del Monte),* ½ cup 4.0
frozen *(Frosty Acres),* 3 oz. 5.0
frozen, cut *(Seabrook),* 3 oz. 5.0
Wax gourd, boiled, drained, cubed, ½ cup 2.6

Welsh rarebit:
canned *(Snow's)*, ½ cup.. 10.0
frozen *(Stouffer's)*, 5 oz.. 9.0
Wendy's, 1 serving:
burgers and sandwiches:
   bacon cheeseburger, Jr. 33.0
   Big Classic... 44.0
   cheeseburger, Jr.. 34.0
   cheeseburger, Kid's Meal... 33.0
   cheeseburger deluxe, Jr.. 36.0
   chicken, grilled 35.0
   chicken, breaded, or chicken club............................... 44.0
   fish 42.0
   hamburger, single, plain.. 31.0
   hamburger, single, with everything 36.0
   hamburger, Jr. 34.0
   hamburger, Kid's Meal 33.0
   steak, country fried 45.0
chicken nuggets, 6 pieces.. 12.0
nuggets sauces, 1 packet:
   barbecue... 11.0
   honey 12.0
   sweet mustard... 9.0
   sweet and sour.. 11.0
chili, small, 8 oz. 21.0
chili, large, 12 oz... 31.0
baked potato:
   plain 69.0
   bacon and cheese.. 75.0
   broccoli and cheese... 77.0
   cheese 74.0
   chili and cheese 80.0
   sour cream with chives 71.0
salads and side dishes:
   breadstick... 24.0
   Caesar salad, side... 18.0
   chicken salad, grilled, to go 9.0
   fries, Biggie.. 62.0

Wendy's, salads and side dishes *(cont.)*
- fries, medium...50.0
- fries, small 33.0
- garden salad, deluxe, to go...9.0
- side salad, to go...6.0
- taco salad, to go 70.0

dressing, 2 tbsp.:
- bacon and tomato, reduced calorie................................5.0
- blue cheese ....<1.0
- blue cheese, reduced fat/calorie...................................1.0
- celery seed 6.0
- French...6.0
- French, sweet red..9.0
- *Hidden Valley Ranch* 1.0
- Italian, golden 6.0
- Italian, reduced fat/calorie...2.5
- Italian Caesar...1.0
- ranch, fat free 8.0
- Thousand Island 3.0

desserts:
- chocolate chip cookie 39.0
- frosty, dairy, small...57.0
- frosty, dairy, medium...76.0
- frosty, dairy, large..95.0
- pudding, chocolate, ¼ cup..12.0
- pudding, butterscotch, ¼ cup 11.0

Western dinner, frozen *(Swanson),* 11.5 oz. 43.0
Western entree, frozen *(Banquet Meals),* 9.5 oz. 30.0
Wheat, whole-grain:
durum, 1 cup...136.6
hard red:
- spring, 1 cup 130.6
- spring or winter *(Arrowhead Mills),* 2 oz........................41.0
- winter, 1 cup..136.7
soft red, for pastry *(Arrowhead Mills),* 2 oz........................41.0
soft red, winter, 1 cup 124.7
hard white, 1 cup..145.7
soft white, 1 cup...126.6

Wheat, parboiled, see "Bulgur"
Wheat, sprouted, 1 cup 45.9
Wheat bran (see also "Cereal"):
crude, 1 oz. 18.3
crude, 2 tbsp. 4.5
toasted *(Kretschmer)*, 1 oz. or ⅓ cup 14.8
Wheat flakes *(Arrowhead Mills)*, 2 oz. 42.0
Wheat flour:
pastry *(Arrowhead Mills)*, 2 oz. 41.0
whole-grain:
  1 cup 87.1
  (Gold Medal), 1 cup 78.0
  (Pillsbury's Best), 1 cup 80.0
  blend *(Gold Medal)*, 1 cup 84.0
  stone ground *(Arrowhead Mills)*, 2 oz. 40.0
white, all-purpose:
  1 cup 95.4
  (Ballard/Pillsbury's Best), 1 cup 87.0
  regular or unbleached *(Gold Medal)*, 1 cup 87.0
  unbleached *(Pillsbury's Best)*, 1 cup 86.0
white, bread *(Gold Medal Better for Bread)*, 1 cup 83.0
white, bread *(Pillsbury's Best)*, 1 cup 83.0
white, cake, 1 cup 85.1
white, presifted *(Pillsbury Shake & Blend)*, 2 tbsp. 11.0
white, presifted *(Wondra)*, 1 cup 87.0
white, self-rising:
  1 cup 92.8
  (Pillsbury's Best), 1 cup 84.0
  (Gold Medal), 1 cup 83.0
  tortilla mix, 1 cup 74.5
Wheat germ:
(Kretschmer), 1 oz. 12.3
crude, 1 oz. 14.7
honey crunch *(Kretschmer)*, 1 oz. 15.2
raw *(Arrowhead Mills)*, 2 oz. 26.0
toasted, 1 oz. 14.1
Wheat gluten, vital *(Arrowhead Mills)*, 1 oz. 9.0
Whelk, meat only, raw, 4 oz. 8.8

Whey:
acid, dry, 1 oz. 20.8
acid, fluid, 1 cup 12.6
sweet, dry, 1 oz. 21.1
sweet, fluid, 1 cup 12.6
Whipped topping, see "Cream" and "Cream
  topping, nondairy"
Whiskey, see "Liquor"
Whiskey sour mixer:
bottled *(Holland House),* 3 fl. oz. 27.0
instant *(Holland House),* .56 oz. dry 16.0
White bean mix*, and rice *(Fantastic* Italiano), 10 oz. 40.0
White beans:
dry, boiled, ½ cup 22.6
dry, small, boiled, ½ cup 23.2
canned, with liquid, ½ cup 28.7
White Castle, 1 serving:
cheeseburger 15.5
chicken sandwich 20.5
fish sandwich, without tartar sauce 20.9
hamburger 15.4
sausage sandwich 13.3
sausage with egg sandwich 16.1
side dishes:
   french fries 37.7
   onion chips 38.8
   onion rings 26.6
White sauce mix:
1¾-oz. packet 25.1
(McCormick/Schilling McCormick Collection), ¼ cup* 3.0
Whitefish, fresh or smoked, without added
  ingredients 0
Whiting, without added ingredients 0
Wiener, see "Frankfurters"
Wild rice:
raw, 1 oz. 21.2
cooked, 1 cup 35.0
(Fantastic Foods), ½ cup 18.0

precooked, cooked *(Master Choice Texmati)*, ½ cup 16.0
Wild rice dishes, see "Rice dishes"
Wine, 1 fl. oz.:
dessert or aperitif[1], 1 fl. oz. 2.3
dry or table[2], 1 fl. oz. 1.2
Wine, cooking:
marsala *(Holland House)*, 1 fl. oz. 2.3
red *(Holland House)*, 1 fl. oz. 1.5
sherry *(Holland House)*, 1 fl. oz. 1.2
vermouth or white *(Holland House)*, 1 fl. oz. .... <1.0
Wine cooler:
Premium *(Bartles & Jaymes)*, 6 fl. oz. 14.0
Premium light *(Bartles & Jaymes)*, 6 fl. oz. 12.0
berry *(Bartles & Jaymes)*, 6 fl. oz. 16.8
berry, light *(Bartles & Jaymes)*, 6 fl. oz. 16.0
cherry, black *(Bartles & Jaymes)*, 6 fl. oz. 16.1
peach *(Bartles & Jaymes)*, 6 fl. oz. 16.8
sangria, red *(Bartles & Jaymes)*, 6 fl. oz. 14.9
strawberry *(Bartles & Jaymes)*, 6 fl. oz. 16.2
tropical *(Bartles & Jaymes)*, 6 fl. oz. 18.6
tropical, light *(Bartles & Jaymes)*, 6 fl. oz. 16.8
Wine marinade:
herb, garden, or hot & spicy *(Holland House)*,
  1 fl. oz. 5.0
lemon & herb *(Holland House)*, 1 fl. oz. 2.0
red wine & herb *(Holland House)*, 1 fl. oz. 3.0
teriyaki *(Holland House)*, 1 fl. oz. 6.0
Winged beans:
fresh, raw, sliced, ½ cup 1.0
fresh, boiled, drained, ½ cup 1.0
dried, raw, ½ cup 38.0
dried, boiled, ½ cup 12.8
Winged bean leaves, trimmed, 1 oz. 4.0

---

[1] *Includes fortified wines containing more than 15% alcohol (sherry, port, vermouth, etc.).*
[2] *Includes table wines containing less than 15% alcohol (Burgundy, Chablis, Champagne, rosé, etc.).*

Winged bean tuber, trimmed, 1 oz.............................. 8.0
Wolf fish, without added ingredients......................... 0
Wonton wrapper:
(Azumaya), 1 oz.. 15.9
(Frieda's), 1 piece... 7.0
(Nasoya), 1 piece... 20.0
Worcestershire sauce:
(Heinz), 1 tbsp... 1.0
regular or hickory *(French's),* 1 tbsp........................ 2.0
regular or white wine *(Lea & Perrins),* 1 tsp................ 1.0

Y

Food and Measure	Carbohydrate Grams

Yam:
baked or boiled, ½ cup 18.8
canned or frozen, see "Sweet potato"
Yam, mountain, Hawaiian:
raw, cubed, ½ cup 11.1
steamed, cubed, ½ cup 14.4
Yam bean tuber:
raw, sliced, ½ cup 5.3
boiled, drained, 4 oz. 10.0
Yard-long bean:
fresh, sliced, raw, ½ cup 3.8
fresh, sliced, boiled, drained, ½ cup 4.8
dried, raw, ½ cup 52.0
dried, boiled, ½ cup 18.1
Yeast, baker's:
(*Fleischmann's* Active Dry/RapidRise), ¼ oz. 3.0
(*Red Star* Active Dry), ¼ oz. 2.7
fresh (*Fleischmann's*), .6 oz. 2.0
household (*Fleischmann's*), .5 oz. 2.0
Yellow bean, dried, boiled, ½ cup 22.2
Yellow squash, see "Crookneck squash"
Yellowtail, without added ingredients......................... 0
Yogurt:
plain:
(*Bison* Lowfat), 1 cup 17.0
(*Bison* Nonfat), 1 cup 16.0
(*Breyers* Lowfat), 1 cup 16.0
(*Colombo*), 8 oz. 13.0

Yogurt, plain *(cont.)*
  (Colombo Nonfat Lite), 8 oz. 17.0
  (Friendship Lowfat), 1 cup 17.0
  (Knudsen), 8 oz. 16.0
  (Knudsen Lowfat), 8 oz. 17.0
  (Yoplait Fat Free), 8 oz. 17.0
  (Yoplait Original, 98% Fat Free), 6 oz. 15.0
all fruit flavors:
  (Bison Nonfat), 6 oz. 13.0
  (Colombo Fruit on the Bottom), 8 oz. 36.0
  (Colombo Nonfat Fruit on the Bottom), 8 oz. 33.0
  (Light n' Lively Free), 4.4 oz. 8.0
  (Yoplait Custard Style), 6 oz. 30.0
  (Yoplait Fat Free), 6 oz. 32.0
  (Yoplait Light), 6 oz. 13.0
  (Yoplait Original, 99% Fat Free), 6 oz. 33.0
  (Yoplait Parfait Style), 6 oz. 34.0
  except lemon *(Bison* Lowfat), 1 cup 44.0
  except strawberry *(Knudsen* Lowfat), 8 oz. 43.0
apple crisp granola *(Bison Astro),* 4.4 oz. 24.0
berry, mixed:
  (Yoplait Breakfast Yogurt), 6 oz. 39.0
  crunch *(Bison Astro),* 4.4 oz. 28.0
  or blueberry *(Breyers* Lowfat), 8 oz. 48.0
blueberry:
  (Knudsen Cal 70), 6 oz. 11.0
  (Light n' Lively), 8 oz. 46.0
  (Light n' Lively 100 Calorie), 8 oz. 15.0
cherry:
  almond *(Yoplait Breakfast Yogurt),* 6 oz. 41.0
  black *(Breyers* Lowfat), 8 oz. 49.0
  black *(Knudsen Cal 70),* 6 oz. 12.0
  black *(Light n' Lively),* 8 oz. 44.0
  black *(Light n' Lively* 100 Calorie), 8 oz. 17.0
chocolate fudge crunch *(Bison Astro),* 4.4 oz. 27.0
coffee *(Bison* Lowfat), 1 cup 33.0
coffee *(Friendship* Lowfat), 1 cup 35.0
date-walnut-raisin *(Bison* Lowfat), 1 cup 44.0

fruit, tropical *(Yoplait Breakfast Yogurt)*, 6 oz. 41.0
grape *(Light n' Lively)*, 4.4 oz. 24.0
lemon:
    (Bison Lowfat), 1 cup 33.0
    (Knudsen Cal 70), 6 oz. 12.0
    (Light n' Lively 100 Calorie), 8 oz. 16.0
oat bran raisin *(Bison Astro)*, 4.4 oz. 27.0
peach:
    (Breyers), 8 oz. 48.0
    (Knudsen Cal 70), 6 oz. 11.0
    (Light n' Lively), 8 oz. 46.0
    (Light n' Lively 100 Calorie), 8 oz. 16.0
peanut butter or pecan toffee crunch *(Bison Astro)*,
    4.4 oz. 29.0
pineapple:
    (Breyers Lowfat), 8 oz. 50.0
    (Knudsen Cal 70), 6 oz. 12.0
    (Light n' Lively), 8 oz. 47.0
raspberry, red:
    (Knudsen Cal 70), 6 oz. 11.0
    (Light n' Lively), 8 oz. 43.0
    or strawberry *(Breyers* Lowfat), 8 oz. 48.0
    or strawberry *(Light n' Lively* 100 Calorie), 8 oz. 15.0
strawberry:
    (Colombo), 8 oz. 29.0
    (Knudsen Cal 70), 6 oz. 11.0
    (Knudsen Lowfat), 8 oz. 45.0
    (Light n' Lively), 8 oz. 45.0
    fruit basket *(Knudsen Cal 70)*, 6 oz. 11.0
    fruit cup *(Light n' Lively)*, 8 oz. 47.0
    fruit cup *(Light n' Lively* 100 Calorie), 8 oz. 15.0
strawberry-almond *(Yoplait Breakfast Yogurt)*, 6 oz. 38.0
strawberry-banana:
    (Breyers Lowfat), 8 oz. 50.0
    (Knudsen Cal 70), 6 oz. 12.0
    (Light n' Lively), 8 oz. 52.0
    (Light n' Lively 100 Calorie), 8 oz. 15.0
    (Yoplait Breakfast Yogurt), 6 oz. 40.0

Yogurt *(cont.)*
vanilla:
  (Bison Lowfat), 1 cup 33.0
  (Colombo French/Nonfat Lite), 8 oz.............................. 30.0
  (Friendship Lowfat), 1 cup 35.0
  (Knudsen Cal 70), 6 oz.. 11.0
  (Knudsen Lowfat), 8 oz. 43.0
  (Yoplait Custard Style/Yoplait Original, 99% Fat
    Free), 6 oz. 30.0
  (Yoplait Fat Free), 8 oz. 34.0
  bean *(Breyers* Lowfat), 8 oz. 41.0
Yogurt, frozen:
all flavors:
  (Borden/Meadow Gold), ½ cup 19.0
  soft serve *(Bresler's* Gourmet), 1 oz. 5.5
  soft serve *(Bresler's* Lite), 1 oz. 6.0
almond praline *(Edy's Inspirations),* ½ cup 22.0
banana nut chocolate chunk *(Colombo* Gourmet),
  3 fl. oz.. 17.0
banana split *(Colombo* Gourmet), 3 fl. oz. 20.0
banana-strawberry *(Häagen-Dazs),* ½ cup.................... 27.0
Black Forest cake *(Swensen's),* ½ cup............................ 21.0
boysenberry-vanilla swirl *(Edy's Inspirations),* ½ cup........ 19.0
Brownie Nut Blast (Häagen-Dazs Exträas), ½ cup............. 29.0
cappuccino coffee bean *(Colombo* Gourmet),
  3 fl. oz. 19.0
caramel fudge sundae *(Colombo* Gourmet), 3 fl. oz. 21.0
caramel pecan chunk *(Colombo* Gourmet), 3 fl. oz........... 19.0
Cheesecake Craze, Strawberry (Häagen-Dazs
  Exträas), ½ cup 31.0
cheesecake, wild raspberry *(Colombo* Gourmet),
  3 fl. oz... 18.0
cherry:
  black *(Sealtest Free),* ½ cup 24.0
  black-vanilla swirl *(Edy's Inspirations* Nonfat),
    ½ cup.. 19.0
  Bordeaux *(Swensen's),* ½ cup 21.0
cherry-almond chunk *(Colombo* Gourmet), 3 fl. oz. 17.0

chocolate:
   (Edy's Inspirations/Edy's Inspirations Nonfat),
      ¹/₂ cup.. 18.0
   (Häagen-Dazs), ¹/₂ cup.. 26.0
   (Sealtest Free), ¹/₂ cup.. 24.0
   brownie chunk *(Edy's Inspirations)*, ¹/₂ cup..................... 20.0
   chunk, Bavarian *(Colombo* Gourmet), 3 fl. oz. 18.0
   sundae *(Edy's Inspirations)*, ¹/₂ cup................................ 21.0
   white, almond *(Colombo* Gourmet), 3 fl. oz. 19.0
chocolate chip, strawberry *(Edy's Inspirations)*,
   ¹/₂ cup 21.0
citrus heights *(Edy's Inspirations)*, ¹/₂ cup 20.0
coffee *(Häagen-Dazs)*, ¹/₂ cup 28.0
cookies'n cream *(Edy's Inspirations)*, ¹/₂ cup 22.0
Heath bar crunch *(Colombo* Gourmet), 3 fl. oz. 19.0
Heath bar crunch *(Edy's Inspirations)*, ¹/₂ cup.................... 20.0
marble fudge *(Edy's Inspirations)*, ¹/₂ cup............................ 20.0
mocha chip *(Swensen's)*, ¹/₂ cup.. 20.0
mocha Swiss almond *(Colombo* Gourmet), 3 fl. oz........... 17.0
Orange Tango (Häagen-Dazs Exträas), ¹/₂ cup 26.0
orange-vanilla swirl *(Edy's Inspirations)*, ¹/₂ cup................. 19.0
peach:
   (Blue Bell Lowfat), ¹/₂ cup.. 22.0
   (Edy's Inspirations), ¹/₂ cup... 19.0
   (Häagen-Dazs), ¹/₂ cup.. 26.0
   (Sealtest Free), ¹/₂ cup.. 23.0
peanut butter cup *(Colombo* Gourmet), 3 fl. oz................. 16.0
Praline Pandemonium (Häagen-Dazs Exträas), ¹/₂ cup 33.0
raspberry:
   (Edy's Inspirations), ¹/₂ cup... 19.0
   (Edy's Inspirations Nonfat), ¹/₂ cup................................. 20.0
   (Häagen-Dazs Raspberry Rendezvous Exträas),
      ¹/₂ cup.. 26.0
   red *(Sealtest Free)*, ¹/₂ cup 23.0
raspberry-vanilla swirl *(Edy's Inspirations)*, ¹/₂ cup............. 19.0
strawberry:
   (Blue Bell Nonfat), ¹/₂ cup.. 20.0
   (Edy's Inspirations), ¹/₂ cup... 18.0

Yogurt, frozen, strawberry *(cont.)*
  (Edy's Inspirations Nonfat), ½ cup 20.0
  (Häagen-Dazs), ½ cup 27.0
  (Sealtest Free), ½ cup 22.0
  passion *(Colombo* Gourmet), 3 fl. oz. 18.0
vanilla:
  (Edy's Inspirations), ½ cup 19.0
  (Edy's Inspirations Nonfat), ½ cup 18.0
  (Häagen-Dazs), ½ cup 26.0
  (Sealtest Free), ½ cup 23.0
  dream *(Colombo* Gourmet), 3 fl. oz. 16.0
vanilla almond crunch *(Häagen-Dazs),* ½ cup 29.0
vanilla-chocolate swirl *(Edy's Inspirations* Nonfat),
  ½ cup 19.0
"Yogurt," tofu:
apple, spiced *(Stir Fruity),* 6 oz. 29.5
berry, mixed *(Stir Fruity),* 6 oz. 26.0
blueberry *(Stir Fruity),* 6 oz. 25.7
cherry, black *(Stir Fruity),* 6 oz. 25.1
lemon chiffon *(Stir Fruity),* 6 oz. 25.9
orange, mandarin *(Stir Fruity),* 6 oz. 25.7
peach *(Stir Fruity),* 6 oz. 25.8
piña colada *(Stir Fruity),* 6 oz. 27.6
raspberry *(Stir Fruity),* 6 oz. 27.5
strawberry *(Stir Fruity),* 6 oz. 24.8
vanilla *(Stir Fruity),* 6 oz. 22.8
Yogurt bar, frozen:
all flavors *(Frozfruit* Nonfat), 1 bar 20.0
cherry chocolate fudge *(Häagen-Dazs),* 1 bar 28.0
crunch, vanilla/chocolate *(Häagen-Dazs),* 1 bar 23.0
crunch, chocolate/coffee *(Häagen Dazs),* 1 bar 24.0
orange passion, tropical *(Häagen-Dazs),* 1 bar 21.0
peach or raspberry *(Häagen-Dazs),* 1 bar 19.0
piña colada *(Häagen-Dazs),* 1 bar 21.0
strawberry daiquiri *(Häagen-Dazs),* 1 bar 20.0
Yogurt shake, frozen, chocolate *(Weight Watchers*
  Sweet Celebrations), 7.5 fl. oz. 44.0
Yuca, boiled, drained *(Frieda's),* 4 oz. 38.6

Z

Food and Measure | Carbohydrate Grams

Ziti dinner, frozen:
ribbed *(Swanson Hungry Man)*, 17.25 oz. 51.0
ribbed, in meat sauce *(Swanson)*, 11 oz. 45.0
Ziti dishes, frozen, in marinara sauce *(The Budget
  Gourmet Side Dish)*, 6.25 oz. 23.0
Ziti entree, frozen, with zesty tomato sauce *(Healthy
  Choice Pasta Classics)*, 12 oz. 59.0
Zucchini:
fresh:
  raw, sliced, ½ cup 1.9
  raw, baby, 1 large, 3⅛″ long, ⅝″ diameter 5
  boiled, drained, sliced, ½ cup 3.5
  boiled, drained, mashed, ½ cup..................................... 4.7
canned, Italian style *(Progresso)*, ½ cup............................. 8.0
canned, with tomato juice, ½ cup 7.8
frozen:
  (Seabrook), 3.3 oz. 3.0
  battered *(Stilwell)*, 8 sticks 17.0
  breaded *(Ore-Ida)*, 3 oz. 17.0
  breaded *(Qwik Krisp)*, 6 pieces...................................... 20.0
  breaded *(Stilwell)*, 8 sticks 18.0